SMARTER WORKOUTS

THE SCIENCE OF EXERCISE MADE SIMPLE

Pete McCall, CSCS

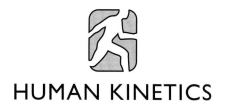

HUMAN KINETICS

Library of Congress Cataloging-in-Publication Data

Names: McCall, Pete, 1972- author.
Title: Smarter workouts : the science of exercise made simple / Pete McCall.
Description: Champaign, IL : Human Kinetics, [2019] | Includes
  bibliographical references.
Identifiers: LCCN 2018042399 (print) | LCCN 2018048692 (ebook) | ISBN
  9781492572602 (epub) | ISBN 9781492567899 (PDF) | ISBN 9781492567882
  (print)
Subjects: LCSH: Exercise. | Physical fitness.
Classification: LCC RA781 (ebook) | LCC RA781 .M3853 2019 (print) | DDC
  613.7--dc23
LC record available at https://lccn.loc.gov/2018042399

ISBN: 978-1-4925-6788-2 (print)

This publication is written and published to provide accurate and authoritative information relevant to the subject matter presented. It is published and sold with the understanding that the author and publisher are not engaged in rendering legal, medical, or other professional services by reason of their authorship or publication of this work. If medical or other expert assistance is required, the services of a competent professional person should be sought.

The web addresses cited in this text were current as of September 2018, unless otherwise noted.

Senior Acquisitions Editor: Michelle Maloney; **Developmental Editor:** Anne Hall; **Managing Editor:** Dominique J. Moore; **Copyeditor:** Marissa Wold Uhrina; **Permissions Manager:** Martha Gullo, **Graphic Designer:** Whitney Milburn; **Cover Designer:** Keri Evans; **Cover Design Associate:** Susan Rothermel Allen; **Photograph (cover):** MichaelSvoboda/E+/Getty Images; **Photographs (interior):** © Rob Andrew; **Photo Asset Manager:** Laura Fitch; **Photo Production Coordinator:** Amy M. Rose; **Photo Production Manager:** Jason Allen; **Senior Art Manager:** Kelly Hendren; **Illustrations:** © Human Kinetics; **Printer:** Premier Print Group

Human Kinetics books are available at special discounts for bulk purchase. Special editions or book excerpts can also be created to specification. For details, contact the Special Sales Manager at Human Kinetics.

Printed in the United States of America   10 9 8 7 6 5 4 3 2 1

Human Kinetics
P.O. Box 5076
Champaign, IL 61825-5076
Website: www.HumanKinetics.com

In the United States, email info@hkusa.com or call 800-747-4457.
In Canada, email info@hkcanada.com.
In the United Kingdom/Europe, email hk@hkeurope.com.

For information about Human Kinetics' coverage in other areas of the world,
please visit our website: **www.HumanKinetics.com**

E7329

This book would not be possible without my amazing wife, Monica, who not only taught me how to teach group fitness but also has provided the support, guidance, and encouragement that have allowed me to flourish as an educator; I love you, thank you for putting up with me. To my daughters, Parker and Ryan, thank you for the opportunity to study and learn more about human movement. I love you both more than words can say.

Contents

PART I The Science and Why It Matters   1

Understand the physiology and the methodology of exercise to help shape your workouts.

1 How Exercise Changes Your Body   3

2 Movement and Intensity in Practice   27

PART II Exercises and Workouts   47

Cover all your bases with a full range of workouts using a variety of equipment to maximize results.

3 Mobility Training   49

4 Core Strength Training   113

5 Metabolic Conditioning   183

Exercise Finder

BODYWEIGHT EXERCISES				
Exercise	Mobility	Core Strength	Metabolic Conditioning	Page Number
Alternating lateral lunges with reach			X	196
Glute bridge		X		127
High plank		X		125
Hip bridge	X			60
Kneeling thoracic spine mobility	X			67
Lateral crawling			X	201
Lateral lunge with trunk rotation		X		129
Multiplanar kneeling to standing	X			64
Offset quadruped rocking	X			61
Plank to knee tap			X	197
Quadruped shoulder rotation	X			66
Reverse lunge with overhead reach		X		130
Rollerblader (ice skater)			X	200
Side plank		X		126
Single-leg balance with arm reach		X		128
Slow-motion burpee	X		X	63/202
Speed squat			X	198
Spider-Man stretch	X			62
Squat with forward reach		X		131
Step-through			X	199
Supine hip circle	X			59

(continued)

STABILITY BALL EXERCISES				
Exercise	Mobility	Core Strength	Metabolic Conditioning	Page Number
Ball pass crunch			X	212
Child's pose	X			69
Crunch		X		140
Diagonal lift			X	208
Full body extension	X			74
Hip bridge to hamstring curl		X	X	133/205
Hip roll to knee tuck		X		138
Knee tuck			X	204
Kneeling chest stretch	X			71
Kneeling cross-body reaching	X			70
One-leg squat		X		139
Pike		X		136
Prone hip roll			X	206
Reverse back extension			X	209
Roll-out			X	207
Russian twist		X	X	137/210
Seated adductor stretch	X			73
Seated hip opener	X			72
Stir-the-pot		X		134
Supine hip rotation		X		135
Supine lateral roll	X			75

MEDICINE BALL EXERCISES				
Exercise	Mobility	Core Strength	Metabolic Conditioning	Page Number
Child's pose cross-body reach	X			77
Diagonal low-to-high lift		X		146
Full-body crunch			X	221
Hip bridge with pullover		X		142
Kneeling with overhead reach	X			78
Lateral lunge with trunk rotation and reach	X			81
Lateral skater with forward reach			X	222
Offset kneeling with trunk rotation	X			79
Push press to bounce catch			X	218
Reverse crossover lunge with reach			X	220
Reverse lunge to chop (over forward leg)		X		147
Reverse lunge with overhead lift			X	223
Romanian deadlift		X		143
Rotational lunge with reach to ground	X			82
Squat to forward press			X	217
Standing rotation		X	X	144/216
Straight-arm slam			X	214
Transverse plane lunge with lift		X		148
Trunk rotation with overhead reach	X			80
Vertical chop		X		145

SANDBAG EXERCISES				
Exercise	Mobility	Core Strength	Metabolic Conditioning	Page Number
Crunch with resistance			X	225
Forward lunge with reach to ground	X			90
Forward to reverse lunge with overhead lift			X	228
Half Turkish get-up			X	232
Hip hinge with offset stance	X			88
Hip thruster	X			86
Kneeling hip flexor stretch with overhead reach	X			87
Lateral lunge with forward press		X		155
Lateral lunge with shoulder carry	X			89
Lying spinal rotation	X			85
One-arm bent-over row		X		154
One-leg hip bridge		X		150
Pullover	X			84
Push press throw to catch			X	226
Reverse crossover lunge with reach			X	231
Reverse lunge with rotation (over forward leg)		X		152
Reverse overhead slams			X	230
Single-leg Romanian deadlift		X		153
Swing (alternating hands)			X	229
Transverse plane lunge reach to ground with overhead press		X		156
V-sit with press		X		151

TWO-ARM RESISTANCE TUBING EXERCISES				
Exercise	Mobility	Core Strength	Metabolic Conditioning	Page Number
Alternating punches			X	258
Fast band pull			X	241
High-to-low band chop		X		159
Kneeling lift	X			96
Lateral lunge to band chop			X	240
Lateral lunge with straight-arm pull-down			X	239
Leg-raise hamstring stretch	X			92
Lunge to one-arm pull		X		160
Lying hip stretch	X			93
One-arm press		X		164
Overhead squat	X			97
Split squat with trunk rotation		X		161
Squat-to-row		X	X	163/235
Standing chest opener	X			94
Standing crunch (facing away from anchor point)		X		158
Standing pull and punch	X			95
Straight-arm pull-down			X	236
Transverse lunge with pull			X	237
Two-hand forward press		X		162

(continued)

DUMBBELL EXERCISES				
Exercise	Mobility	Core Strength	Metabolic Conditioning	Page Number
Alternating-arm bent-over row		X	X	170/243
Cross-body rotating shoulder press			X	246
Hip press		X	X	167
Lateral lunge reach-down to overhead press		X		169
Lateral lunge to overhead press			X	244
Lateral lunge with reach to ground	X			100
Pullover to crunch		X		166
Romanian deadlift to biceps curl		X		168
Rotating shoulder press	X			102
Rotating uppercut		X	X	171/245
Single-leg alternating biceps curl			X	248
Single-leg sword draw		X		173
Split squat with single-arm overhead press	X			101
Squat to overhead press		X		172
Supine pullover	X			99
Sword draw	X			103
Transverse plane lunge with reach to ground	X		X	104/249
Triceps extension			X	249

KETTLEBELL EXERCISES				
Exercise	Mobility	Core Strength	Metabolic Conditioning	Page Number
Goblet squat		X	X	178/251
Halo	X			108
One-arm bent-over row		X		180
One-arm clean			X	255
One-arm high pull			X	252
One-arm overhead press		X		179
One-arm push press			X	256
Pullover to crunch		X		175
Reverse crossover lunge with reach to ground			X	253
Reverse lunge in racked position	X			107
Reverse lunge to balance with offset weight		X		176
Reverse lunge with one-arm overhead carry		X		181
Reverse lunge with trunk rotation	X			109
Supine rollover with single-arm press	X			106
Transverse plane lunge with reach to ground			X	257
Trunk rotation with single-arm press	X			110
Two-hand swing			X	254
Windmill		X		177
Windmill low hold	X			111

Foreword

The road to success is always under construction.

—Lily Tomlin

The fitness industry has always been a unique community; most people who get into this business do so because they have a genuine desire to share the gift of movement with others. When it comes to success in fitness, some people focus only on what they see in front of them, without fully recognizing what it takes to get there. Not everybody becomes a high-profile fitness expert; one question I'm always asked is, "How can I get to where you are?" In this field, the focus is often on quick fix exercise solutions, and that mentality seems to have trickled into the mindset of aspiring trainers. With the rise of social media platforms, overnight success has taken on a whole new meaning; the right photos combined with the luck of tapping into a digital zeitgeist can result in becoming an almost instant sensation. Yes, social media can increase visibility; without science and knowledge to stand on, though, even social media success can be short lived.

As a young girl, I was heavily influenced by watching my father jog every night after work. My father knew that regular exercise was important for good health, and he would come home from work, change his clothes, and go for a run before we had dinner. Most nights, as my father finished his run, I'd be at the end of the driveway waiting for him so we could run around our street together. Looking back on it, his behavior probably had the greatest influence on me, because he showed me that regular exercise is an important part of life and that it is truly a gift to be able to move your body.

Over the course of my career in fitness, amazing things have occurred: developing my teaching technique (the Stoked Method), garnering a devoted following of Stoked athletes, working with celebrity clients, becoming a key resource for top media outlets, landing magazine covers, making frequent television appearances, leading sold-out workouts across the country, representing brands in national media campaigns, and creating a platform to share my approach to fitness with the world. I give this brief review of my background not to brag about my accomplishments but to emphasize the point that movement matters—and success takes work and adaptability to change.

This brings me to why I am so delighted to see Pete McCall's book *Smarter Workouts*. It features the same approach to exercise that I have found works for my clients. In my more than 20 years of being a trainer, I have found that teaching my clients how to improve their movement skills can help them learn how to enjoy exercise, which has been the key ingredient to the changes they have been able to achieve. Pete and I have had many conversations about how exercise should focus on movement instead of independent muscle actions. The top professionals in our industry share a similar approach to the workouts we design for our clients: Exercise is a function of movement.

I first met Pete when we both worked for the same health club company; besides being a personal trainer and group fitness instructor there, he was a member of the team who educated the fitness staff. Over the years, Pete has pursued his passion of teaching and educating other fitness professionals, and it has been fun to watch him become one of the most influential thought leaders in our industry. And he sticks to this philosophy: The key to learning how to enjoy exercise is first learning how to move properly. If you want long-lasting results from your workouts, then understanding how to work smarter—not harder—is the way to go.

All goals are constantly under construction. There's no magic pill to achieving any long-lasting goal. (Even if you hit a lucky break, you still have to work to maintain the success.) In this book you will find the key building blocks to help build your own path to success while understanding that *smarter workouts* are the ones you are constantly learning from—the ones always under construction.

—Kira Stokes

Preface

In Greek mythology, Sisyphus, a deceitful king who displeased the gods, was punished for his treachery by being sentenced to an eternity of pushing a boulder up the side of a mountain, only to have it roll down, forcing him to start all over again. This is actually a fitting analogy for how many people approach their fitness programs: They invest a tremendous amount of physical effort but are not always able to experience the desired outcomes toward which they are working. They are pushing the proverbial rock up a mountain, only to watch it roll back down because they're not getting the results they want.

Here's a little story that will help you understand the purpose of this book. A number of years ago, my wife and I bought a condo in downtown Washington, D.C. It was our first home, and after making the down payment, we didn't have any money left to hire a contractor. It was up to us and some family members to do the painting and make a few small repairs before moving in. Now, as a self-admitted gym rat, I can walk into almost any fitness facility in the world and feel comfortable almost immediately. But walking into one of the oversized do-it-yourself hardware stores? Ugh. In my experience, it can be scary and overwhelming. That's when it occurred to me that how I felt walking into a super-sized hardware store is how many people feel when walking into a health club or fitness facility: uncomfortable and out of place. Whether it's a large commercial health club, a nonprofit recreation center, a boutique fitness studio, or a weightlifting gym, just walking through the doors can be an extreme act of courage for many people. Once inside, the different equipment and machines can range from confusing to intimidating, even for those of you who may have some experience. Maybe you've participated in a conditioning program for a sports team; followed a workout program from a book, Internet site, or magazine; or even worked with a personal trainer. However, getting results from an exercise program doesn't require using all the equipment in a gym; you only have to know how to use one piece of equipment properly to have an efficient and effective workout. Reading this book will give you the know-how to use just one piece of exercise equipment at a time to perform an effective workout for improving mobility, enhancing core strength, or burning calories through metabolic conditioning.

For the better part of two decades, I have been working directly with individual personal-training clients, teaching group fitness classes, educating personal trainers, and writing articles and blogs about how to apply the science of exercise to design workout programs that work. This book is a culmination of this body of knowledge (pun intended), which can help you identify the best exercise solutions for your needs. Whether you want to reap the health benefits of exercise or simply desire to improve your physical appearance, from my professional experience I've found that many people like you are motivated to exercise but just don't know what to do to get started. For those of you who choose to exercise at home, you will learn how to create your own workouts using easily available and affordable fitness equipment.

When it comes to exercise there are no shortcuts, but knowing the underlying science of how exercise affects the human body can help you identify what will work best for your needs. Exercise does not have to be hard to be effective, but it is necessary to know how to perform different types of exercise to produce the results you want.

The primary purpose of this book is to be a resource to help you learn how to perform time-efficient, effective workout programs using only one piece of equipment at a time in either a commercial fitness facility or from the comfort of your own home. You will learn exercise programs based on the idea of working smarter so that you can achieve results without a tremendous amount of unnecessary effort. The pieces of exercise equipment selected for this book are dumbbells, a kettlebell, a medicine ball, a stability ball, a sandbag, and a two-armed resistance band. These were chosen because they are often found in fitness facilities and are affordable enough to be purchased by those of you who want the ability to exercise at home.

Dumbbells have long been a standard piece of fitness equipment but are often only used for working one muscle group or body part at a time; exercises that involve a number of different muscles can help burn more calories while increasing the strength of all of the involved muscles. Medicine balls and kettlebells were found in the first commercial fitness centers of the late nineteenth century and are still popular today because they are easy to use, but you have to know how to use them properly to get the best results. With a little creativity, a stability ball can be used to improve core strength as well as provide other fitness benefits in a relatively small amount of space. Cable machines are a staple feature of fitness facilities that can be used for a number of different exercises; however, due to their size, they are not practical for home use. Instead, a two-arm resistance band can be used to replicate many moves performed on a cable machine in a home setting. Sandbags, or sand-filled discs such as Sandbells, deliver a challenging workout by requiring you to stabilize the weight as the sand shifts.

This book covers three categories of fitness that will help you get results. *Mobility* refers to the ability of muscles to produce and control movement through a joint's available range of motion. Mobility is an essential component of an exercise program that is often overlooked in favor of muscular development or aerobic conditioning. However, it is probably the most important component when it comes to improving coordination, movement skill, and overall quality of life. Like strength, mobility is a specific trait that can be developed with the proper exercise program. Each piece of equipment in this book can be used to enhance your body's mobility and, as a result, improve your overall balance, dexterity, and coordination—skills often lost through the biological aging process.

Cardio training is an often-misused term in the context of exercise. Are you breathing right now? Good, then you're technically doing cardio because your heart is working to deliver oxygenated blood to your muscles while returning deoxygenated blood to the lungs, where it receives a new supply of oxygen. When it comes to exercise, it is more appropriate to identify which one of the body's metabolic pathways is being facilitated to generate the energy to fuel muscular contractions. Each piece of exercise equipment featured in this book can be used for a metabolic conditioning workout that will have you sweating and burning calories while simultaneously improving your body's ability to turn food into energy for muscular activity.

Core training is another misused term that usually means a focus on using the abdominals and other muscles of the midsection. This book will teach you how to do exercises that effectively integrate movements of your hips and shoulders, which is how the muscles of our body are designed to function. Each piece of exercise equipment featured in this book can help you develop the muscles that control your body's center of gravity, not only to help you to look better but, more importantly, to help you move better and be able to enjoy more of your favorite activities.

The first two chapters will provide a brief overview of exercise physiology related to mobility, core strengthening, and metabolic conditioning. Chapter 1 addresses how exercise changes the human body. Chapter 2 discusses how to design exercise programs to make desired changes to your body. Chapters 3, 4, and 5 feature specific exercise programs to enhance mobility, develop core strength, and improve metabolic conditioning, respectively, using only one piece of equipment for each workout. You may have a favorite piece of equipment that you like to use, or even a favorite workout that you love, but one challenge of exercise is that after a certain amount of time, the body will adapt to whatever type of work it is being required to perform. Long-term success in an exercise program requires the knowledge of how to structure workouts so they are constantly challenging the body with different tasks. In that light, the final two chapters introduce different ways to plan and organize your workouts so that you can continually challenge your body in different ways throughout the course of a year and over one's lifetime.

As someone who has worked full time in the fitness industry for almost 20 years, I often see people expend a lot of effort yet become frustrated because they're not getting the results they want. The simple truth is that achieving results from an exercise program is truly a function of working smarter as opposed to working harder. This book will help you understand how the body responds to exercise and how to use one piece of equipment for effective and time-efficient workouts that can improve mobility, burn calories, or improve strength so that you have the time and ability to enjoy the things you really want to do in life.

Acknowledgments

Over the course of a career, when serving others it can be extremely difficult to identify only one or two individuals who have had a significant impact. Many people have motivated, encouraged, and supported me during my career as a personal trainer, fitness instructor, and educator; in some way, each of you has been a part of the inspiration for this book. While many of my friends and colleagues have helped me develop into the fitness professional I am today, I want to say a special thank you to Cedric Bryant, Fabio Comana, Todd Galati, Jessica Matthews, and Christine Ekeroth. It's hard to put into words how much I appreciate working with each of you; it was our time together at the American Council on Exercise that put me on the journey of becoming a fitness writer. To my parents, thank you for buying me my first weight set. I never had any idea it would lead to an amazing career where I have the opportunity to travel the world sharing my passion for fitness. To my fellow trainers and instructors in Washington, DC, thank you for helping me get started in the industry; I cherish our days grinding on the gym floor. To all of the fitness professionals I have worked with over the years, your energy, enthusiasm, and passion inspire me to be my best every time I step in front of a group, thank you. To all of my clients and group-fitness-class participants I have had the privilege of serving over the years, you may not realize it, but every single one of you has played a role in encouraging me to learn more about how exercise changes the human body. Thank you for trusting me with the most precious assets in your life—your body and your time. To my fellow fitness educators, master trainers, and presenters: your pursuit of knowledge and dedication to our profession motivate me to work hard; thank you for your support and encouragement over the years. Finally, to Michelle and the team at Human Kinetics, thank you for the opportunity to share my experience and put my thoughts on paper.

Introduction

Yes, you have heard that regular exercise is important. Yes, you know that you should probably be doing more of it. But short of that, how much do you really know about exercise and how it affects your body? You may have a number of questions: What is exercise? Why is it so important? How do different types of exercise create changes in the body? What types of exercise should I be doing? How can I identify the best type for my needs? How often should I be exercising and how hard? Where is the best place to achieve the recommended amount of exercise? Do I need to pay for a costly health club or buy lots of expensive exercise equipment that I'm not going to know how to use?

As someone who has been a personal trainer for 20 years and in the business of educating other personal trainers for most of the past 15, including being a media spokesperson for the American Council on Exercise, these questions come up all the time from people I meet in health clubs and from fitness reporters working on stories for consumer magazines. Yes, it can be difficult to sort through all the information to find accurate, reliable, evidence-based information; all too often marketers promote a new exercise fad or gimmick without explaining how it works to change your body. If you take the time to learn why exercise is important, the basic science of how various types of exercise apply different kinds of stimuli to your body, and, most importantly, which types you should be doing to help improve your health and achieve the specific results you want, then you will have the tools you need in order to make exercise an integral part of your life.

Here's a startling reality: Each and every single individual will have a different response to exercise. *No one* who makes a living as a personal trainer, strength coach, group fitness instructor, or health coach can guarantee with 100 percent certainty that exercise will deliver specific results. If anyone ever promises or guarantees that you can get a specific outcome from following their workout program, then your first exercise is to run away, because it is virtually impossible to guarantee specific results. The results you experience from any exercise program will vary based on the types of exercise that you do as well as a number of other lifestyle habits, such as nutrition, sleep, and overall stress levels.

The only thing that is known about exercise and the human body is that regular exercise can promote good health and significantly lower the risk of developing a number of chronic health conditions, while lack of regular exercise and a sedentary lifestyle can reduce life expectancy. Aging is unavoidable, and the normal biological aging process affects all systems in the human body. Evidence suggests that adults with a sedentary lifestyle can expect to experience a more rapid degradation of bodily functions and face a greater risk of premature death than those who make exercise a regular habit (Candow et al. 2011; Taylor and Johnson 2008). If you want to maintain good health and add years to your life while giving you the ability to enjoy all of the things that you love to do, then it is necessary to learn how to make exercise a regular habit.

Exercise and Health

We are all busy with work, family, and other activities that occupy our time. Today's overstimulated and automated society presents limited opportunities for physical activity, which is unfortunate because the evidence proves that a lack of regular physical activity can lead to a number of adverse health conditions and preventable diseases (Skinner et al. 2015). The 2008 Physical Activity Guidelines for Americans acknowledges that "all Americans should engage in regular physical activity to improve overall health and to reduce risk of many health problems . . . Regular physical activity over months and years can produce long-term health benefits. Realizing these benefits requires physical activity each week" (US Department of Health and Human Services 2008, 1). This is an important statement because in it, the federal government acknowledges that regular exercise can be an essential component of experiencing a healthy life with a reduced risk of developing a costly, debilitating, and potentially fatal disease. The guidelines suggest that a minimum of 150 minutes of moderate exercise or 75 minutes of vigorous exercise every week can provide health benefits.

OK, so you know you can benefit from exercise, and maybe you have tried to start making it a habit but have stopped for a variety of reasons. One of the more common reasons why many people stop exercising is that they simply do not enjoy it because it is perceived as difficult and uncomfortable. Finding exercises that you actually enjoy, that fit your lifestyle, and that produce results that enhance your overall quality of life can be a challenge. Here's some really good news: You don't have to do any specific type of exercise, nor does it have to be extremely difficult; it just has to be consistent. Right now, you are holding in your hands a number of simple solutions that can help you learn how to enjoy exercise and make it a part of your regular life.

Exercise for basic health purposes can help improve the efficiency at which your lungs place oxygen into your bloodstream while strengthening your heart to move that oxygenated blood around your body. In addition, you will be increasing your overall activity to help expend energy, a necessary component of managing a healthy body weight. If time is a challenge for you, keep in mind that it's not necessary to do all the exercise at the same time. Adding 20 to 30 minutes of exercise a day in 10-minute increments could have a positive impact on your health. If you're not that active at the present time, adding a 10-minute walk in the morning, at midday, and in the evening can be the literal first step toward improving your health and making exercise a healthy habit. This could be as simple as a walk around the block before getting into the car in the morning, a walk around your building or the block of your worksite during the day, and another walk around the block when you get home. When it comes to enhancing your overall health, remember this simple saying: Any activity is better than no activity at all.

Over the past few years, fitness professionals—the catchall term for personal trainers, group fitness instructors, and small-group training coaches—have become instrumental in helping people learn how to do the right exercises for their needs. If you have had the opportunity to work with a good fitness professional, then you know the benefits he or she can provide, including helping you establish an exercise program for your particular needs. The first thing the fitness professional should do is establish why you want to exercise and what your specific expectations are by asking a series of questions:

- Why are you starting an exercise program?
- What are you doing right now for exercise?
- What are the exact things that you want to achieve from an exercise program?
- Where will you be doing the workouts?
- When can you make time for exercise?
- How are you going to make exercise a regular part of your daily life so you can achieve and maintain good health?

One of the most important steps when starting an exercise program is establishing clear expectations for what you want to achieve. It is important that your desired outcomes match the amount of time and energy you can dedicate to the process of reaching them. Setting a challenging goal like losing a specific amount of weight or achieving a certain type of appearance can certainly be one way to motivate yourself to be more active. But if you don't have the time to dedicate to the work it takes to reach those goals—and it takes a lot of work—then establishing more realistic expectations can help you learn how to enjoy the process of exercise instead of punishing yourself because you failed to achieve a certain result.

No one wants to spend part of their day being uncomfortable or in pain, and many people mistakenly have an association between exercise and physical discomfort. Yes, there are times when exercise should be challenging, but it should not be extremely uncomfortable or painful, because pain is a signal that something is going wrong in your body. In addition, exercising to the point of pain could establish negative feelings about the experience, with the end result being that you will find other things that bring you pleasure or enjoyment to occupy your time. The best exercise program is the one you enjoy, because you will be more likely to incorporate it as a consistent part of your lifestyle. This book will help you learn how to remove the complexity from exercise so that you can identify the types that are effective and, most importantly, enjoyable. That should be your expectation from exercise: Learn how to make it fun so it becomes an activity you actually look forward to doing.

PART I

The Science and Why It Matters

1

How Exercise Changes Your Body

Joining a health club or going to a fitness studio is a common first step when starting an exercise program, but identifying the best type of exercises for your needs can be difficult. Many common exercise programs are derived from bodybuilding workouts, which creates some confusion surrounding what to do for exercise. The focus of a bodybuilding program is usually muscle isolation exercises involving only a single joint or muscle group at a time, meaning that the individual body parts are worked as separate, discrete units. An example is the knee extension machine, which requires you to be in a seated position as you move a weight by straightening your legs. Yes, this action can strengthen the larger muscles of your upper thigh, but those muscles are designed to work with both your hip and knee while you're standing on your feet, not while sitting down.

A muscle isolation approach promotes maximum hypertrophy, the technical term for muscle growth, for individual muscle groups; although it is necessary for the sport of bodybuilding, it's not necessarily the most effective method when designing a workout program for the purpose of improving health or maintaining a healthy body weight. It's necessary to point out that in addition to doing exercises for only one or two body parts at a time, bodybuilders also spend many hours a week implementing nutrition and supplement strategies to achieve their desired levels of muscle size and definition, without which it can be hard to achieve the same appearance. Following a bodybuilding approach to exercise can create inefficiencies that lead to frustration for the average person.

Drawbacks to Muscle Isolation

Muscle isolation training can help improve overall aesthetic appearance but at the expense of exercises that improve your coordination or that burn calories efficiently.

Planes of Motion

Many of the strength training machines and free weight exercises traditionally used for bodybuilding focus on movement in a single plane of motion, like the aforementioned knee extension. However, during upright activities such as walking, the human body uses several muscles at the same time to create movements and joint motions that occur through multiple planes of motion simultaneously.

Alignment

The muscles of the body behave like spokes in a bicycle wheel. If one or two spokes become too tight or too loose, the wheel will fall out of alignment and could be damaged. Isolation training loads physical forces into specific sections of muscle, which is like overtightening one or two spokes on a bicycle wheel. If some muscles are used more than others, this could create an imbalance of forces and, just as a wheel that falls out of alignment could damage a bike, a muscle that changes its alignment because it is overused could lead to injury. If an exercise program causes injury due to muscle imbalances, you may have to quit before any significant changes to the body can occur.

Calorie Expenditure

Your body will expend approximately five calories of energy to use one liter of oxygen. The more muscle tissue that you can involve with an exercise, the more oxygen your body will consume, resulting in more calories being burned. Because they only use small sections of muscle at a time, isolation exercises require only a limited amount of oxygen, making them a poor choice if you want to burn a lot of calories in a short amount of time. If you are following a program featuring muscle-isolation exercises to manage weight by trying to get rid of unwanted calories, you will not be receiving a maximal return on your investment of time.

Movement Patterns

The body is made to move. As babies we learned how to roll over, crawl, and walk before we could talk. The systems of our body naturally learn how to perform complicated movement patterns before we develop the skill for effective communication; it is how our nervous system is wired. The seemingly simple act of walking is in itself a complex pattern of movement that occurs in all three dimensions and involves all of our muscles and joints working as a complete system to create efficient movement. Therefore, an isolation approach to exercise is contrary to how the body actually functions.

Muscle Alignment

The structures of the human body—including muscle, the fascia and connective tissue that surround it, and bones—are all aligned to be the most mechanically efficient when we're standing upright to move over the ground, so to use exercises that move only a single joint or involve only one muscle group at a time is working against our fundamental physiology. Because multiple systems function together to create and control movement, effective exercise programs should be based on developing and enhancing the fundamental patterns of movement as opposed to using only isolated muscle actions.

Realistic Expectations for Exercise

Regular exercise can provide a wide variety of outcomes based on the types and amount you do. Exercise can be described as existing on a continuum, from low-intensity movement such as walking for the purpose of improving basic health to high-intensity performance training to enhance athletic skills. There is no one, single right way to exercise. The important thing is that it becomes a consistent habit. To help you establish realistic outcomes and expectations for your exercise program, identify the area of the continuum that best reflects your specific needs and the amount of time you may have to commit to an exercise program. (Be honest with yourself.)

The types of activity that can improve movement skill or enhance muscular strength and appearance require exercises designed specifically for how your body moves. Many traditional exercises focus on using one body part or muscle at a time; however, during many of the movements you perform on a daily basis, multiple muscles work together to control how your body moves. When studying movement, it is very easy to see that the only time a muscle works in isolation is during an exercise focused specifically on a single muscle or body part. For example, a seated chest press machine is designed with a linear path of motion and single axis of rotation that places all of the force into the muscles of the chest, shoulders, and upper arms while a push-up uses those muscles along with all of the core muscles responsible for stabilizing the spine and hips. The result is that because it recruits and uses numerous muscles at the same time, a push-up can require you to do more actual work than using a seated chest press machine, which will use only a limited amount of muscles. Many exercises like the chest press are designed specifically so that only one muscle or muscle group does the work; however, producing and controlling human movement involves numerous systems of the body, including the muscular, skeletal, nervous, and metabolic, working together simultaneously. If you only have a limited amount of time, why not focus on dynamic movement patterns that involve these systems and multiple muscles working at the same time? Here's the great news: Relatively short workouts that involve a number of muscles working together and challenging your body to move in multiple directions can help you to move better while expending more energy, which is a win-win combination essential for desired outcomes such as losing weight, looking better, or simply improving overall health.

Exercise and Physical Change

The human body is a series of systems interacting with one another to produce and control movement. Exercise is physical stress applied to the body. The actual types of stress, how often those stresses are applied, and how your body is allowed to recover once the stresses are removed are all important variables that determine your response to any exercise program. Movement is a skill that can be developed and enhanced with practice, and performing exercise is a function of movement. Learning exercises that enhance your ability to move can be the foundation for learning how to maximize your enjoyment from exercise. As your movements become more efficient and coordinated, you will start feeling better, and before you know it you will start moving more often, which is the real secret for long-term success from exercise.

Change does not occur to your body without a preceding stimulus, and exercise is a physical stress that can be applied to create many changes, including increasing muscle size, boosting definition, reducing body weight, improving aerobic efficiency, and enhancing coordination. If the goal of exercise is to make changes to your body, it is important to work to a point of mild discomfort, not pain. Discomfort means your body is being challenged to work harder than it is used to working, whereas pain is an indication that your body is experiencing an acute overload of stress that could cause an injury. This does not mean that it is always necessary to exercise at an uncomfortably high level of intensity, but it does mean that in order to get results you should be prepared to do some higher-intensity workouts that make you feel uncomfortable while other workouts can and should be at a relatively low or comfortable level of effort. Knowing when and how to place more challenging physical stresses on the body is essential and will be addressed in the following chapters.

Before jumping into the different types of workouts that can deliver the results you want, it's first important to have a general understanding of how exercise affects different structures and systems in your body. These are muscle, fascia and elastic connective tissue, bone (skeletal system), the central nervous system (CNS), the cardiorespiratory system and energy metabolism, and the endocrine system, which is responsible for producing the chemicals that influence change in all of the cells of your body.

Muscle

The mass of the human body can be organized into two general categories of tissue: fat-free mass—which includes lean muscle, connective tissue, skeletal structures, internal organs, skin, and blood—and fat mass—where the body stores surplus energy in adipose tissue. Adults over the age of 25 can expect to lose up to 10 percent of their muscle mass per decade unless they exercise regularly (Taylor and Johnson 2008). Whether you want to alter the appearance of your body or its ability to perform a specific task, one important outcome of exercise is change in both the function and appearance of muscle.

Muscle is composed of different types of tissues (figure 1.1): the contractile element responsible for generating a force and the noncontractile, elastic component that transmits mechanical forces between different sections of muscle (Verkoshansky and Siff 2009).

The contractile element of skeletal muscle transmits information via mechanical forces. When muscles are shortening to exert tension against an external resistance, it's a compressive force, and when a muscle lengthens in reaction to an applied force, it experiences a tensile force (Myers 2014). Exercises to improve muscular strength can either rely on the body's own weight, such as push-ups, or use external resistance, such as dumbbells, a medicine ball, or a kettlebell. Strength training is the application of external forces to skeletal muscle tissue for the purpose of making it stronger and capable of generating higher levels of force. Strength training can increase the amount of lean muscle mass as well as enhance a particular muscle's ability to produce force, which can help change appearance, burn calories, and improve the ability of the heart to pump blood around the body.

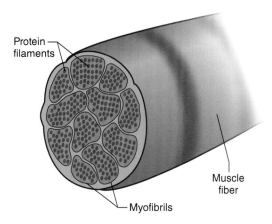

Figure 1.1 A muscle includes two types of tissue: the contractile element that generates force and the elastic component that can store and release mechanical energy.

A common misperception about exercise is that if you stop strength training your muscle will turn into fat. Here is why this is a complete myth: Muscle and fat are two extremely different types of tissue. Muscle is a use-it-or-lose-it tissue. When you exercise regularly, especially strength training, you can increase muscle volume. But without the forces from resistance training, muscle will atrophy, meaning that the individual fibers will become smaller and the overall size of a particular muscle will shrink. Aerobic exercise such as walking, running, or swimming can help improve your body's ability to move blood to the working muscles, but these types of exercise may not put enough force into muscles to stimulate growth or significantly change appearance. Strength training, with external resistance or your own body weight, can be the most effective way to change your muscles, whether by adding size or improving the ability to perform a variety of functions.

Understanding the basic premise of how muscle adapts to strength training gives you the ability to determine the most effective type(s) of exercise for your needs. Research can provide a guide to how your body may respond to strength training, but the reality is that even when following the exact same exercise program every person can experience slightly different outcomes. This means that you will need to do a little trial and error to identify which method of exercise or type of equipment works best for you and your needs. This book will help you in that quest.

Muscle Growth Stimulus

If you have read any popular fitness magazines or received advice from other fitness enthusiasts, you may be familiar with the concept that strength training damages muscle tissue and that because of that damage, muscles repair themselves to become stronger and, in some cases, bigger. That is a relatively accurate but incomplete description of the mechanisms responsible for muscle growth. There is absolutely no dispute that strength training causes muscle growth; however, identifying the most effective type of stimulus to cause that growth is a little more nuanced. This is because strength training introduces two specific types of stress—mechanical and metabolic—each of which can provide the necessary stimulus for muscle growth (Bubbico and Kravitz 2011). A high-intensity load in the form of an extremely heavy weight applies a mechanical stress to muscle, whereas performing a high number of repetitions to the point of momentary fatigue creates a significant metabolic stress (Schoenfeld 2016).

Mechanical stress refers to the physical forces imposed on the structures of a muscle fiber. Strength training imposes mechanical forces that cause microtrauma to muscle fibers, which, in turn, signal the biochemical reaction to produce the new satellite cells necessary for repairing the mechanical structure of the muscle tissue (Schoenfeld 2010, 2013). Mechanical loading of the contract element can initiate signal changes within a muscle that create hypertrophy (Spangenburg 2009). When muscles generate mechanical force, the structure of the tissues and how they perform changes.

One thing is certain: Strength training with progressively heavier weights causes muscles to grow and become stronger. What is not 100 percent understood, however, is whether these changes are the result of mechanical or metabolic overload. Both the amount of weight used and exercising to a point of momentary fatigue can impose the stresses that initiate adaptations. Dr. Brad Schoenfeld, a researcher who studies how muscles adapt to strength training, observed, "Mechanical stress is unquestionably a primary driving stimulus in post-exercise muscle growth. There is compelling evidence that metabolic stress may also contribute to hypertrophic adaptations. . . . A problem with the research is that mechanical and metabolic stress occur in tandem which can make it difficult to tease out the effects of one from the other" (Schoenfeld 2013, 99).

Muscle Fiber Types

Your body has different types of muscle fibers, which are classified by how they function: type I (slow-twitch) and type II (fast-twitch). Understanding how muscle fibers differ from one another and the functions they are best suited to perform can help you understand how different types of exercise can produce specific results.

Slow-twitch muscle fibers are also known as aerobic muscle fibers because of their ability to create energy from oxygen, allowing them to sustain force over an extended period of time. Tonic stabilizers are the muscles responsible for producing and maintaining good posture and are composed of mostly type I fibers. Type I muscle fibers are activated by type I motor units, the end point of the nervous system attached to a bundle of muscle fibers. When a muscle is required to generate a force, the central nervous system (CNS) will recruit type I motor units and muscle fibers first; once they fatigue, other motor units and muscle fibers are recruited to generate the necessary amounts of force (Zatsiorsky and Kraemer 2006).

There are different classifications of type II (fast-twitch) muscle fibers: type IIb, which produces energy without the presence of oxygen (anaerobic), and type IIa, which, depending on the training stimulus and need for energy, takes on characteristics of either type I or type IIb fibers. Both classifications of type II muscle fibers, referred to as phasic muscles, are responsible for creating the higher levels of force necessary to produce human movement.

All muscle fibers are activated by the motor neuron, which is the connection between the CNS and individual muscle fibers. A motor unit, which functions like a light switch for your muscles, is the motor neuron and the individual muscle fibers attached to it. When a light switch is turned on it completes an electrical circuit, causing the light to shine. When a motor unit receives the appropriate command from the CNS it sends the signal to its attached muscle fibers, causing them to contract and shorten. When the body needs force from a particular muscle or group of muscles the CNS sends a signal to the appropriate motor neurons to initiate the necessary contractions to perform a specific task.

Motor units can be classified as fast-twitch or slow-twitch based on the individual fibers to which they are attached. Slow-twitch motor units and the attached muscle fibers have a low threshold for activation, low conduction velocities, and are engaged for long-duration activity requiring minimal force. Fast-twitch motor units, on the other hand, attach to the type II muscle fibers that can produce more force in shorter periods of time, have a higher activation threshold, are capable of conducting signals at higher velocities, and are better suited to strength- and power-based activities. Motor units are activated according to the all-or-none theory, which postulates that when a motor unit is activated, it shortens all of its attached muscle fibers (Zatsiorsky and Kraemer 2006).

Type II muscle fibers have a larger diameter than type I fibers and are responsible for increasing the size and definition of a particular muscle. In addition to increasing the efficiency at which type II motor units function to generate force, strength training initiates a number of important adaptations in type II muscle fibers, including increasing the quality and quantity of the muscle proteins and anaerobic enzymes that affect the structure of a muscle. Specific structural changes include increasing the quantity of enzymes necessary for anaerobic metabolism, elevating the amounts of energy substrates such as phosphagen and glycogen stored in muscle, as well as increasing the contractile proteins of myosin and actin; specifically, the myosin heavy chains become thicker, which allows muscle contractions to occur with more velocity and greater amounts of force (Haff and Triplett 2016).

If your fitness goals involve toning up or enhancing muscle definition, the only way to achieve this is by activating the type II motor units and muscle fibers. (Note: The term *tonus* refers to a state of semi-contraction of a muscle and is the basis for the phrase *muscle tone*.) There are two ways to activate type II motor units: One is to use a heavier resistance, which recruits more motor units in order to generate higher levels of force; the second is to work until a moment of fatigue, which indicates the muscle has reached its limit to generate force. No matter which method you choose, the higher-threshold type II motor units and muscle fibers responsible for definition will not be engaged unless a muscle is exercised to the point of momentary fatigue.

You may regularly participate in physical activities such as walking, hiking, running, swimming, or yoga—all of which can provide important health benefits—but those activities involve primarily your cardiorespiratory and metabolic systems. When it comes to achieving and maintaining an optimal level of fitness, strength training should be an important component of your long-term exercise plan because it can ensure that you maintain the muscle mass and force production abilities to perform your favorite activities with a much lower risk of injury.

Without a consistent application of mechanical forces, the type II fibers of your muscles can atrophy and lose the ability to generate force. Strength training to the point of fatigue will engage a greater number of type II motor units and muscle fibers, helping you maintain strength and lean muscle mass well into your later years. If you want to develop definition without increasing size it may be tempting to use only light weights, but here's an important consideration: One definition of insanity is repeatedly doing the same thing but expecting a different result. Constantly using the same weights for the same exercises simply won't produce the results you want from your workouts. The best way to make changes to your body is by challenging it to work in different ways with a variety of movement patterns using different types and amounts of resistance. Exercise to a moment of fatigue is necessary to increase strength, maintain muscle mass, and improve definition.

Fascia

Exercise affects all of the tissues in your body, not only your muscles, which are just the most visible. Within the human body is a complex network of muscle, fascia, and elastic connective tissue organized into one single, integrated system responsible for maintaining a constant equilibrium of forces. Fascia, the noncontractile elastic component of muscle tissue, can be broadly defined as the soft, fibrous connective tissue interwoven between all of the cells and organs within the human body (and should be considered an organ in its own right). Research suggests that noncontractile connective tissue is the richest sensory organ in the human body, containing many nerve endings and sensory receptors when compared to the fibers of the contractile element of muscle (Schleip et al. 2012). As important as fascia is to the proper function and appearance of your body, how many times have you started a workout thinking, "Today is my fascia training day"?

Mechanotransduction describes how mechanical force initiates chemical changes to the cells that are the building blocks for various tissues in the body, including bone, muscle, fascia, and elastic connective tissue of the body. The architectural term *tensegrity* is a combination of tension and integrity and refers to a structure that is self-supporting through a combination of tensile (lengthening) and compressive (shortening) forces. Muscles shorten (compress) and lengthen (stretch); the entire myofascial system is a balance of compression and tension (Scarr 2014; Myers 2014; Ingber 2003). In response to the competing forces of compression and tension, fascia and the elastic connective tissue maintain a constant balance between the synthesis of new cells and the remodeling of existing ones.

The concept of tensegrity allows us to consider the extensive myofascial network as a single, integrated system responsible for maintaining a constant equilibrium of forces where sections of tissue communicate with one another as forces are transferred from one area to the next (Myers 2014; Schultz and Feitis 1996). It is estimated that mechanical vibrations moving through the myofascial network move three times faster than the signals sent by the CNS. On the macro level, force is distributed between the different segments of muscle, fascia, and elastic connective tissue, while on the micro level mechanotransduction initiates chemical reactions that change the structure and biophysical properties of individual cells (Scarr 2014; Langevin 2006; Vogel and Sheetz 2006; Ingber 2003, 2004). Multidirectional movement patterns that place mechanical loads on fascia and elastic connective tissues can help strengthen the entire system.

Fascia envelopes every single muscle fiber and organizes numerous fibers into bundles that are commonly recognized as individual muscles (figure 1.2). The epimysium is a layer of fascia responsible for attaching various bundles of muscles to one another and becomes the tendon connecting the contractile element of muscle tissue to skeletal structures. The fascia and connective tissue surrounding an individual muscle are responsible for transferring forces between different sections of neighboring muscle. This system, easily visible on the macro scale with the naked eye, repeats itself on the micro level with the endomysium distributing load between individual muscle fibers by forming a latticework that connects every single cell in the human body to one another (Schleip et al. 2012). Connective tissue is directly responsible for organizing how mechanical forces are distributed throughout the human body (Myers 2014; Vogel and Sheetz 2006; Ingber 2004).

The myofascial network functions most efficiently when it is moved in all directions at a variety of different velocities. Lifestyle habits such as maintaining a sed-

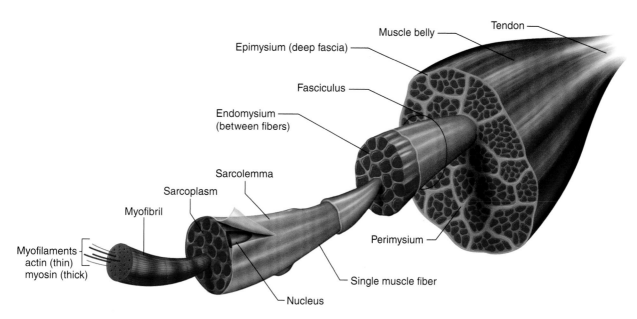

Figure 1.2 The skeletal muscles that generate the force for movement are organized into many layers, with each individual fiber surrounded by fascia and elastic connective tissue.

entary position for multiple consecutive hours can adversely affect the hydration and, ultimately, the elasticity of fascia and connective tissue. A lack of multiplanar movement and proper hydration can cause layers of fascia to bind to one another, changing the body's ability to move in multiple directions. On the cellular level, force regulation can change the physical properties and biochemical function of a cell, affecting the structure of muscle tissue from the smallest unit to the largest (Schleip et al. 2012; Vogel and Sheetz 2006; Ingber 2004).

The physical changes you can experience from exercise are the result of mechanical forces applied to your body. As a result, the whole of the body functions synergistically to become much stronger than the sum of its individual parts (Ingber 2003). If the system is not properly balanced, forces such as compression, tension, torsion, or shear can change the architecture of cellular structures and the overall function of the body. Chronic stresses from repetitive movement patterns, exercises performed with poor technique, or a lack of multidirectional movement in general affects the body on many different levels and can have a significant impact on the results you can expect to experience from an exercise program. Understanding how various forces, on both the macro and micro scales, affect the structures of the body from the cellular level on up to initiate changes can help you identify the types of exercise that can be most beneficial for your particular wants and needs.

While some movement is better than none, exercise in a single plane of motion, the feature of many common muscle-isolation exercise programs, will primarily engage the contractile element of muscle fibers, whereas moving an external load in different directions will involve more fascia and elastic connective tissue. With this knowledge you can easily see why it is important to perform both types of exercise in a workout program: Linear movements, which engage the contractile element, generate force, and multidirectional movements strengthen the fascia and connective tissue between every single muscle fiber. Workouts to strengthen the contractile element of muscle require either heavier amounts of weight or work to a moment of fatigue. Workouts for the fascia and elastic connective tissue focus on multidirectional movements that lengthen muscle and fascia under resistance using only body weight or lighter loads in order to increase the tensile strength of the tissues, which can help reduce the risk of many common injuries. "If one's fascial body is well trained, that is to say optimally elastic and resilient, then it can be relied upon to perform effectively and at the same time offer a high degree of injury prevention" (Schleip et al. 2012, 465).

Skeletal System

Another component of the body that is directly affected by exercise yet is often overlooked in traditional exercise programs are the bones of the skeleton. The skeletal system is the support system for the human body; the bones create a structural framework to protect internal organs while allowing for multidirectional movements generated by the muscle, fascia, and elastic connective tissues. A joint is an intersection where two bones come in proximity to one another but do not touch. Joints that allow movement around a fluid-filled cavity are called synovial joints. All joints serve a purpose: to either allow mobility through a structural range of motion or limit motion to provide stability. Efficient movement is an integrated coordination of unrestricted motion at the mobile joints combined with structural support created by the stable ones.

Other than the bones themselves, the structures of the skeletal system include the articular cartilage at the end of a bone, the connective tissue forming the joint capsule, fibrous membranes, such as the menisci in the knees, and the synovial fluid enclosed within the joint capsule. All together, these structures ensure that the ends of two separate bones do not touch as joints move through their designated paths of motion. Some joints, such as the hip (a ball-and-socket joint), are designed to move, while other joints, such as the sutures of the skull, are not. Because they provide the attachment points for the muscles through the fascia and tendons, bones can themselves be considered a form of connective tissue and, like other tissues in the body, will grow and remodel themselves in response to applied forces (Neumann 2010). Strength training with external resistance helps develop denser, stronger bones and joint structures capable of resisting physical damage, such as fractures or breaks.

The structural design and placement of bones within the skeletal system help dissipate both internal and external forces. According to Wolff's law, stimulation precedes structural change, meaning that the skeletal system adapts to the physical forces applied to it through exercise or the lack of movement related to a sedentary lifestyle. Mechanotransduction applies to skeletal structures as well. For example, poor posture can cause structural changes to the bones that make up joints, such as the intervertebral segments of the spine or the intersection of the upper leg and pelvis. Forces consistently applied to the body can change the position of bones, which, in turn, alter the structure of a joint, ultimately changing the motion and function of that joint (Neumann 2010).

The muscle, fascia, and elastic connective tissue surrounding a joint function to create both the necessary stability for controlling joint position while it is in motion and the force to move the joint through its path of motion. Optimal mobility allows a joint to experience full, unrestricted motion while controlling the constantly changing axis of rotation. Regular exercise and physical activity can ensure that a joint maintains a volume of synovial fluid as well as the elasticity of the attached connective tissues to safeguard functional performance over the course of the human lifespan.

Just like muscle, fascia, and elastic connective tissue, the structures of the skeletal system operate in a use-it-or-lose-it relationship with movement efficiency; lack of consistent multidirectional movements combined with the repetitive stress from poor posture or sedentary habits can change the position of bones. This alters the ability of joints to perform their designated functions, increasing the likelihood of injury.

Ligaments connect bone to bone, provide structural support to joints, and are pliable to allow motion to occur, yet, unlike muscles and tendons, are not elastic (i.e., they are not designed to lengthen). An imbalance of tensile and compressive forces from muscle caused by bad posture or poor exercise technique can change a joint's position as well as its structure and ability to either allow motion or provide a platform for stability. A chicken-and-egg relationship exists between muscle imbalances and the faulty joint motions that could cause an injury. Over time, repetitive motions or a lack of movement can cause adjustments to the length–tension relationships of muscles, fascia, and connective tissue restricting normal joint motion. Likewise, continuing to maintain poor posture while in sedentary positions can change joint structures, which subsequently changes the length-tension relationships of the muscles surrounding a joint. It's not clear which comes first, poor posture that causes a muscle to shorten or a shortened muscle causing bad posture, but a failure to address either cause could increase the risk of injury during physical activities because when joint structure and motion change, it alters the ability of the muscle, fascia, and elastic connective tissue around that joint to efficiently produce, reduce, and control force.

The three segments of the body that allow the greatest mobility are the foot and ankle complex (actually a number of joints but are organized into one structure for the purpose of this discussion), the hip, and the intervertebral segments of the thoracic spine (again, actually a number of separate joints that function together in one unit). The joints comprising these three segments of the body provide important mobility in all three planes of motion that is essential for optimal movement efficiency of the gait cycle. The loss of mobility at one joint in these segments, even the loss of mobility in a single plane of motion, can affect the structure and function of the entire body. If a joint loses mobility, it could affect joints above or below it, greatly altering their ability to function.

Mechanical forces affect all tissues in the body, especially muscle, fascia, and elastic connective tissues as well as the bones of the skeleton, and can change both their structure and function. Regularly changing the type of exercises you perform and using different types of workout equipment ensure that you are subjecting your body to a wide variety of forces, which is essential for developing the physical structures that can help you achieve and maintain optimal fitness.

Central Nervous System

You've been learning about how exercise affects various structures within the human body. Now it's time to learn how the various systems of the body are organized to function as a single, integrated unit. Muscles receive the input to shorten, lengthen, and control force from the sensory receptors of the CNS. Movement happens as the result of muscles working together as a coordinated system around a joint; as muscles on one side of a joint shorten to initiate movement, the muscles on the other side lengthen to allow the limb to move through its structural range of motion. Think about a movement that you do every day, such as putting your keys in your car or walking from one room to another. What does it take to perform that movement? How many muscles are involved? How many joints work together to allow your body to go through that movement? When you execute that movement, do you tell your brain to activate specific muscles, or do you just go directly into the learned range of motion (ROM) of the movement, known as the movement pattern?

When you move, your CNS doesn't think of the specific muscles involved in movement; rather, it identifies a movement pattern, then activates and coordinates all of the muscles necessary to complete that pattern. Many of the daily movements we perform happen as a result of these subconscious, reflexive actions. One of the benefits of an exercise program based on movement patterns (as opposed to isolated muscle actions) is that it helps develop and refine the integration between your CNS and muscular systems so that efficient movement skill becomes a subconscious reflex, allowing your conscious mind to focus on other things as you participate in your favorite activities.

The CNS works to feel what is happening in your environment so that it can select the appropriate muscles to generate the proper amounts of force required to create movement. This is called *proprioception*. The CNS, muscular system, and skeletal system are independent from one another, yet they must operate interdependently to create efficient movement. Sensory receptors—often nerve endings—in ligaments, joint capsules, muscles, and connective tissue provide specific information about the position of a joint and its rate of change as it moves through a ROM. In addition, sensory nerves operate within muscle and fascia to detect whether a compressive force is needed or a tensile force should be allowed. Optimal movement efficiency means that the CNS receives the inputs, allowing a muscle to lengthen rapidly as the muscles on the opposite side of a joint shorten, resulting in unrestricted joint motion.

The sensory information is communicated through the spinal cord to the brain to determine the most effective motor output to produce mobility and control a joint through its entire ROM (figure 1.3). For example, you can feel the difference between walking on hard asphalt or loose sand: Because your CNS can detect that the sand is unstable, more muscles are recruited to help your body maintain stability; thus, your body works a lot harder. All of the information written about exercise comes down to the fact that muscles will not function properly without the appropriate input from the CNS. Uploading the right types of information into the CNS is critical for achieving the desired results of an exercise program.

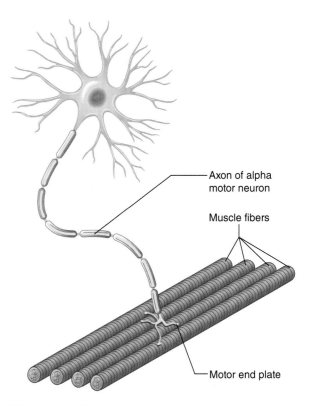

Figure 1.3 The central nervous system communicates via electrical impulses that are responsible for initiating muscle contractions. Shown here is a muscle motor unit, the motor neuron, and the individual fibers it is attached to and responsible for contracting.

Axon of alpha motor neuron

Muscle fibers

Motor end plate

Role of the CNS in Controlling and Improving Movement

Think about how you use your body every day. When is your balance challenged? When do you have to move quickly to change directions? If you have to pick things up off the floor or balance on one leg to reach up on a shelf, balance should be a critical part of your training plan. Likewise, if you have young children who are a bundle of energetic, unpredictable movement, or you live in an urban community where you have to navigate crowded subways and sidewalks, adding exercises for mobility, dynamic balance, and agility can help improve your ability to change direction rapidly while maintaining control of your body.

How many times have you walked into a gym thinking, "I'm going to train my coordination and dynamic balance today"? Probably not very often. It can be a challenge to improve these skills, which is why many people avoid doing it. However, the good news is that with the proper exercise program you can improve these skills almost immediately.

Coordination is a combination of dynamic balance and agility. Dynamic balance is the ability to maintain your body's center of gravity, which in itself is a critical component of the core region, over a constantly moving base of support—your legs and feet. Agility is the ability to rapidly decelerate, change direction, and reaccelerate while maintaining control of your center of gravity. Improving skills such as dynamic balance and agility is simply a function of uploading the right sensory information into the CNS and is a critical reason why following a movement-based exercise program is so important: You are uploading a tremendous amount of information as well as the mechanical forces that ultimately influence adaptation and growth of the muscles.

For an exercise program to be successful, all systems must work together. The CNS will detect what is happening around you and will select an appropriate motor response for the muscles to produce the corresponding movement. Muscles will then work to move the structural support system of the skeleton. Skills such as agility, dynamic balance, and strength are not discrete components of human movement but instead rely directly on one another to allow you to achieve an optimal mechanical efficiency and maximize movement skill during any physical activity, whether exercise or activities of daily living.

The CNS and Strength Gains

Strength, or muscle force output, is a function of the number of individual muscle fibers involved in producing the force for a movement. Intramuscular coordination is the efficiency at which the CNS recruits and activates individual fibers within a particular muscle and is based on three separate components:

1. *Muscle fiber recruitment*: The lengthening phase stimulates muscle spindles to activate muscle motor units within a specific muscle.
2. *Synchronization*: The simultaneous activation of more motor units to increase the force output.
3. *Rate coding*: The speed at which motor units are activated by the CNS. Faster firing rates of muscle motor unit recruitment result in an increase of muscle power or the ability to generate force at a rapid velocity.

What the Science Says:
The Body Functions Like a Computer

A computer provides an accurate analogy for how various body systems function together to generate movement. A computer is a collection of different pieces of hardware, specifically plastic, metal, glass, wires, and circuits. When wired together into an integrated system, this hardware is relatively useless unless there is an operating system to organize how it all functions together as a single unit capable of performing a variety of functions, from writing documents to searching the internet.

The muscle, fascia, elastic connective tissue, and skeletal structures are the hardware of the human body. Just like the individual components of a computer, the various structures of the human body need a central operating system to initiate the commands for performing specific functions. The CNS plays the role of the operating system, which organizes the signals to the hardware to initiate movement. Unlike a computer, which needs specific instructions from software telling it what functions to perform, the CNS is a self-learning system, constantly receiving a variety of inputs that determine the outputs that result in the execution of specific movements.

Sensory receptors are the components of the CNS that receive information from both inside and outside the body in order to determine the proper motor response from the muscular system. Sensory receptors located alongside individual muscle fibers, in ligaments, tendons, joint capsules, and joint linings, can determine the rate of length change as a muscle experiences a tensile force as well as identify the rate at which a joint changes position during movement. These positional changes are used to determine how much force is needed from specific sections of muscle to execute an appropriate motor response, which results in a movement.

From the moment we begin to learn how to wiggle, extend our spine, roll over, and ultimately crawl, the sensory receptors of the CNS are gathering data from gravity and ground reaction forces to develop the motor programs that instruct the muscles how to generate the forces that ultimately result in our ability to walk and move upright on our feet. We are made to move; our CNS is constantly upgrading its operating system to improve our ability to move as long as we are feeding the appropriate information into it. The secret to developing a successful training regimen is to improve the software's ability to move the hardware. In other words, train your nervous system to select the necessary muscles to execute a specific movement in a fluid and graceful manner.

Intermuscular coordination is the ability to activate many muscles at the same time in an effort to elevate the maximal force output for a specific movement. The CNS is responsible for increasing both intra- and intermuscular coordination, which can ultimately enhance the rate of force production or total force output for a particular movement. Co-contraction is the simultaneous activation of muscles on both sides of a joint, traditionally referred to as the agonist and the antagonist for a particular movement. Increasing the neural efficiency of muscles can allow an antagonist to relax at a faster rate during an agonist muscle action, leading to an increased rate of force production and a faster movement velocity (Verkoshansky and Siff 2009).

A muscle in a constant state of tension will not be able to shorten effectively to produce a force and will not be able to lengthen to allow motion to occur. When muscle, fascia, and connective tissue are in a constant state of tension, collagen fibers may bind between the layers of tissue to create rigidity and impede joint mobility. The CNS plays an essential role in supporting optimal mobility. Sensory nerves detect changes to mechanical loading and positioning of body segments. The nervous system has sensory receptors located in the contractile element of muscle, mechanoreceptors in fascia and joint capsules, and the ability to monitor movement of skeletal structures. For every sensory nerve in muscle, there are up to 10 in fascia and connective tissue (Schleip et al. 2012). The high level of sensory nerve endings in fascia makes it a huge influence on the signals the nervous system sends to create and organize effective motion. Exercise programs need to follow an appropriate progression of movement complexity and intensity in order to allow the CNS to develop efficient motor timing to control compression and tension within the muscle and fascia network.

Cardiorespiratory System

The cardiorespiratory system consists of the heart, lungs, and blood vessels (arteries, veins, and capillaries). The lungs bring oxygen into the body, and the heart pumps deoxygenated blood to the lungs, which place oxygen into the blood before it is pumped back to the heart and around to the rest of the body. Your breathing rate increases when the intensity of exercise becomes more challenging because the lungs need to work faster to bring more oxygen into the body and push carbon dioxide out while the heart beats faster to move blood around the body. A tachometer measures the revolutions per minute (RPM) of your car's engine, which indicates how hard the engine is working to maintain driving speed; the faster you drive your car, the higher the RPM. Your heart works in a similar fashion: The harder you work during exercise, the greater the levels of oxygen needed for the muscles and the faster the carbon dioxide needs to be removed. This, in turn, causes the heart to beat faster to facilitate this process, making heart rate an effective metric for measuring exercise intensity.

Cardiorespiratory exercise, often referred to simply as *cardio*, consists of activities that elevate the heart rate for extended periods of time. However, this can be somewhat of a misnomer, because if you are breathing (which you are hopefully doing while reading this), you are doing cardio as you pull oxygen into your body in an effort to help fuel the activity of staying awake to read this page. Your body's metabolism produces the necessary energy to sustain physical activity and is a function of various systems, including the cardiorespiratory, digestive, circulatory, endocrine, and muscular systems. Physical activities, including exercise, use two types of energy to fuel physical activity: chemical and mechanical. Adenosine triphosphate (ATP) is the form of chemical energy created from the nutritional substrates of fat, carbohydrates, and, in some cases, protein, which is then used to fuel muscle contractions. Mechanical energy is stored during the rapid lengthening of the elastic fascia and connective tissue then released during the shortening phase of muscle action. A more accurate way to describe the type of exercise that elevates your heart rate and helps to improve the efficiency at producing energy is *metabolic conditioning*.

Both steady-state (maintaining the same intensity for an extended period of time) and interval training (alternating between periods of high- and low-intensity activity) exercise increase the demand for chemical energy, ATP. Your body will produce ATP in one of three ways: lipolysis, breaking down fatty acids with oxygen to sustain low- to moderate-intensity activities for an extended duration of time; glycolysis, metabolizing glycogen into ATP either with or without oxygen; and ATP stored in the muscle cell. The intensity and duration of exercise determine the amount of oxygen required as well as the substrates used to generate ATP.

Metabolic conditioning has become a term used to describe high-intensity exercise; however, all exercise is a form of metabolic conditioning, because the body metabolizes substrates into ATP to fuel muscle activity. Higher-intensity exercise requires more oxygen and higher levels of ATP. Therefore, a better way to think of metabolic conditioning is energy-expensive exercise; more muscle tissue involved in a workout will create a higher demand for oxygen, thereby expending more energy.

When you are at rest or working at lower exercise intensities, your type I muscle fibers use oxygen to help metabolize ATP from fatty acids. As exercise intensity increases, type II muscle fibers either use stored ATP or convert glycogen (stored carbohydrates in muscle cells) to ATP with or without the presence of oxygen. Aerobic glycolysis is the production of ATP from glycogen while using oxygen. Anaerobic glycolysis is how glycogen is processed into ATP without the use of oxygen.

During rest and low-intensity exercise, ATP is provided through aerobic metabolism. However, the energy for high-intensity exercise is produced by the phosphagen and glycolysis energy pathways, placing a significant demand on the involved muscle tissue and the circulatory system to rapidly deliver the ATP required to fuel muscle activity (figure 1.4). It doesn't matter whether it is resistance training or cardiovascular conditioning; one of the outcomes of high-intensity exercise is an extreme amount of metabolic stress responsible for initiating changes in the systems used for producing and fueling movement.

Fatty acids require oxygen and take longer to convert to ATP, making them an inefficient source of energy during high-intensity exercise. Carbohydrates are converted to glycogen in the liver, and when muscles need energy rapidly, carbohydrates are

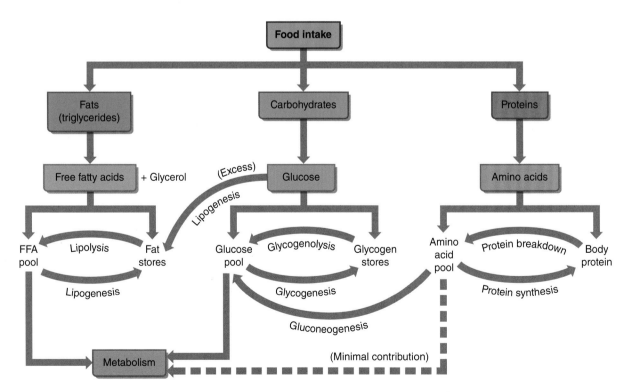

Figure 1.4 Cellular metabolism.

used in the type II muscle fibers, where they are converted to ATP with or without oxygen. The intensity and duration of the exercise will influence which substrates are used and whether oxygen is required to convert them into ATP. When high-intensity exercise persists for an extended period of time and no more glycogen is immediately available to create ATP, the body will convert amino acids, the building blocks of protein, to ATP during gluconeogenesis.

High-intensity exercise programs are popular because they produce results, but they require a lot of energy and generate a lot of mechanical forces, causing stress to both the mechanisms in muscle cells responsible for producing ATP and the mechanical structures of muscle fibers, respectively. These metabolic and mechanical stresses are responsible for initiating the mechanisms leading to muscle growth, but it is important to understand that doing high-intensity exercise too often or for too long, or both, could result in damage to cellular structures that could keep you from reaching your fitness goals (Kenney, Wilmore, and Costill 2015).

During low- to moderate-intensity exercise your body does not need a significant amount of oxygen, so you should be able to hold a conversation because your breathing rate will not interfere with the ability to speak. As exercise intensity increases, your body needs more oxygen, so your breathing rate will increase, limiting your ability to say more than a few words at a time. During low-intensity exercise, your body does not need a lot of energy, nor does it need it that quickly, so your breathing rate remains relatively consistent and should allow you to talk. If you can speak comfortably, you are working below the first ventilatory threshold (VT_1), identified as the exercise intensity at which the body shifts from metabolizing fat as the primary source of energy to relying on carbohydrates stored in muscle cells as glycogen to produce ATP.

Exercising at an intensity above VT_1 restricts speaking to only short phrases or a few words because you are burning primarily carbohydrates, stored in muscle cells as glycogen, for energy. A by-product of carbohydrate metabolism is carbon dioxide (CO_2) and is one reason why you start breathing faster when exercising at higher intensities: Your body is attempting to get rid of higher levels of CO_2. Another reason for a faster breathing rate is that you are trying to draw in as much oxygen as quickly as possible to help generate energy. Monitoring your ability to talk can help you determine whether you are using your aerobic or anaerobic energy pathways during exercise. Some workouts feature steady-state training just below VT_1, while others follow an interval training model with the work intervals above VT_1 and the recovery intervals below. As your fitness levels improve, try to remain at an aerobic steady state for longer periods of time, and when you do interval training, you can either push harder to get out of breath quicker or spend a longer time above VT_1, where breathing is challenging, combined with less time below for recovery.

After a period of high-intensity exercise, which depletes available ATP stores, muscles need to rest or work at a lower intensity in order to allow the accumulated hydrogen ions to be removed as well as to replace spent ATP. This is the basic science behind interval training: During a period of lower-intensity exercise or rest, the body will use oxygen to help produce and replace the ATP used during the higher-intensity interval. The more oxygen the body uses both during exercise to fuel activity and afterward to help with the recovery process, the more calories will be spent.

After you are finished with a high-intensity workout you will continue to breathe at a faster rate than normal because your body still needs additional oxygen to help with the postexercise recovery process. Oxygen is used during the recovery period after exercise to support a number of physiological functions, including production of new ATP; conversion of lactate (a by-product of energy metabolism) into glycogen to replace what was used during exercise; restoration of oxygen levels in venous blood, skeletal muscle blood, and myoglobin; repair of muscle proteins as well as other tissue damaged during the workout; and restoration of body temperature to normal, resting levels. Commonly referred to as the *excess postexercise oxygen consumption* (EPOC), this phenomenon is also known as the *oxygen debt*. It is the intensity of exercise, not the duration, that determines the magnitude of the EPOC effect.

Endocrine System

The CNS organizes the electrical impulses that control muscle actions; however, structural changes to muscle, fascia, and elastic connective tissues are influenced by hormones, chemicals that control many cellular functions. The endocrine system regulates the production of hormones and is directly responsible for many of the physiological adaptations to exercise. Hormones only work with specific receptor sites in a cell and can affect cellular functions in different ways. Hormones control a number of physiological reactions in the body, including energy metabolism, tissue growth, hydration levels, synthesis and degradation of muscle protein, reproductive processes, and mood. Hormones are responsible for both building new muscle and helping metabolize fat into energy. Therefore, it is important to understand which ones are released in relation to exercise as well as the physiological functions they influence. The chances are that you have probably never started a workout thinking, "Today is my endocrine system training day," yet anytime you exercise you are engaging the endocrine system to produce specific changes in your body.

The type of exercise you do, the intensity at which you do it, and how well you allow yourself to recover afterward will influence production of hormones, which can create either an anabolic response to build new tissues such as muscle and fascia, or a catabolic response that will metabolize fat, carbohydrate, and sometimes protein into energy. Anabolic hormones are responsible for supporting the protein synthesis necessary for muscle growth, while catabolic hormones play an important role in the energy expenditure required for weight loss.

There are three major classifications of hormones: steroid, peptide, and amines (modified amino acid hormones), each of which has a unique chemical structure that determines how it interacts with specific receptors. Steroid hormones interact with receptors in the nucleus of a cell. Peptide hormones are composed of amino acids and work with specific receptor sites on the cell membrane. Amines contain nitrogen and influence the sympathetic nervous system, which is responsible for, among other functions, initiating the processes to produce energy for exercise.

Polypeptide hormones are composed of amino acids and are capable of binding to receptors in blood or to receptors located on the cell membrane. Insulin and human growth hormone (HGH) are two examples of polypeptide hormones. All steroid hormones are fat soluble, allowing them to passively diffuse across the sarcolemma of a muscle fiber. Steroid hormones are produced in the adrenal cortex and gonads and are derived from a common precursor, cholesterol. Steroid hormones include the male sex hormone testosterone (T) and the female sex hormone estrogen.

High-intensity exercise can cause mechanical damage and metabolic stress, such as acidosis, to muscle tissue. The response is an increase in the anabolic hormones responsible for repairing and building new muscle proteins or the collagen used in fascia and elastic connective tissues. Among other functions, the hormones HGH, insulin-like growth factors (IGF-1), and T help repair damaged muscle proteins, essential for increasing muscle size and force production. If your goal is to increase lean muscle mass, this becomes one of the most important benefits of high-intensity training. However, it is also a reason why simply relying on a scale for body weight as a measure of progress is not necessarily a good thing. As a hormone like HGH helps to metabolize fat for fuel, it also helps to grow new muscle tissue. This means you may not lose much net weight, but you could experience a different body composition with higher levels of muscle and lower levels of excess body fat.

Like HGH, T is an important hormone that stimulates muscle protein synthesis, making it an integral component of increasing lean muscle mass. Increased T levels are an acute response to strength training, especially when it is performed to a point of momentary fatigue, indicating both metabolic and mechanical overload. As you add lean muscle mass, you are increasing your resting metabolism and elevating the amount of calories you burn at rest. A pound of muscle will expend approximately five to seven calories per day to sustain normal function, so adding five pounds of muscle could elevate resting metabolism by 25 to 35 calories per day. The human body expends approximately 100 calories to walk or run one mile, so over the course of a week, adding five pounds of muscle provides the energy expenditure equivalent of walking almost two miles without taking a single step!

Other hormones include the catecholamines of epinephrine and norepinephrine, which increase the catabolism of fat and carbohydrate molecules to produce the chemical ATP, used to fuel muscle contractions. Epinephrine, produced by the adrenal gland, also influences the nervous system by facilitating increased motor unit activity. An accumulation of lactate is related to an increased release of GH and IGF-1 used to repair damage to the involved tissue. Exercises that elevate IGF-1 are also linked to an elevation in brain-derived neurotrophic factors (BDNF), the neurotransmitter associated with building new neurons in the brain and improving cognition function.

While the body produces hormones responsible for myriad physiological functions, the ones listed in this section are directly influenced by physical activity in general and exercise in particular. Therefore, they play essential roles in helping the body adapt to the imposed physical demands of exercise. Currently, many fitness professionals understand that the nervous and muscular systems play important roles in determining the outcomes of an exercise program. However, the reality is that hormones influence many of the physiological adaptations to physical activity, meaning that the appropriate response to many questions about how the human body responds to exercise is, "It's all hormones nowadays" (Haff and Triplett 2016; Kenney, Wilmore, and Costill 2015).

Insulin

A peptide hormone produced by the pancreas, insulin regulates carbohydrate and fat metabolism. When blood sugar is elevated, insulin is released to promote the storage and absorption of glycogen and glucose. Insulin helps reduce levels of glucose in the blood by promoting its absorption from the bloodstream to skeletal muscles or fat tissues. As it relates to physical activity, it is important to know that insulin can cause fat to be stored in adipose tissue instead of being used to fuel muscle activity. When exercise starts, the sympathetic nervous system suppresses the release of insulin. As a result, it is important to avoid foods with high levels of sugar (including sports drinks) before exercise because they can elevate insulin levels and promote glycogen storage instead of allowing that glycogen to be used to fuel physical activity. Wait until the body has started sweating before using any sports drinks or energy gels.

Glucagon

Released in response to low levels of blood sugar, glucagon is produced by the pancreas to stimulate the release of free fatty acids (FFAs) from adipose tissue as well as increasing blood glucose levels, both of which are important for fueling exercise activity. As glycogen levels are depleted during exercise, glucagon releases additional glycogen stored in the liver.

Cortisol

Cortisol is a catabolic steroid hormone produced by the adrenal gland in response to stress, low blood sugar, and exercise. Cortisol supports energy metabolism during long periods of exercise by facilitating the breakdown of triglycerides and proteins to create the glucose necessary to help fuel exercise. Cortisol is released when the body experiences too much physical stress or is not sufficiently recovered from a previous workout. While cortisol helps promote fat metabolism, exercising for too long can elevate levels of cortisol to catabolize muscle protein for fuel instead of conserving it to be used to repair damaged tissues.

Epinephrine and Norepinephrine

These amine hormones play an important role in helping the sympathetic nervous system (SNS) produce energy and regulate the body's cardiorespiratory function during exercise. Classified as catecholamines, epinephrine and norepinephrine are separate but related hormones. Epinephrine is often referred to as adrenaline because it is produced by the adrenal gland. Epinephrine elevates cardiac output, increases blood sugar to help fuel exercise, promotes the breakdown of glycogen for energy, and supports fat metabolism. Norepinephrine performs a number of the same functions as epinephrine as well as constricting blood vessels in parts of the body not involved in exercise.

Testosterone

Testosterone is a steroid hormone produced by the Leydig cells of the testes in males and the ovaries in females, with small amounts produced by the adrenal glands of both sexes. Testosterone is responsible for muscle protein resynthesis, the repair of muscle proteins damaged by exercise, and plays a significant role in helping grow skeletal muscle. Testosterone works with specific receptor sites and is produced in response to exercise that damages muscle proteins.

Human Growth Hormone (Somatotropin)

HGH is an anabolic peptide hormone secreted by the anterior pituitary gland that stimulates cellular growth. Like all hormones, HGH works with specific receptor sites and can produce a number of responses, including increasing muscle protein synthesis responsible for muscle growth, increasing bone mineralization, supporting immune system function, and promoting lipolysis (fat metabolism). The body produces HGH during the REM cycles of sleep and is stimulated by high-intensity exercise such as heavy strength training, explosive power training, or cardiorespiratory exercise at or above the onset of blood lactate (OBLA, the second ventilatory threshold).

Insulin-Like Growth Factor

Insulin-like growth factor (IGF-1), also commonly referred to as *mechano growth factor*, has a molecular structure similar to insulin. IGF-1 is an important hormone stimulated by the same mechanisms that produce HGH. IGF-1 is a peptide hormone produced in the liver. It supports the function of HGH to repair protein damaged during exercise, making it an important hormone for promoting muscle growth.

Brain-Derived Neurotrophic Factor

Resistance training may seem like a relatively simple type of exercise, and weight-lifters often face a stereotype related to a lack of intelligence, but when it comes to making changes in the body, resistance training initiates a series of chemical, neurological, and structural reactions that ultimately lead to muscle growth and can actually enhance cognitive function. Brain-derived neurotrophic factor (BDNF) is a neurotransmitter that helps stimulate the production of new cells in the brain. The production of BDNF is closely related to the production of HGH and IGF-1. The same exercises that create metabolic or mechanical overloads responsible for elevating the levels of those hormones also increases amounts of BDNF. High-intensity exercise can stimulate anabolic hormones for muscle growth while simultaneously increasing the productions of BDNF.

Hormones have both short- and long-term responses to exercise; understanding how exercise influences the hormones that control physiological functions can help you develop effective exercise programs to meet your goals. In the acute phase immediately postexercise, T, HGH, and IGF-1 are produced to repair damaged tissue. Over the long-term there is an increase in the receptor sites and binding proteins, which allow T, HGH, and IGF-1 to be used more effectively for tissue repair and muscle growth. Exercise performed to a point of momentary fatigue will generate high levels of both the mechanical and metabolic overload that damage muscle proteins and, in turn, initiate the production of T, HGH, and IGF-1 to repair the damage, resulting in muscle growth. The concentration of anabolic to catabolic hormones can be used as a marker to identify signs of overtraining and accumulation of fatigue (Kraemer and Ratamess 2005). As the catabolic hormone cortisol accumulates during periods of rest and recovery, an individual is at risk of becoming underrecovered. The concentration of these hormones is affected by the intensity and duration of each individual exercise session. Research indicates that organizing the volume and intensity of a training session to feature short bursts of extremely high-intensity exercise combined with shorter rest periods can lead to an increase in the production of the anabolic hormones responsible for promoting muscle growth (Schoenfeld 2016; Kraemer and Ratamess 2005).

Putting It All Together

Exercise is much more than working up a sweat; when done properly it can change the function and structure of the human body. Mobility training can improve movement efficiency and strengthen the fascia and elastic connective tissues, helping them to be more resistant to injury. In addition to enhancing aesthetic appearance, strength training and metabolic conditioning can be used to improve the ability to

What the Science Says:
Apps That Control Functions

To take the analogy of the human body as a computer a step further, it is necessary to look at the various software programs or apps that control how the body functions. In a computer, the software determines how efficient the machine is at performing various functions. An app on a computer provides the necessary information for how the components of the machine work together to perform a specific function. For example, a bookkeeping app can help you organize your finances to keep track of income and expenses.

GIGO is an old software programming term standing for "garbage-in, garbage-out," which means that if the software used to perform a function isn't well-written, it will be inefficient or unable to properly perform the assigned task.

Using this analogy, it can be easy to see how traditional muscle-isolation exercises can be considered faulty software because they upload garbage commands, telling only one or two muscles at a time to work while a joint is held in a relatively stable position. This approach to exercise works directly against the inherent learning capabilities of the human operating system, the CNS, which self-learns how to control movement by sending commands to a number of muscles working together to move various joints to learn and refine specific patterns.

One app that helps control the function of various components of the body's hardware is the endocrine system, which produces the chemicals—more specifically, hormones—responsible for initiating and controlling the functions of individual cells such as those of muscle, fascia, and bone. After a strength training workout that results in a mechanical overload on the structures of muscle fibers, the endocrine system will signal the production of testosterone and other anabolic hormones to help promote the protein synthesis required to repair the damaged fibers.

One tip for developing a successful exercise program is to improve your operating system's ability to move the hardware. In other words, use a variety of different movement patterns to upload new information into your CNS in order to control how your muscles, fascia, and connective tissue work more efficiently as a completely integrated system. The specific patterns of hip-hinging, squatting, lunging, pushing, pulling, and rotating can themselves be considered complex software programs capable of dictating how the hardware components of muscle, fascia, and bone work together to produce coordinated movement. These movements are often considered the basic patterns of human movement and should likewise be the foundation for any exercise program created to improve mobility, core strength, and metabolic conditioning.

convert food to energy, change hormone levels, and increase muscle force output, all of which are critical for performing your favorite pastimes or essential activities of daily living. Using exercise to achieve these and other desired results relies on a number of different variables, including sex, age, resistance-training experience, genetics, sleep, nutrition, hydration, and emotional and physical stressors. Each of these influences how your physiological systems adapt to exercise in general or resistance training specifically; for example, too much stress at work or a lack of sleep may significantly reduce your ability to grow muscle.

An exercise is a movement, and movement is a skill that requires practice to master. It may be tempting to change exercises frequently; however, maintaining some consistency with the same exercises over a period of six to eight weeks can help improve coordination and movement skill as well as muscular strength. Efficient movement patterns require synergistic coordination between all systems of the human body. Exercise programs that emphasize using movement patterns use a number of muscles at the same time, which can make the workouts more metabolically challenging, helping you burn more calories, which is essential for maintaining a healthy body weight.

To create and sustain the energy for dynamic, multidirectional movement patterns, the different components of the body need to develop the ability to function as a single system controlled by the CNS. Compared to the limitations of traditional muscle isolation exercises, using only one piece of equipment to challenge the body to move in all directions can result in a more creative, engaging, effective, and fun workout experience. Multijoint movements such as squats to shoulder presses with dumbbells, lifts with a medicine ball, or kettlebell swings are all examples of exercises that involve large amounts of muscle tissue and, in turn, challenge the heart to pump blood to keep the muscles fueled, which can provide a number of health-promoting benefits.

2

Movement and Intensity in Practice

When it comes to exercise, having consistent habits is important. However, staying with a routine that you've been following for an extended length of time may actually work against you, because performing the same exercise program for too long can lead to a plateau where no more physiological changes occur. While any form of regular physical activity provides *some* benefits and is better than doing nothing at all, changing your workouts on a regular basis can help ensure that you continue to see results. To get the best results, it's important that an exercise program is challenging but not too hard, because exercise that is too intense or increases in difficulty too quickly could cause an injury.

The General Adaptation Syndrome, identified by endocrinologist Hans Selye, describes how the physiology of the body adapts to a physical stimulus such as exercise. When beginning an exercise program, an initial alarm phase of one to three weeks occurs during which the body recognizes that a new stimulus is being applied. This is followed by an adaptation phase of 4 to 16 weeks during which the body adapts to the stimulus and becomes more efficient at tolerating it. Finally, after an extended period, up to 12 to 16 weeks, the body reaches what is called the exhaustion phase during which the stimulus no longer has a significant effect (Haff and Triplett 2016).

Many different methods of exercise are touted with the promise to help you achieve results. Which is the best for *you*? You want to find an exercise program that works and doesn't make you waste energy on frivolous efforts, so how can you filter through all of the marketing blather to select the right type(s) of exercise for your needs?

When creating your own workout program, the biggest challenge can become how to identify and perform the most effective exercise from each category for your particular needs. There are three general modes of exercise:

1. Mobility is a combination of reducing muscle tightness, increasing tissue extensibility, and improving joint range of motion (ROM).

2. Core strength training enhances the force production and coordination of the muscles that control the body's center of gravity, enabling them to perform greater amounts of physical work.

3. Metabolic conditioning uses the cardiorespiratory system to place oxygen in the bloodstream and pump it, along with the energy substrates, to working muscles.

Mobility exercises can reduce muscle tension and improve joint ROM, both of which are essential for enhancing overall movement efficiency. Mobility training can improve coordination and dynamic balance as well as reduce the risk of injury from repetitive movements or lack of movement.

Strength training improves the ability of the core muscles to generate force, which both expends energy (burns calories) and results in better looking, more aesthetically pleasing muscles. Strength training exercises help improve muscle force output, which can elevate resting metabolism (the ability to burn calories while at rest), enhancing functional performance in a variety of activities and preventing the risk of developing a number of chronic diseases and health conditions.

Metabolic conditioning enhances the ability to move oxygen and nutrients to working muscles as well as remove metabolic waste, thereby allowing muscles to continue to perform a particular activity. The benefits of metabolic conditioning include increasing energy expenditure for weight loss and improving the efficiency at which the heart pumps blood around the body to working muscles.

Exercise is a function of integrated movement patterns that require numerous muscles to coordinate their actions, not separate, isolated, or discrete muscle actions. The human body is designed to move, and one of the most important benefits of consistent exercise is that it will improve your ability to move without any physical discomfort. Most likely this improvement will create the desire to move more often, which is the foundation of making physical activity a lifelong habit and achieving and maintaining optimal health.

A well-designed exercise program will include all three methods, but if you want to improve muscle definition, your primary focus should be on strength training. If your goal is to improve flexibility to avoid a number of repetitive stress injuries while enhancing movement skill, the focus should be on mobility training. Finally, if you're exercising for the purpose of specific endurance training, like participating in a race, or weight loss, you will want to emphasize metabolic conditioning to improve your cardiorespiratory efficiency. Metabolic conditioning at a lower, steady-state intensity will draw on aerobic pathways that primarily metabolize fats for fuel. Higher-intensity metabolic conditioning, either interval or steady state, will use the anaerobic pathways and help you increase the length of time you can exercise before fatigue sets in.

Mobility Training

Improving mobility first before doing higher-intensity exercises for core strength or metabolic conditioning can help establish the foundation for long-term success. If you're not doing mobility or flexibility training regularly, it's probably because you either don't have the time or don't know how to do the exercises in a way that will make a difference in your body.

There are a variety of stretching techniques. The one you are most likely familiar with is static stretching: holding a stretch for 30 seconds or so, causing the muscle to relax and lengthen. Static stretching can help reduce tension, but it does so by reducing nervous system activity in the muscle fibers, which is not necessarily the best thing to do prior to being active; it is best saved for the end of a workout. While stretching does provide benefits like reduced soreness and improved joint motion, a workout consisting only of static stretching would be relatively dull, and if it's dull, it's unlikely that you would make it a regular habit.

Proper mobility training, on the other hand, challenges the CNS by using movement patterns that integrate motion in both the upper- and lower-body segments together, which improves contraction of the motor units while lengthening both the contractile component of muscle as well as the elastic connective tissues. The resulting exercises provide numerous benefits such as enhancing the ability of the CNS to activate muscles, increasing circulation to the working muscles, reducing tension in tight muscles, and improving joint ROM. Mobility exercises can provide low- to moderate-intensity workout solutions that can be used to improve movement skill or promote recovery the day after really hard exercise that leaves you sore.

Remaining in sedentary positions for an extended time or restricting movement patterns to predictable, repetitive motions could lead to significant loss of elasticity from fascia and elastic connective tissue, which can greatly change the function of a joint and reduce its ROM. Likewise, repetitive, cyclic actions performed in a single, linear plane of motion could cause collagen adhesions that restrict extensibility (the ability of muscle, fascia, and elastic connective tissues to lengthen and shorten), limiting joint motion and reducing mobility. Injuries related to the loss of joint mobility are preventable because the superficial layers of fascia have a loose density, and fibers respond to multidirectional forces by layering and aligning in multidirectional patterns. The dense, thick ligaments and tendons that connect to bony structures are organized in a unidirectional pattern. Many common injuries restricting joint mobility can be related to fascia and connective tissue being loaded repetitively beyond its existing capacity (Schleip and Bayer 2017; Schleip et al. 2012).

For example, individuals who spend a large portion of their time seated can develop collagen adhesions between the layers of the large major muscles responsible for flexing the hip (picking the knee up to waist height when in a standing position). In this case, the tightness from the hip flexors can limit the ability of the femur to extend behind the hip by reducing the nervous system activity to the muscle motor units of the gluteus maximus (the primary muscle responsible for hip extension), changing the function of the muscle and the mobility of the joint. However, physical activities, including exercise, that require multidirectional movements at a variety of speeds can create more elastic, resilient fascial structures that allow for optimal loading of mechanical energy while improving joint mobility. The ability of fascia and elastic connective tissue to lengthen allows a joint to move through a complete ROM, supporting optimal joint mobility. If joints designed to be mobile allow unrestricted freedom of movement, it can reduce stress across the entire system and lower the risk of injury. "If one's fascial body is optimally elastic and resilient then it can be relied upon to perform effectively while offering a high degree of injury prevention" (Schleip et al. 2012, 465).

Like the spokes of a wheel, muscle, fascia, and elastic connective tissue establish a balanced transfer of forces throughout the entire skeletal structure (figure 2.1). Fascia is organized between each individual muscle fiber or bundles of fibers, known as fascicles, to accommodate three-dimensional forces, mitigate stresses, and create equilibrium to establish an efficient structure in the human skeleton. Fascia possesses an ability to adapt and recreate its structure relative to applied forces; compressive and tensile forces from exercise and other physical activities ultimately determine whether fascia has a linear or multidirectional structural pattern. Repeated application of strain and tensile forces can increase the density of fascia, enhancing its ability to dissipate these forces. Because they remodel their architecture in response to applied stresses, even to the microscopic level of individual cells, fascia and elastic connective tissue play an important role in adapting to the applied demands of exercise to enhance physical activity (Ingber 2003, 2004; Vogel and Sheetz 2006; Schleip and Bayer 2017).

During extremely cold weather, it is common practice to allow your car to warm up so that the engine can function properly. Your body is the same way; in order to properly prepare for activity, performing a series of mobility exercises can warm up and prepare your body to function its best during the more strenuous parts of a workout. Exercises based on integrated movement patterns are a form of active stretching because your muscles actively take the joint through its entire ROM. This can be an effective strategy to enhance mobility prior to a workout because mobility exercises can elevate the body temperature, increase the blood flow, and activate the motor neurons of the muscles and tendons about to be used; for the same reasons, mobility-specific workouts are great for the days after a high-intensity strength or metabolic conditioning workout to help reduce soreness and promote recovery.

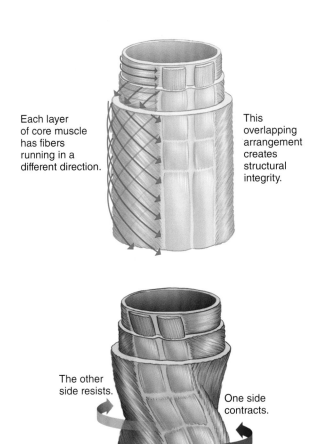

Each layer of core muscle has fibers running in a different direction.

This overlapping arrangement creates structural integrity.

The other side resists.

One side contracts.

Figure 2.1 Fascia surrounds all muscle tissue down to the individual muscle fiber; it is responsible for transferring force between different sections of muscle.

Mobility training features bodyweight exercises that integrate the upper- and lower-body segments together to learn efficient movement patterns and are an excellent option when you want to move in a way that does not put too much stress on the body or want to promote recovery from a strenuous workout. Because mobility exercises are specifically designed to help increase joint ROM, tissue extensibility, dynamic balance, and coordination without working to a point of fatigue or discomfort, they should be considered low to moderate intensity.

Here's an important takeaway: Exercise does not have to be hard or crush you to be effective. Yes, if you want to make changes to your body it is necessary to do some extremely challenging workouts that create a metabolic or mechanical overload, either of which can leave you feeling exhausted and drained; however, it's also completely appropriate to do some workouts that focus only on low-intensity movements that use your muscles for work but that are below the intensity thresholds that cause mechanical or metabolic fatigue. Mobility exercise programs can also be done during periods of high stress or a busy schedule when you want workouts that help you feel invigorated and more energetic as opposed to fatigued and crushed.

Core Strength Training

Core training is paradoxically one of the most popular yet misunderstood phrases in the fitness world today. For some, core training means doing crunches until the abs cramp in exhaustion; for others, core training means doing all sorts of complicated moves on various pieces of equipment that look better suited for a circus than a fitness facility. It can seem as if every fitness instructor or YouTube star has a different approach to core training, some derived from academic research and others based on pure fiction or opinion.

With all of this information, it can be difficult to determine the most effective core training program for your needs. If you really want muscle definition so you can show off your abs, pay heed to the phrase, "Abs are made in the kitchen," because it's absolutely correct. We all have a six-pack; some of us, however, are keeping it in a cooler. Extra energy is stored as fat cells in adipose tissue, which also functions to provide insulation to muscles and organs, and for a number of people, extra fat is stored in the adipose tissue of the abdominal cavity. Developing definition in muscles is as much a function of eating the proper amounts of the right types of nutrients as it is expending energy through exercise.

As you begin to develop your exercise program, think about when you use your core strength. Do you use a higher amount of core strength when lying on the ground or when you're standing on your feet and moving in multiple directions? For an effective core training program that can increase caloric expenditure while enhancing strength and reducing the risk of injury, it will become necessary to start thinking of any exercise done standing on your feet as a core exercise. The right exercises for improving and enhancing core strength provide many benefits, from changing aesthetic appearance to reducing lower-back soreness. By simply learning how to brace the multiple layers of your abdominal muscles while on your feet, you will help the muscles activate and do their job to stabilize your body through the hips, spine, and pelvis. Knowing the best types of core exercises that can increase strength while improving dynamic balance and movement skill first requires understanding how the core muscles actually function during upright movement patterns.

A lot of the confusion surrounding this topic stems from the fact that there is not one specific core muscle, nor is there a specific region of the core. Any muscle that attaches the legs to the pelvis or the pelvis to the spine and rib cage, controls motion of the shoulders on top of the spine, or simply runs along the spine can influence motion at your center of gravity, which, in most adults, is just below the belly button; these can be considered a core muscle. Lying on the floor for core training can be effective for some exercises in the initial stages of developing strength, but whether you are in a face-down or face-up position you will not be fully integrating the muscles of the hips, abdominals, and lower back to function as a single system. For example, performing numerous crunches while lying on the back is a traditional approach to core exercises that causes excessive amounts of spinal flexion and possibly leads to the muscle imbalances that are often a source of injury (Contreras and Schoenfeld

2011). Some of the most effective strategies for strengthening core muscles require you to be in an upright standing position with your feet planted on the ground.

To fully understand how the muscles of the core are designed to function all we need to do is observe the human gait cycle. The structures of the human body operate most effectively when standing upright while reacting to the downward forces caused by gravity and the upward forces of ground reaction created as the foot impacts the ground when walking or running. You're no doubt familiar with gravity; its downward pull places a constant force on the body that your muscles have to work to overcome. However, you're probably not that familiar with the ground reaction forces that occur every time your foot hits the ground. As your foot impacts the solid ground, the ground doesn't absorb the force of your body weight and instead pushes back against your foot. Normal walking can place about 1.5 times your body weight in each leg as your foot hits the ground. When you run, the ground forces are higher; at top sprint speeds, you could experience up to six times your body weight in reaction forces (Haff and Tripplet 2016).

The body is designed to function most efficiently while using gait, either walking or running, as the primary means of locomotion, with the muscles aligned to take advantage of gravity and ground reaction forces to generate mechanical energy. Most strength training exercises that take place in a standing position with your feet on the ground *are* core exercises. According to a comprehensive review of the research literature on exercise for the core muscles, Contreras and Schoenfeld wrote, "Most training can be considered 'core training' . . . With respect to program design, basic core strength and endurance will be realized through performance of most non-machine-based exercises such as during squats, deadlifts, chin-ups and push-ups" (Contreras and Schoenfeld 2011, 14).

Stuart McGill, PhD, is professor emeritus of kinesiology at University of Waterloo in Waterloo, Canada, where he ran the Spine Biomechanics Laboratory for thirty-two years. Dr. McGill has conducted an extensive amount of research and has published numerous academic articles and textbooks on spinal mechanics featuring the evidence-based exercise programs for improving core strength. Dr. McGill defines the core as "composed of the lumbar spine, the muscles of the abdominal wall, the back extensors and quadratus lumborum. Also included are the multi-joint muscles, namely, latissimus dorsi and psoas that pass through the core linking it to the pelvis, legs, shoulders and arms" (McGill 2010, 33).

Rather than rolling on the ground like a turtle stuck in its shell, an effective core conditioning workout should be based on strength training exercises featuring a variety of upright movements using different loads to ensure optimal strength of postural stabilizers combined with maximal force production from the muscles responsible for moving the body. For example, the hips should be able to move and produce force in all three dimensions in order to accomplish a number of ADLs or recreational sports like golf or tennis. If the muscles around the hips lose the ability to generate force in all three planes, it could increase the forces directed into the lumbar spine or knees and significantly increase the risk of injury at the joints. According to McGill's observations, "People rarely flex their rib cage to the pelvis

Movement and Intensity in Practice | **33**

shortening the rectus abdominis in sport or everyday activities. Rather they stiffen the abdominal wall while loading the hips or using the shoulders" (McGill 2010, 38). When it comes to enhancing movement skill, improving dynamic balance, and increasing levels of muscular strength, the concept of core training should be expanded to include all of the muscles that help the body walk or run.

Metabolic Conditioning

Your metabolism is how your body converts the macronutrients—carbohydrates, fats, and proteins—you consume through your diet into the chemical adenosine triphosphate (ATP) used to fuel muscle contractions. Your body produces ATP either with oxygen or without oxygen via specific metabolic pathways. Muscle cells use oxygen to help produce the energy to fuel contractions. As stated previously, you will use approximately five calories of energy to consume one liter of oxygen; therefore, the more oxygen you consume during (and after) exercise, the more calories you will burn.

Calories Explained

A calorie is a unit of energy. More accurately, a kilocalorie is the energy used to increase the heat of one liter of water by one degree centigrade (Haff and Tripplet 2016). Just like a gallon of gas should provide your car with enough energy to travel a certain distance (measured in miles per gallon), when a piece of food is estimated to have a certain amount of calories, that is how much energy it delivers to your body. According to the first law of thermodynamics, energy is neither created nor destroyed, but is merely transferred. The macronutrients of protein, carbohydrate, and fat provide four, four, and nine calories per gram, respectively. If a piece of food has 10 grams of protein, 20 grams of carbohydrate, and 5 grams of fat, it should provide approximately 165 calories worth of energy. When you consume energy through macronutrients, your body will use some of it immediately for tissue repair, energy, and other vital functions. The energy is doesn't use will be stored as fat for use at a later time.

The human body requires energy for a variety of functions, including repairing and replacing damaged tissues, digesting food, and performing physical activity. As it relates to expending energy for physical activities, your body will burn calories in two specific ways: activities of daily living (ADLs), which include such mundane tasks as brushing your teeth, cleaning the house, or walking to the car, and exercise that is physical activity for the purpose of improving the body's ability to perform specific tasks or simply expending excess energy.

Physical activity, whether ADLs or exercise, is an important component of managing a healthy body weight because it is how you expend excess energy. Managing consumer credit can provide an analogy to help you understand what is required for healthy weight management.

When you have a credit card, it is not a good idea to spend more than you earn because you will end up in debt. On the other hand, if you make smart decisions with your income, spend only what you need for expenses, limit impulse purchases to only what you can afford, pay off your credit cards every month, and place any extra income in a savings account, you will end up with a surplus of money.

Replace money with calories. If you consume more calories in a day than you expend through various types of physical activity, you will end up with a surplus of calories in "savings." While it is a good idea to place extra money in a savings account, we generally want to avoid accumulating a surplus of unused energy in the body because it is stored as fat. Increasing physical activity, through both ADLs and exercise, can help you spend as many, if not more, calories than you consume. While deficit spending can lead to credit card debt, which is something you want to avoid, when it comes to exercise this is how we can eliminate surplus energy and is what you should be working toward. This is the one time in your life when you are allowed to spend more than you earn; spending more energy through physical activity than you consume through caloric intake is a key component of weight loss.

Over the course of the normal biological aging process, adults who are sedentary for extended periods of time and do not participate in any types of physical activity could accumulate excess amounts of energy (stored as fat) as well as experience the loss of balance, mobility, and muscle mass. A decline in muscle mass reduces your body's resting metabolism, the ability to burn calories without actually doing any activity, and could result in a loss of strength, reducing your ability to perform many essential ADLs. An age-related loss of muscle strength is a predictor of diminished physical function, balance impairments, and overall frailty, resulting in an increased risk of falls or other incapacitating injuries. It's true that a relatively sedentary lifestyle can result in a loss of functional capacity that severely impacts the over-all quality of life; however, long-term participation in a strength training program can reduce the loss of age-related muscle mass, maintain or increase muscle force production, and enhance the ability to successfully perform most ADLs, allowing you to remain functionally independent well into the later years of life. In addition, even if you get a late start, consistently following an exercise program to enhance mobility, strength, and metabolic efficiency can help you maintain a high level of physical performance and good health well into old age.

Understanding the Calorie

For years, we've been told that we need to pay attention to calories both in how many we consume and how many we expend through physical activity. What is a calorie and why does it matter how many we consume or burn when we exercise?

Weight gain happens when you have a surplus of calories because you consume more calories than you expend. Think about that for a moment. If you are eating a couple thousand calories a day but doing just a minimal amount of physical activity, you are taking in excess energy that will be stored as fat in adipose tissue. Having excess body fat means that you are carrying around extra energy, which is like driving around with extra tanks of gas in your car. It's just not necessary, and if you have too much, it becomes potentially dangerous. Carrying too much gas in your car increases the risk of a fire; carrying too much extra energy on your body in the form of fat can lead to a number of negative health outcomes. A pound of fat provides approximately 3,500 calories of energy. The human body expends about five calories of energy to consume one liter of oxygen; during exercise, muscles use oxygen, so if you are carrying extra fat on your body, doing movement-based workouts that use numerous muscles at the same time will help you turn that stored energy into kinetic energy.

Role of the Heart

The heart is a muscle that functions as a pump to circulate blood through the body to carry nutrients and oxygen to muscles to create the ATP required to perform physical activity and remove metabolic by-products (the "exhaust" from muscular contractions), which can either be recycled into new ATP or excreted from the body (figure 2.2). Any form of exercise that elevates the heart rate is helping it become a stronger, more efficient pump. The harder you work, the faster the heart has to pump to do its job of delivering the good stuff and removing the bad stuff from the working muscles. The heart rate (HR) is measured in beats per minute (BPM). The most effective way to determine the intensity of cardiovascular exercise is to pay attention to the HR by measuring its BPM. When the exercise becomes too intense, the body is not able to efficiently remove metabolic by-products—hydrogen ions and lactic acid—from the muscle, so it begins to accumulate, leading to acidosis, which means the blood has become more acidic, thus creating that sensation of the muscle burning when you're working really hard.

A common gym belief claims that in order to burn fat and lose weight, it is necessary to perform an extensive amount of cardiorespiratory exercise, often shortened to just *cardio*. While not wrong, this is an incomplete explanation of what is happening during exercise that elevates the heart rate. As mentioned earlier, anytime you are breathing, you are bringing oxygen into your body, and your lungs are placing it into your blood, which is then pumped to the muscles that need it. But when it comes to exercise, your body needs to produce energy to fuel the activity that you are doing; therefore, it is more appropriate to refer to this type of exercise as *metabolic conditioning* in order to identify the specific pathway or pathways that will be used to create energy during a workout.

To help you understand why this is important, consider sport-specific training. Metabolic conditioning for a specific sport should focus on how the body moves

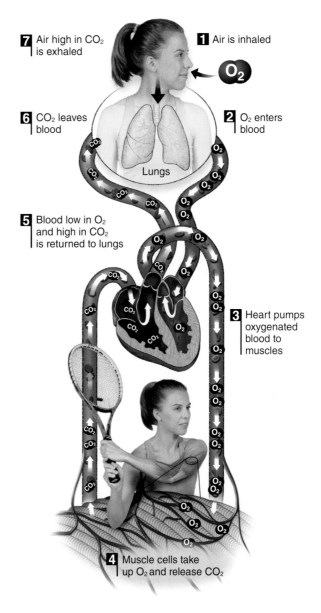

Figure 2.2 The heart is a muscle responsible for pumping blood through the body. The heart rate, measured in beats per minute, is a good indicator of exercise intensity; when your muscles work harder, the heart has to beat faster to supply oxygen and remove metabolic by-product.

in the sport as well as the pathways that will produce and deliver the energy for that activity. For example, endurance runners will focus on aerobic metabolism for long-term energy for the legs, while athletes in sports such as football, rugby, or basketball will focus on training the anaerobic pathways to be more efficient at producing energy for the explosive movements required for their respective sports. Metabolic conditioning for the purpose of promoting good health and maintaining a healthy body weight should focus on exercises that are energy-expensive—that is, those exercises that expend a number of calories in a relatively short time.

Aerobic metabolism requires oxygen and uses either fats or carbohydrates to produce energy during low-intensity activities, yet this is considered slow; anaerobic metabolism converts carbohydrates to ATP when energy is needed quickly. During anaerobic glycolysis one molecule of glycogen (how a carbohydrate is stored in muscle or transported in blood) can provide two to three molecules of ATP. Aerobic glycolysis can yield up to 39 molecules of ATP from one molecule of glycogen. When energy is produced during aerobic lipolysis one molecule of FFA yields approximately 129 ATP. At the start of physical activity, during extremely high-intensity activities that last a brief period of time, or during the transition from low to higher intensities, energy is supplied by ATP stored in muscle cells, which can provide up to approximately 20 seconds or so of energy.

Similar to how a car's engine remains warm after being turned off, once a workout is over and you're back in your daily routine, your body's metabolism can remain elevated, burning more calories than when at complete rest. This physiological effect is called the *excess postexercise oxygen consumption* (EPOC). EPOC is the amount of oxygen required to restore your body to its normal, resting level of metabolic function (called *homeostasis*) and explains how your body can continue to burn calories for a period of time after you've finished your workout. Exercise that places a greater demand on the anaerobic energy pathways during the workout can increase the need for oxygen after the workout, enhancing the EPOC effect.

When the need for anaerobic ATP increases it also creates a greater demand on the aerobic system to replenish that ATP during the rest intervals as well as the postexercise recovery process. Strength training using compound, multijoint movement patterns in a circuit format, alternating between upper- and lower-body actions with minimal rest periods between exercises, places a greater demand on the involved muscles for ATP from the anaerobic pathways and can result in an elevated EPOC. Exercising to the point of momentary fatigue combined with shorter recovery intervals can increase the demand on the anaerobic energy pathways during exercise, resulting in a greater EPOC. The EPOC effect is real, but it has been overemphasized by well-meaning but ill-informed fitness professionals. When compared to being in a normal, rested state, your body will burn more calories after high-intensity exercise, but it is not a significant amount of calories, so it is still important to make smart nutrition choices if your primary reason for working out is weight management.

The Physics of Exercise

How the body consumes, stores, and expends energy is a function of both dietary intake and physical activity. Identifying how Newton's laws of physics apply to exercise can help you understand why regular exercise is so important for maintaining a healthy body weight. Exercise is the application of these basic laws of physics. It is simply performing work and expending energy to accomplish physical tasks.

Inertia or Momentum

Inertia refers to how a body at rest will stay at rest unless acted on by an external force. Momentum refers to how a body in motion will remain in motion unless acted on by an external force. Applied to exercise, this law explains how a mass, whether your body weight or an external weight, will remain at a constant state of rest until another force, like one from a muscle shortening action, is applied to create motion.

Force = Mass × Acceleration

Force is the product of a mass and its rate of acceleration. When a muscle contracts, it is generating force to accelerate that mass. In exercise, force can be manipulated one of two ways: use a heavier mass to challenge muscles to generate greater magnitudes of force, or use an object with a light mass and move it at a faster rate of acceleration.

Work, measured in joules, is a product of force and distance ($W = F \times D$). It is the amount of muscular force required to move a mass a quantifiable distance, which can be how far a body segment moves with each repetition. Power, measured in watts or joules per second, is the rate of doing work and measures the amount of work performed per unit time ($P = W/T$). Another way to describe power is that it is the product of force and velocity ($P = F \times V$). Either way, the faster an object can be accelerated, the greater the amount of power generated.

If you have only a limited amount of time for exercise—say, 30 minutes—increasing your speed of movement, as is done during fast-paced metabolic conditioning exercises, can increase your overall work rate and your net caloric expenditure.

For Every Action, There Is an Equal and Opposite Reaction

Applied to exercise, this law supports the SAID principle of exercise program design, which states the body will adapt (react) to the physical demands imposed on it (action). For example, when you use a strength training machine that dictates the movement, the body reacts by becoming strong specifically for the motion allowed by that machine.

If you perform only a minimal amount of physical activity throughout the day, you will not expend the energy (calories) being consumed through your diet, which can lead to weight gain.

The overload principle states that achieving results from exercise requires challenging a physiological system to perform a greater amount of physical work than it is currently able to perform (Haff and Triplett 2016). An effective method for improving muscle strength is to apply a physical stimulus to the muscles at a greater intensity than they are accustomed to receiving. Exercising with weights like medicine balls, dumbbells, kettlebells, or sandbags stimulates specific neural and structural adaptations that can improve the size and force production capacity of skeletal muscle. Applied correctly, an overload can improve the efficiency at which the muscle communicates with the CNS as well as leading to an increase in the size and structure of the involved fibers and connective tissue—for example, by activating more muscle motor neurons and their attached muscle fibers.

A different way to apply an overload is to challenge your coordination by using patterns that move your body in a variety of directions. Exercises to strengthen the core should integrate motion of the hips, trunk, and shoulders to efficiently distribute the forces created when moving in multiple directions. Forces applied to the human body, whether external from resistance-training equipment or internal in response to muscle contractions, can change the shape and function of tissues, specifically fascia, muscle, and bone. Optimal movement efficiency relies on the integrating of muscle, fascia, and the CNS, which uses sensory input to coordinate the appropriate motor response, ultimately leading to improvements in coordination and movement skill.

Organizing Workout Variables

The human body is extremely efficient at conserving energy. The more often you perform a certain exercise with the same amount of weight or run the same distance, the more efficient your body will become at performing that work, and you could experience a reduced training effect. Workout programs based on learning and performing movement patterns can provide you with more options for how to exercise, which can ultimately lead to greater results. Whether it's exercise to improve muscular strength, enhance metabolic efficiency, or increase mobility, exercise programs contain the same basic elements known as the variables of exercise program design, which are exercise selection, intensity, repetitions, tempo, rest interval, sets, and frequency of exercise sessions. How these variables are organized and applied will determine the results from an exercise program.

Designing a Workout Is Like Cooking a Meal

Simply throwing a bunch of stuff in a pan and hoping that it turns into an appetizing and edible meal is not an effective way to cook. Likewise, hopping from one piece of equipment to the next, bouncing around between different fitness trends or doing exercises only for specific muscles are not effective methods of exercising. The first step of cooking is determining exactly what to make. In a similar fashion, the first step in designing an exercise program is determining the specific outcome you are trying to achieve. In cooking, the dish you want to prepare will determine the ingredients, the utensils used for preparing the food, and finally the best pots and pans for doing the actual cooking. Your fitness goal will determine the best equipment to use, the specific exercises you do, and how often you do them.

To prepare a successful meal it is important to know how to organize the ingredients, how much of each to use, the order in which they're added, and finally the optimal temperature and length of time in the oven. Using too much or too little of a specific ingredient, the wrong temperature, or wrong length of time can drastically change the outcome of a dish. Exercise is very much the same way; performing exercises that are not relevant to your goal, using too much or too little resistance, or doing too many or too few repetitions could drastically change the outcome of the workout. The variables of exercise program design (table 2.1) can be applied based on what you want to achieve from an exercise program. Add muscle? Lose excess body weight? Enhance athletic performance? Improve health? The variables can be adjusted to provide the appropriate mechanical or metabolic overload in a manner that creates a safe yet effective stimulus to meet your objectives.

Table 2.1   **Variables of Exercise Program Design**

Variable	Description	Example
Exercise selection	The exercises performed during a workout. A program that favors some exercises or muscles over others could cause the muscle imbalances that are a potential source of injury. The CNS is extremely efficient at coordinating individual muscle firing patterns to perform integrated movements. For best results, exercises should be based on movement patterns that require the integration and coordination of many muscles working together to generate the forces needed for joint motion. The workouts in this book organize exercise selection based on the five basic patterns of human movement: • *Squatting or hinging patterns*: The hips flex and extend with both feet in contact with the ground. • *Lunging or single-leg patterns*: One foot leaves the ground and makes contact in a pattern similar to the actions that occur during the gait cycle. • *Pushing movements*: The hands move away from the body either to the front or to an overhead position. • *Pulling movements*: The hands move toward the body from the front or from an overhead position. • *Rotational movements*: Either the thoracic spine or pelvis rotate to provide motion. Effective exercise programs select the appropriate movements and organize them in a progressively more challenging sequence to ensure the necessary overload to make the desired changes.	Kettlebell goblet squat Dumbbell reverse lunge Push-up Single-arm dumbbell row Medicine ball lift
Intensity	The specific amount of weight or external resistance used for strength training. Often, intensity refers to the amount of weight used with traditional equipment, such as barbells, dumbbells, or machines. In general, heavier weights for increasing core strength require fewer repetitions and place a mechanical overload on the muscles, while using a light weight or body weight means doing more repetitions to apply a metabolic overload.	10 lb (4.5 kg) medicine ball 22 lb (10 kg) dumbbells 53 lb (24 kg) kettlebell
Repetition	A single, individual action of movement at a joint or series of joints that involves three phases of muscle action: muscle lengthening, a momentary pause, and muscle shortening. Repetitions and intensity have an inverse relationship; as the intensity increases, the number of repetitions able to be performed decreases. Heavier weights can induce mechanical overload in only a few repetitions, while lighter loads or bodyweight exercises can be done for a relatively high number of repetitions to create metabolic overload. Repetitions can also be performed for a specific amount of time. If this is the case, the goal is to perform as many as possible in the available period of time.	8 to 10 reps of a core strength exercise 30 sec of a metabolic conditioning exercise 10 to 12 reps of a mobility exercise
Set	The number of repetitions or length of time a specific exercise is performed before a rest interval to allow recovery. The exact number of sets in each workout is based on the available amount of time and your focus (core strength, metabolic conditioning, or mobility).	3 or 4 sets of a core strength exercise 2 to 4 sets of a metabolic conditioning exercise 1 to 3 sets of a mobility exercise

(continued)

Table 2.1 *(continued)*

Variable	Description	Example
Tempo	The speed of movement for an exercise. Time under tension (TUT), the length of time muscle fibers are under mechanical tension from a resistance-training exercise, is another way to describe this variable. Along with intensity, TUT is critical for creating the desired stimulus of either mechanical or metabolic overload. A slower TUT can induce more mechanical overload; a faster tempo can create a greater metabolic response.	Moderate-paced tempo for a core strength exercise Fast-paced tempo for a metabolic conditioning exercise Slow tempo for a mobility exercise
Rest interval	Time between exercise sets. A rest interval allows replenishment of ATP stores in the involved muscles and recovery from neural fatigue. Proper rest intervals are essential for increasing muscular strength and allowing for optimal metabolic conditioning.	Resting for 30 sec between exercises Resting for 90 sec after completing a circuit of different exercises
Frequency	Number of workouts or exercise sessions within a specific period of time, such as a week or month. Too many high-intensity workouts without proper recovery in between each workout could lead to an overtraining injury.	2 high-intensity workouts 2 or 3 moderate-intensity workouts 2 or 3 low-intensity workouts a week
Recovery	Following exercise, the body needs time to repair damaged tissues and replace spent energy; the time between workouts is when your body restores the muscle glycogen used during exercise and initiates the protein synthesis to repair damaged muscles. Exercise is the application of a physical stimulus; it is the period afterwards when the body actually experiences physiological changes.	After a high-intensity metabolic conditioning workout, 2 low- to moderate-intensity workouts are done to allow for optimal recovery before another challenging, high-intensity workout.

Finding the Motivation to Exercise

Lack of time is one of the most popular excuses for avoiding exercise. Another reason for skipping exercise is that there is almost too much information available, making it hard to identify the types that you should be doing for the results you want. These two reasons alone demonstrate why it's easy to find other things to do instead of exercise; you'd rather spend your limited free time doing something you enjoy instead of something that feels awkward or uncomfortable. Most importantly, you probably just want to know how to exercise in a manner that will provide the greatest amount of benefits without an extensive time or cost commitment.

First, exercise is something you do in your free time, so it should be an activity that you at least *don't mind* doing. (*Enjoy* doing would be more preferable, but it's necessary to set realistic expectations.) To identify the types of exercise that can bring you the greatest amount of enjoyment, think back to the types of activities that brought you the most pleasure. Understanding just a little about muscle fiber physiology can help you identify the types of exercise activities that will feel right for your body. If you've always gravitated toward endurance sports such as running, cycling, or swimming for long distances, you may have more type I muscle fibers, which are extremely efficient at aerobic metabolism. However, if you've found that you enjoy field sports such as soccer or football, court sports such as tennis or basketball because of the fast-paced running and rapid changes of direction, sprinting, or dancing, you probably have higher levels of type II muscle fibers, which are responsible for creating the powerful muscle contractions needed for those activities.

If you have been struggling to follow an exercise program consistently for the long term, maybe your focus is in the wrong area. Rather than placing all of the emphasis on the outcome of exercise, why not adjust your thinking and focus on the process? You are better off choosing activities that are easily accessible and that you enjoy doing as opposed to workout programs that you think you should do even if you don't look forward to them and especially if it is at an out-of-the-way location that can be difficult to get to.

Principles of Exercise Program Design

Understanding how the different systems function as discrete components can help you identify the best methods for synergistically coordinating their actions to produce the desired results from an exercise program. Participation in a regular exercise program is essential for achieving and maintaining good health, which can help you avoid having to pay expensive medical costs as you age. Exercise provides numerous health benefits, including increased bone mineral density, improved blood lipid profiles, elevated mitochondrial density, increased aerobic capacity, lowered blood pressure, and improved glucose tolerance. All these benefits help reduce the risk of developing chronic diseases while providing various cognitive benefits, such as improving memory recall, making exercise as important for your brain as it is for your muscles. Exercise should engage all of the physiological systems reviewed in chapter 1, with a specific emphasis on enhancing mobility, strengthening the core, and improving metabolic efficiency. Identifying the best exercise program for your particular needs first requires a basic understanding of how exercise changes the human body.

The SAID principle (specific adaptations to imposed demands) states that the type of exercise stimulus placed on the body will determine the expected physiological outcome. Changes to the structures and systems of the human body do not occur without a preceding stimulus. The body is very adaptable and adjusts to any physical stimulus it is exposed to regularly. Each physiological system—neural, endocrine, metabolic, fascial, muscular, and skeletal—will respond and adapt to the specific physical demands applied through a progressively more challenging exercise program.

According to the SAID principle, an individual who performs only muscle-isolation exercises can expect to strengthen the specific muscles used during exercise but may not achieve the intermuscular coordination necessary to improve skills such as coordination and dynamic balance.

Applying the Variables to Design Your Workouts

One thing most top fitness professionals agree on is that an effective exercise program doesn't need to be overly complicated. It's not necessary to do overly complicated moves or change the exercises you do every workout; only five basic movement patterns determine the exercises you should do during the workout. Simply changing one or two of the variables, like the amount of intensity, number of repetitions, or length of the rest interval, can significantly change the demands imposed on your body. As you get started with your exercise program, you should be aware that research can provide some general insights about how fitness may affect your body, but there are many factors besides the variables of exercise program design, like nutrition, sleep patterns, and overall stress levels, that will determine your specific response.

Inducing metabolic and mechanical stress in the gym does help promote muscle growth; however, what you do in the gym is only one component of the equation for achieving results. T and GH are produced during the REM cycles of sleep, meaning that after a hard workout, a full night's rest is essential for promoting muscle growth and achieving optimal recovery. Insufficient rest does not allow for optimal muscle protein synthesis to repair tissues damaged during exercise, nor does it allow for adequate replenishment of the muscle glycogen used to produce ATP and could lead to an accumulation of energy-producing hormones such as epinephrine and cortisol, which can reduce the ability to generate new muscle tissue. Loss of sleep, loss of appetite, lingering illness, and cessation of gains from exercise are all symptoms of overtraining, which can significantly affect your ability to achieve your fitness goals.

The postworkout recovery period is often the most overlooked variable of any exercise program. Whether it is mechanical or metabolic stress that provides the stimulus for muscle growth is not as important as allowing the time for T, GH, and IGF-1 to promote muscle protein synthesis after the exercise is over. Exercise is when a physical stimulus is applied to a muscle and is only part of the equation responsible for muscle growth. Adequate recovery is important to allow the trained muscles sufficient time to replace muscle glycogen and the physiological process to repair and rebuild new tissue (Bishop, Jones, and Woods 2008; Hausswirth and Mujika 2013). The frequency of your workouts will depend on a number of factors, including your specific training goals, overall exercise experience, level of physical conditioning, and the amount of time you have available. After a higher-intensity core strength or metabolic conditioning workout, an appropriate recovery period is approximately 48 to 72 hours before training at the same intensity. Lower-intensity mobility workouts can be performed the next day to either expend the energy for weight management goals or as a form of active recovery.

Structuring Your Workouts

When it comes to workouts to enhance core strength or improve metabolic conditioning, repeatedly performing the same exercises with the same amount of weight could limit the amount of mechanical or metabolic stress placed on the involved tissue, which then minimizes the training effect. It's important to change workouts on a regular and consistent basis. Changing too often will not allow your body time to adapt, and following the same program for too long could result in a plateau. (The specifics of how and when to adjust your workouts will be covered in chapter 6.) To produce the desired results, the acute variables of exercise program design must be applied in a structured, systematic manner that either imposes a mechanical stress on the muscle, fascia, and elastic connective tissue or creates a sizable metabolic demand.

Increasing exercise intensity can be done a couple of ways: performing a strength exercise to a point of momentary muscle fatigue or increasing the work rate by moving at a faster speed to challenge the metabolic energy pathways that fuel the muscles. Valdimir M. Zatsiorsky and William J. Kraemer identify three specific types of strength training, two of which can be applied to improve core strength or enhance metabolic conditioning with only one piece of exercise equipment. The three methods are the maximal effort method, the dynamic effort method, and the repeated effort method. The maximal effort method, as the name suggests, is for enhancing maximal muscle force output using extremely heavy amounts of weight, which, while a worthy outcome, is not relevant to workouts that can easily be done with one piece of equipment at home or a fitness facility. The other two methods, the repeated effort and dynamic effort methods, can be adapted to use only one piece of equipment, making them efficient and effective solutions regardless of where you work out (Zatsiorsky and Kraemer 2006).

Repeated Effort Method

The repeated effort (RE) method of strength training requires the use of a non-maximal load performed until momentary muscle failure (the inability to perform another repetition) to ensure proper stimulation of the motor units and depletion of energy stores. Applying the RE method of exercise requires performing the final few repetitions per set in a fatigued state in order to stimulate all of the involved muscle fibers. The RE method is an effective means to stimulate the adaptation of increasing lean muscle mass. This method uses slower motor units for the initial repetitions; as these motor units begin to fatigue, the muscle will recruit type II high threshold motor units to sustain the necessary force production.

One limitation to the RE method is that as the type II motor units are activated, they fatigue quickly, leading to the end of the set. If the load is not sufficient or the set is not performed to fatigue, it will not stimulate the fast motor units most responsible for changing muscle definition.

One significant benefit of this method is that as anaerobic type II fibers are recruited, they create energy through anaerobic glycolysis, which produces metabolic waste such as hydrogen ions and lactic acid, changing blood acidity. Research suggests that acidosis, the change in blood acidity due to an accumulation of blood lactate, is associated with increases in GH and IGF-1 to promote tissue repair during the recovery phase (Schoenfeld 2010).

The RE method provides two key advantages when using just one piece of exercise equipment: It has a greater impact on the metabolic function of the muscle, provoking greater levels of growth, as well as involving a significant number of motor units, leading to strength gains.

Dynamic Effort Method

The dynamic effort (DE) method of strength training uses nonmaximal loads with the highest attainable velocity of movement to apply the muscle motor unit stimulation. Vladimir M. Zatsiorsky and William J. Kraemer suggest that the DE method is an effective means of increasing the rate of force development and developing explosive strength, but when using a submaximal load for bursts of high-intensity movement speed, it can be an effective means of metabolic conditioning as well (Zatsiorsky and Kraemer 2006).

The DE method activates the contractile element of muscle to create an isometric contraction and place tension on the bodywide network of fascia and elastic connective tissue. When the contractile element shortens, it loads the fascia with elastic mechanical energy, which, when rapidly shortened, creates an explosive shortening action to generate movement.

When using the DE method with one piece of equipment for metabolic conditioning, the goal is to perform a move at an explosive or fast pace until either becoming out of breath or feeling the sensation of burning in the involved muscles, both of which are important markers of a metabolic overload.

Effective Equipment for Developing Mobility, Core Strength, and Metabolic Conditioning

One inside tip that many fitness professionals know is that it's *not* the actual equipment you use, but *how* you apply it that leads to physical changes. Yes, different types of exercise equipment place different stresses on the body, resulting in slightly different adaptations. And, yes, to some degree weight is weight: A medicine ball that weighs 10 pounds is the same weight as two 5-pound dumbbells. However, the movements you do during an exercise plus the way you apply the other variables of program design, such as sets and rest intervals, actually determine the changes that will happen to your body. Staying with the example of the medicine ball and two dumbbells, even though they weigh the same amount, the way they are used in a workout will result in completely different outcomes. A medicine ball is held in both hands while the dumbbells allow each arm to move independently, imposing a number of stresses on the various systems of the body.

The equipment selected for the workouts in this book (table 2.2) was chosen specifically because they are capable of imposing the appropriate demands for mobility, core strength training, or metabolic conditioning as well as being very affordable and easy to use in a home setting where space may be limited. In addition, the equipment selected can be found in most commercial health clubs or fitness facilities. Learning to use one piece of equipment for an effective workout gives you options for when you want the convenience of exercising at home or when both space and equipment are in short supply at the gym. When you make it to the gym only to see that all of the equipment is being used and people are waiting in line to take their turn, you can smile knowing that you'll still get a great workout. All you need to do is grab a single piece of equipment, secure a little space, and have at it. You'll be sweating and working toward your goals in no time!

Movement is exercise and exercise is movement. Knowing how to move with the pieces of equipment listed above, along with knowing how to organize the variables of an exercise program, can help ensure that you are doing workouts that will produce the results you want. All of the top fitness instructors know that exercise is both a science and an art: The science can provide insights on how the human body will adapt to specific types of overload, but the art comes from finding the best types of exercise that feel right for your particular needs. One piece of equipment, like a kettlebell, can be used for mobility, core strength training, *or* metabolic conditioning based on how the variables of exercise program design are applied. The next chapters show you dozens of exercises to help you get the results you want, simply and effectively.

Table 2.2 **Exercise Equipment**

Equipment	Description	Benefits
Bodyweight	Bodyweight exercises use the body you were born with, comprised of upper, core, and lower regions. The CNS organizes various systems, including the muscles, fascia, and elastic connective tissue, to work together in coordination to create movement.	Bodyweight training is effective for all mobility, core strength, and metabolic conditioning. Bodyweight exercises can be done anywhere in only a limited amount of space. With the exception of a stretch mat, timer, or heart rate monitor, bodyweight exercises do not require any special equipment.
Kettlebell	Resembling a bowling ball with a handle, a kettlebell is a weighted ball with the handle outside the center of mass.	Originally kettlebells were popular in the 19th century but have experienced a resurgence in the modern fitness market because they provide numerous benefits for mobility, core strength, and metabolic conditioning. The unique design of the handle and mass allows it to be used for explosive exercises such as kettlebell swings, which are perfect for metabolic conditioning, or for unique exercises such as the windmill, which can improve both mobility and core strength. Kettlebells can be purchased from a variety of sporting goods stores or online retailers. There are a variety of kettlebells, from traditional to rubber-coated to adjustable weight. The two types of kettlebells recommended for these workouts are either traditional or competition-style. Pick the one that works best for you.
Dumbbells	Dumbbells have a handle in the center of mass. Dumbbells are designed to be used with one in each hand but also can be used one at a time when held with both hands, and they come in a variety of styles, sizes, and weights.	Dumbbells allow for complete freedom of movement in all planes of motion to improve task-specific muscular strength or to challenge metabolic conditioning. You control the path of motion as you move through multiple planes or directions. The amount of force can change as a joint moves through a complete ROM. Each arm can be used independently to create unique loading challenges for mobility training, core strength, and metabolic conditioning exercises. Using one dumbbell allows for a variety of ways to load lower-body or core exercises.
Medicine ball	A medicine ball is a weighted ball made of rubber, leather, or synthetic material. Medicine balls can be lifted in multiplanar movement patterns or thrown. There are different types of medicine balls: • *Live balls*: Usually made of hard rubber; designed to bounce when thrown against a hard surface such as a solid wall or the ground. • *Dead balls*: Made of leather or moldable plastic; soft and designed to not bounce (but may roll) and to stay in place when thrown to the ground. • *Handle balls*: Mostly round but have one or two handles integrated into the design to make it easier to hold during multiplanar, multidirectional movements.	You can control the path of motion and move the resistance in any direction, which could lead to higher levels of mobility and enhanced core strength. Live balls can be thrown repeatedly against the ground or hard wall for upper-body-specific metabolic conditioning. Using a medicine ball can help elevate your heart rate and engage a number of core muscles, providing both metabolic conditioning and core strength training benefits that can be difficult to achieve with other pieces of exercise equipment. Medicine balls are extremely affordable and can be purchased from a number of online vendors or retail sporting goods stores.

(continued)

Table 2.2 *(continued)*

Equipment	Description	Benefits
Stability ball	A stability ball is an inflated, oversized rubber ball that creates a variety of challenges for human movement. A properly sized stability ball should allow you to sit on it so that your knees and hips are both at 90 degrees.	The inherent instability of using a large ball creates a number of challenges to improve the strength and resiliency of muscle, fascia, and elastic connective tissues. The ball can help support your body weight during certain mobility exercises, helping to improve joint ROM. The leverage and positions created by a stability ball create numerous exercises for developing and enhancing core strength.
Sandbag	A sandbag is made of a thick, durable material such as nylon or neoprene filled with sand (or a similar material). A sandbag adjusts position and changes shape during use.	The adjustable and shifting mass is useful for creating leverage for mobility exercises, provides dynamic variety for core strength training, and can be thrown explosively for metabolic conditioning exercises. Different types of sandbags can be purchased from specialty retailers. Some are relatively flat and circular with no handles while others resemble small duffle bags with a variety of handles. It can be easy to make your own sandbag with a little ingenuity and creative engineering.
Two-arm resistance band	A two-arm resistance band can be used at home to recreate a number of exercises traditionally performed on cable machines in commercial fitness facilities.	The band can be attached to a door frame or another solid anchor, such as a fence post or playground jungle gym. The density, thickness, and length of the tubing determine the actual amount of resistance. A resistance band provides a number of exercise options from a standing position, the way the human body is actually designed to function. A resistance band is one of the most important pieces of equipment for developing strong, stable, and functional core muscles.

PART II

Exercises and Workouts

3

Mobility Training

Vern Gambetta, an authority on performance training, defines athleticism as "the ability to execute a series of movements at optimum speed with precision, style and grace" (Gambetta 1998, 19). Mobility, along with the skills of dynamic balance and coordination, is derived from the coordinated integration of the different physiological systems described in chapter 1 but with an emphasis on the central nervous system (CNS) and muscular system. Proper mobility training can improve the communication between the CNS and muscular system to enhance the ability to move with "precision, style, and grace," while simultaneously improving extensibility and joint range of motion (ROM); the end result is that you will move better as well as feel better, a definite win–win.

Take a second look at that description; it identifies movement skill and coordination as prerequisites for being an athlete, not participating in a competition or earning a spot on a team. Think again about how you use your body during your normal ADLs, favorite recreational pastimes, or exercise program. If Gambetta's definition of athleticism can accurately describe how you move, performing multidirectional exercises at a variety of different speeds can help improve mobility and enhance your ability to move with "precision, style, and grace." In other words, you will be improving your athleticism for the game of life.

It is possible to organize exercise into five foundational patterns of movement. Any exercise is either the application of one of these movement patterns or is a specific component of one of these patterns.

- *The hip hinge or bend-and-lift pattern*: Any hip-dominant movement on both legs, including, but not limited to, deadlifts, Romanian deadlifts, squats, or kettlebell swings.

- *The lunge or single-leg pattern*: Any movement on a single leg or alternating one at a time between both legs, including, but not limited to, step-ups, lunges, split-leg squats, or single-leg squats.

- *The push*: Any movement away from the front of the body in either a forward or overhead direction, including, but not limited to, push-ups, shoulder presses, chest presses, or triceps push-downs.

- *The pull*: Any movement toward the body from a position located either overhead or in front of the body, including, but not limited to, bent-over rows, biceps curls, or upper-cuts.

- *Rotation*: Occurs when the thoracic spine or pelvis are moving in a rotational direction either one at a time, moving in the same direction or moving in opposite directions of one another, including, but not limited to, the way the shoulders and pelvis counterrotate when walking or running, rotational chopping patterns, or rotational lifting patterns.

The human body is designed to move, and the movements listed previously occur in almost everything we do, whether playing a sport, doing a chore, or simply taking a walk. Basing an exercise program on these movement patterns means that you will be training like an athlete even though you may never step on a field or court to compete. Traditional gym exercises that focus on a single muscle group or body part can help change your appearance, but how can they improve your athleticism as defined above?

This question is especially relevant when you think about the fact that many traditional gym exercises require you to lift a weight up and down in a linear motion or simply push or pull a lever on a machine. Consider many of the chores and tasks that you perform throughout the course of your normal daily life; don't you often use the entire body to carry or move a mass from one place to another through gravity, not simply against it? Doesn't "precision, style, and grace" apply to *any* movement you might perform on a daily basis? When you do this, it's the network of muscle, fascia, and elastic connective tissue that generates the tension required to control a mass as you move through gravity. Consider these daily activities, chores, or tasks that you may perform on a regular basis:

- Carrying a gym bag, work-related bag, large purse, baby bag, computer bag, or suitcase when traveling
- Carrying laundry
- Walking a dog and bending over to pick up any waste products
- Moving groceries from the store to the car and into the home
- Carrying your young children around the house or picking them up to care for them
- Placing young children in car seats, cribs, high chairs, or strollers
- Digging in a garden to install new plants or remove old ones
- Pushing, pulling, and rotating with a rake or other piece of lawn care equipment
- Navigating a busy urban sidewalk while carrying a bag, holding a cup of coffee, and typing out a text message
- Hustling, with carry-on luggage, as you hurry from one airport terminal to another to make a connecting flight

Once you learn how to perform the foundational patterns of movement, it becomes necessary to learn how to generate and control the muscle forces required to move mass through gravity instead of directly against it. The goal is to perform the foundational patterns often enough so that they become reflexive, meaning that you can execute them flawlessly without any conscious thought. Performing multidirectional movements while carrying loads like groceries, laundry, or even young children are the types of tasks you frequently perform in your daily life but are often omitted from traditional exercise programs. Having the proper joint mobility as well as the ability to move through a ROM without having to think about the movement you are performing makes accomplishing any or all of the tasks listed above easier to handle.

The Role of Mobility in Exercise

The modern fitness era began in the 1970s with the trends of jogging and dance aerobics group fitness classes and has now evolved to the point where health clubs, fitness studios, personal trainers, and group fitness instructors all play integral roles in our culture. It wasn't until the 1970s that the modern version of the membership-based health club became a viable business model. In the 1980s, the health club industry received a significant boost in membership numbers thanks to numerous action movies featuring muscle-bound actors like Arnold Schwarzenegger and Sylvester Stallone vanquishing foes and getting the girl, creating the perception that buff, muscular physiques made life better. To mimic the appearance of the big screen stars, many fitness consumers focused on isolation exercises to maximize the growth and definition of muscles. The exercise equipment sold to gyms was designed to meet the needs of bodybuilders and their desire to focus on only one body part at a time, leading to a variety of machines designed to strengthen individual muscles that you probably didn't even know you had.

In addition to the growth of the health club industry, the '80s also saw the introduction of the field of personal training. Specialists could now be hired by those interested in achieving a specific fitness goal. Fittingly (pun intended), the first personal trainers were bodybuilders hired to help clients achieve a more muscular appearance. In addition, as fitness became more popular, many books and magazine articles about exercise were either written or heavily influenced by bodybuilders; exercise for the sake of exercise became a popular pastime, and workouts using only one or two body parts at a time became the established norm.

The 1990s saw the field of personal training evolve from bodybuilders helping movie stars add muscles for blockbuster movies to a mainstream service offered by many health clubs. At the same time the introduction of the personal training studio created a business dedicated solely to helping clients in a private, more exclusive environment. What had initially been an ancillary service offered to health club members became in the late 1990s a lucrative source of revenue for health clubs and studios and created job opportunities for those who wanted to earn a living by helping others learn how to exercise.

How we exercise has changed more since the turn of the century than it did between the early 1970s and the year 2000. First, fitness has become an established career field no longer dominated by bodybuilders; numerous professional trainers and instructors have degrees in exercise science or kinesiology, while many others have earned professional certifications in a variety of exercise modalities. Second, popular group workout programs like CrossFit, SoulCycle, Orangetheory Fitness, and CorePower Yoga provide a wide variety of options for group workouts, helping to make exercise time an important component of one's social life. Finally, the explosive popularity of social media platforms allow both educated fitness professionals and enthusiastic amateurs alike to easily produce quality exercise videos using only a phone; this has helped promote the benefits of exercise to a wide audience. Each of these factors have helped to propel the fitness lifestyle from a niche hobby to a popular subculture.

As the fitness industry has grown, so has our knowledge about the impact that exercise has on the various systems in the body. Gone are the days of going to the gym to pump up or exercising to the point of pain in the misbegotten hopes that it can bring a desired gain. Yes, numerous people still exercise for the sole purpose of changing their appearance; however, the way they exercise has changed significantly.

Exercise programs have progressed from those that focus only on muscle isolation to workouts based on how we move, often with a specific emphasis on improving the quality of movement as opposed to simply going for the burn. We now have a much better understanding of how exercise can be used to help you move better and, most importantly, the types of exercises that can help you enjoy pain-free movement.

Educated fitness professionals now understand that there are two separate, distinct components of muscle tissue: the contractile element responsible for generating force and the elastic component of fascia and connective tissue that helps distribute forces throughout the entire body (Verkoshansky and Siff 2009). The muscle-isolation workout programs of the past focused almost exclusively on the contractile element of muscle to improve size and definition. However, educated fitness professionals know that if one set of muscles becomes stronger or more developed than others, it could cause an imbalance around a joint and change how that joint functions. As a result, many exercise programs now feature multidirectional movement patterns that involve more of the fascia and elastic connective tissue to enhance mobility and coordination.

Understanding Mobility

When you hear the word *flexibility*, you probably think of static stretching, the practice of holding a specific muscle in a lengthened position in order to help increase its length. The term *flexibility* has often been used to describe the ability of muscles to lengthen in order to allow joint motion, specifically, the ability of a joint to move through its structural ROM. Again, this is not wrong, but it *is* incomplete because static flexibility *can* reduce muscle tension, which can be useful at the end of a workout or in the period between workouts. However, *extensibility* is the better term to describe the mechanical ability of muscle and connective tissue to lengthen and shorten as joint motion is occurring. As muscle, fascia, and elastic connective tissue lengthen and shorten, they control the movement of a limb or body segment through its ROM. Therefore, mobility should be thought of as a combination of flexibility and extensibility: the structure of a joint to allow motion combined with the ability of the involved tissue to lengthen and shorten while controlling that motion without any restrictions.

Static stretches require you to hold a stable position with minimal movement. Now think about how you use your body. Do you need flexibility when you are sitting still or lying down? Probably not, because you're not moving. On the other hand, when you are moving to enjoy your favorite activities or perform essential ADLs, having uninhibited mobility can allow you to complete tasks with minimal risk of injury. Motion at a particular joint is only one component of movement; improving your mobility requires the integration of stability, balance, postural control, coordination, and proprioception between all of the major joints in your body. Learning and controlling efficient movement patterns is predicated on the timing and coordination of muscles to produce and stabilize motion through a series of joints.

Muscle and Fascia: An Interconnected System

When we move, our brains do not think about the actions that individual muscles perform. Instead, we think about a movement that we want to execute, and our muscles react according to this intention. The body is designed to be as mechanically efficient as possible and will move in the path of least resistance. The result is

What the Science Says:
Stability–Mobility Relationships in the Body

The joints of the skeletal system have structures that either provide stability or allow mobility. In reality, many joint structures both create stability and allow mobility, but understanding the basic stability and mobility relationships between major joints in the body can help you understand why mobility training is the foundation of successful exercise programs. Enhancing the ability of the stable joints to provide stability while improving the ability of the mobile joints to allow unrestricted motion is key to a successful exercise program and can be an important step overlooked by many traditional muscle-isolation programs. Some exercises should improve the stability of the stable joints of the foot, knee, lumbar spine, and scapulothoracic joint, while other exercises should be designed to enhance the mobility of the mobile joints of the ankle, hip, thoracic spine, and glenohumeral joints. Focusing on increasing muscle size without first working to improve stability, mobility, and movement skill could lead to the muscle imbalances that are a potential cause of injury.

Joint	Location	Function
Foot	*Note*: The foot has numerous joints that help ensure proper motion. The transverse tarsal joint located between the heel bone (calcaneus) and the bones of the mid-foot plays an important role in helping the foot be both mobile and stable during the gait cycle.	During the gait cycle of walking or running, the foot transitions from being mobile when it hits the ground to a stable structure. As the body passes over the foot the transverse tarsal joint creates a stable lever for propulsion, which helps create force for the next phase of the gait cycle.
Ankle	The distal tibia-fibula joint (the far end of the two bones in the lower leg) and the talocrural joint (the talus bone between the far ends of the tibia and fibula)	Designed to be mobile and experiences its greatest amount of mobility when the foot is on the ground as the body passes over it during the mid-stance phase of the gait cycle.
Knee	The connection between the lower end of the thigh bone (femur) and the upper portion of the tibia bone in the lower leg	A relatively stable joint that helps control motion between the segments of the upper and lower leg.
Hip	Where the femur bone of the thigh connects with the pelvis	Allows mobility in three planes of motion during the gait cycle of walking or running. A loss of motion in any one of these three planes can cause the joints above or below the hip to attempt to allow the lost motion.
Lumbar spine	Intervertebral segments of the lumbar spine	Creates a platform of stability between the mobile joints of the hips and the intervertebral segments of the upper spine.
Thoracic spine	Intervertebral segments of the thoracic spine	Allows mobility for rotation as the arms swing forward and backward during the gait cycle. The intervertebral segments of the cervical and thoracic spine, the neck and mid-back, respectively, allow most of the motion for rotation of the spine, while the structures of the lumbar spine are designed to move primarily forward and backward.
Shoulder blades	Scapulothoracic joints, where the shoulder blades sit on the thoracic spine of the mid- and upper back	Creates a stable platform for movement of the shoulder and arm.
Shoulder joint	Glenohumeral joints, where the head of the humerus, relatively the shape of a ball, rests on the glenoid fossa of the scapula, which creates a socket or cup	One of the most mobile joints in the body, they allow multidirectional movement of the arm.

that if a mobile joint doesn't allow the freedom for uninhibited movement, a nearby stable joint will have to allow that motion to occur. When the stability and mobility relationships between joints becomes altered, it will also change the extensibility of the surrounding muscle and connective tissue, affecting the ability to execute efficient movement patterns (Cook 2010).

Muscles play an important role in creating and controlling mobility; by shortening to create tension on the fascia and elastic connective tissue, muscles generate the internal forces that control movement of the skeletal system. Doing too many repetitive motions or not moving much throughout the day could cause imbalances that disrupt the normal length-tension relationships between muscles. As certain muscles become overused, they can become tight, which restricts their ability to lengthen when the muscles on the other side of a joint shorten. Other muscles can be underused, which results in them losing the ability to generate force properly.

Here is a scary thought: If your exercise programs do not include multidirectional movements at varying rates of speed, your muscle, fascia, and elastic connective tissues could lose the ability to efficiently store and release mechanical energy over the course of the normal biological aging process. Mobility is an important compo-

What the Science Says: Biotensegrity

It is important to consider the network of fascia and connective tissue as a single, integrated system responsible for establishing a constant equilibrium of forces. It can be easy to forget that a human being grows from a single cell in the embryonic form and experiences rapid growth via cell division during the gestation period. This is important because throughout a human being's lifespan, all cells and bodily tissues remain connected (Myers 2014; Schultz and Feitis 1996). *Tensegrity*, which refers to the combination of tension and integrity, is an architectural term used to describe a structure that is self-supporting through a combination of tensile (lengthening) and compressive (shortening) forces. Given that the myofascial system is a balance of compression and tension, *biotensegrity* is an effective term to describe how the body has a natural, structural tendency to balance forces (Myers 2014; Scarr 2014; Ingber 2003).

Traditional anatomy teaches that muscles attach to bones via the tendon; however, following the model of biotensegrity, it is more accurate to say that skeletal structures float within a three-dimensional matrix of muscle and connective tissue (Myers 2011, 2014; Scarr 2014). Fascia is a living tissue that maintains a constant balance between synthesis of new cells and remodeling of existing cells in response to external and internal forces. The primary regulators of tensegrity—tension and compression—influence a cell's biochemical response to stress; the biotensegrity model of human anatomy has been shown to both qualitatively and quantitatively predict mechanical behaviors of human cells (Ingber 2003, 2004).

Understanding the tensegrity model of structural balance in the human body should completely change how you approach exercise. As opposed to simply doing an exercise for a specific muscle or joint, using integrated movement patterns can help remodel the entire myofascial network into a more efficient structure capable of balancing the ever-present forces of compression and tension. Applying the tensegrity model to the human body demonstrates that when forces are introduced at one point in a structure, they will be concurrently transmitted and used in other parts of the same structure. So, when lifting a weight, it's not just the immediate muscles involved and doing the work; a wide network of different muscles will contribute and share in the force distribution.

nent of athleticism because it helps ensure that aging muscle, fascia, and connective tissue remain pliable and elastic to allow joints to articulate through their full ROMs.

The stretch-shorten cycle (SSC) describes how muscle tissue stores mechanical energy during the lengthening phase in order to release it when muscles contract. It is helpful to think of the SSC as a rubber band; if a rubber band is stretched and held in a lengthened position before being released, it won't produce the same amount of explosive force as when the band is rapidly pulled and immediately released. Mobility training can improve tissue extensibility, which then helps reduce the transition time between lengthening and shortening, ultimately increasing muscle force output (Verkoshansky and Siff 2009). The good news is that the right type of exercise program can enhance the elasticity and structural integrity of fascia, restoring the ability of muscle tissue to perform multiplanar movements at any point along the aging process.

Including Mobility in Your Workouts

The human body functions as a more efficient and structurally sound system when performing movement patterns as opposed to exercises that treat the body as a series of individual parts. A primary benefit of a movement-based exercise program is that, because more oxygen is required as a result of all of your muscles working to generate force, it can be more effective for burning calories. A second benefit of the movement-based approach to exercise is that muscles improve their timing and ability to generate appropriate levels of force to execute the patterns with precision and grace. A third benefit is that these exercises can be performed with only one piece of exercise equipment, making it a perfect option whether you want to exercise at home or need quick, effective solutions for when your gym is crowded. Let's face it: Sitting in an exercise machine using only one part of the body is kind of boring, but challenging yourself to learn how to flawlessly execute complicated movement patterns can help make exercise a little more fun. Plus, you'll have a great sense of accomplishment as you can feel yourself performing the movements with greater ease and more coordination.

Mobility training provides the following benefits:

1. Joint capsules and ligament endings contain numerous sensory receptors that measure and identify pressure, movement, and rate of movement of their respective joints. Mobility exercises feature slow, controlled movements through a complete ROM, allowing the nervous system to learn how to control movement through the degrees of freedom allowed in each individual joint, which is essential for helping you improve your coordination and movement skill.

2. Muscle and fascia each contain sensory receptors that sense tension, length change, and rate of length change. The multidirectional movements of mobility training help you learn how to feel where your body is in space and how to control its movements. Mobility exercises engage the sensory receptors in both the contractile and elastic tissues to fully involve the CNS to teach it positional awareness and how to control the muscle actions that move your entire body.

3. As muscles lengthen, the muscle spindles sense the rate of length change and communicate with motor neurons to initiate muscle contractions. Mobility exercises increase CNS activity within muscles, making them more effective at generating force during exercise. In essence, mobility exercises wake up your

CNS and muscles, helping you achieve greater levels of strength and power both during the workout as well as for long-term adaptations.

4. Multiplanar movements at a variety of rhythmic speeds increases heat in the body. As body temperature elevates, it allows muscle and fascia to become more extensible and capable of lengthening and shortening. Mobility exercises are a form of dynamic stretching that can help reduce soreness as well as the muscle tightness that could be a possible cause of injury.

5. If you want to become stronger or faster, you first have to learn how to turn some muscles off so other muscles can turn on more quickly. The term *reciprocal inhibition* refers to the physiological action that occurs when the shortening or contracting of one muscle sends a signal to its functional antagonist (the muscle on the other side of a joint), allowing it to lengthen. The controlled contractions during multidirectional mobility exercises use the principle of reciprocal inhibition to increase the speed at which muscles lengthen in response to contractions by the muscles on the other side of the joint. The speed at which muscles turn off to lengthen in order to allow for rapid contractions by the opposing muscles is an important component of improving strength, power, and movement skill.

6. Establishing a greater degree of freedom during joint motion can help improve overall strength while reducing the risk of injury. Tight muscles can restrict joint motion, causing other joints above or below the altered joint to provide the lost motion. Improving mobility of your hip joints can increase the strength and definition of your hip, thigh, glute, low-back, and oblique muscles that connect your legs to your pelvis as well as your pelvis to your spine. (These muscles are often referred to as your core.) Mobility exercises for the hip joints allow the muscles to experience a greater ROM, which can help activate more individual fibers, giving you more control while increasing overall strength, both of which can help reduce the risk of injury.

7. Having good mobility can help you improve your coordination and ability to react to sudden changes of direction, both of which can help reduce the risk of an accidental fall. Optimal joint mobility and movement skill should be a reflexive action that happens automatically. The good news is that it is not that difficult to improve joint mobility.

Moving in multiple directions at a variety of speeds can enhance circulation and elevate tissue temperature, along with activating the nervous, circulatory, and respiratory systems, which are responsible for controlling and fueling movement. In other words, it involves almost all of the systems that control your body. Mobility training can be an effective way to fully prepare for a tough and physically demanding workout; it can provide a low-intensity way to recover from a hard or challenging workout the previous day; or it can offer a stand-alone workout for those times when you want to move but don't have the time for a long workout or just aren't interested in pushing yourself that hard.

Effective mobility workouts use each of the foundational movement patterns as well as combinations of the patterns; start with slow, controlled, linear movements and gradually progress to challenging, fast-paced, multidirectional patterns. Adding a light weight to the movements can help you move into a deeper and more complete ROM. If you attend almost any elite or professional-level sporting event early enough to see the pregame warmup, you will see many of the athletes use these or similar mobility exercises.

Refer back to Gambetta's quote at the start of this chapter that says that athleticism is a function of precise, coordinated, graceful movements and has nothing to do with actually playing a sport. Even if you have no desire to play a sport, you should borrow workout strategies from the world of professional athletes. If a type of exercise can help an athlete perform his or her best, allowing him or her to earn millions of dollars for playing a sport, then using that same strategy can help you to move, feel, and look your absolute best.

For easier reference, flip to the red-colored tabs on the sides of the pages to help you quickly identify the mobility exercises in this book.

Mobility Workouts

One underlying theme of this book is to dispel the notion that exercise needs to be hard or challenging to be effective. Nothing could be further from the truth. Of course, it is necessary to do challenging workouts; pushing your body to work a little harder than it is used to is absolutely necessary to make physiological changes. However, not every workout needs to be hard. The most important thing about getting results from exercise is consistency—to do a little something every single day. Mobility exercises are, by definition, not designed to be high intensity but rather to help reduce the risk of common injuries such as muscle strains or ligament sprains that can result from muscle imbalances. Many of the mobility exercises in these workouts move your joints through their designed ROM, which lengthen and stretch the muscles and elastic connective tissues that control motion at that joint. Lengthening the muscle and connective tissue while enhancing joint range of motion can help you to reduce muscle tightness as well as move with better control and coordination. If you currently don't have great flexibility, movement skill, or coordination, you might feel as if these exercises can be really difficult, but it's extremely important to remain consistent with them because they can help establish the foundation of successful movement skill.

On the days after a physically demanding workout, lower-intensity mobility exercises can help your body recover from the stresses of the previous day and may be some of the most beneficial workouts that you can do because they can leave you feeling energized, refreshed, recharged, and ready to take on your next task. Depending on your specific goals and overall training schedule, your fitness program should include one to three mobility workouts per week. For best results, pick a workout and do the same one for a period of six to eight weeks so that your body has time to learn and adapt to the movements as you gradually increase the intensity by adding a couple of reps or an additional set every two or three workouts.

Start with 10 to 12 reps (5 to 6 each arm or leg) of each exercise, rest for 30 to 45 seconds, and complete 2 sets before moving on to the next exercise. To increase the challenge, quickly transition between exercises with no rest, rest 2 minutes after all exercises and perform 2 circuits. Gradually add reps until you're doing 20 in a row (10 each arm or leg), then add extra sets until you can do 4 sets of 20.

BODYWEIGHT EXERCISES FOR MOBILITY

Your body is one of the best pieces of fitness equipment ever invented *if* you know how to use it properly. Old-school flexibility exercises have you hold a stretch for a period of time, which can help lengthen the muscle by reducing neural activity (how the CNS activates individual muscle fibers), but does not necessarily train that muscle to shorten and lengthen as its attached joint(s) go through a complete ROM. Mobility exercises using just your body's own weight can create a variety of joint positions and motions to lengthen various muscles that can help stretch the muscles while also increasing neural activity, which is important for enhancing strength in workouts using external resistance. For the bodyweight exercises, start with 2 sets of each exercise, and as you feel your mobility improve, add 2 reps per week until you reach 20 reps per exercise. Once you reach 20 reps per each side, work up to doing 4 sets of each exercise.

Exercise	Sets	Repetitions	Rest interval
Supine hip circle	2	8-12 per side	30-45 sec
Hip bridge	2	8-10 (beginner); 12-15 (advanced)	30-45 sec
Offset quadruped rocking	2	10-12 per side	30-45 sec
Spider-Man stretch	2	5-6 per side (beginner); 10-12 per side (advanced)	30-45 sec
Multiplanar kneeling to standing	2	4-6 each direction (lateral and rotational)	30-45 sec
Slow-motion burpee	2	5-6 (beginner); 10-12 (advanced)	30-45 sec
Quadruped shoulder rotation	2	8-12 per side	30-45 sec
Kneeling thoracic spine mobility	2	4-5 per side	30-45 sec

To increase the level of difficulty, complete all of the exercises in a row with no rest; allow 2 minutes of rest after the entire circuit. Work up to 4 circuits, and then add reps until you can do 20 of each exercise (10 on each arm or leg).

Supine Hip Circle

Benefits

Lying down allows the spine to remain in a neutral position, supported by the ground. This increases mobility and the available ROM in the hips. The exercise can increase tissue temperature and fluid in the joint capsule. Mobilizing one hip while keeping the other hip stable can help improve mobility in each joint. This exercise alone is great after spending an excessive amount of time in a seated position.

Instructions

1. Lie flat on your back with your right hand on your right knee and your left hand on your left knee.
2. Circle both knees by pulling them up to your chest, then pull your right knee out to your right side while pulling the left knee out to the left side; both knees move away from the midline of your body.
3. Perform 8 to 12 circles in this direction, then change directions from the outside of the body, toward the midline, and down away from your torso.
4. Hold the right knee stable, with the left hand on the left knee. Circle the hip 8 to 12 repetitions in each direction, both clockwise and counterclockwise. Then switch hips—hold the left hand on the left knee and circle the right hip for 8 to 12 repetitions in each direction. Start with 2 sets of hip circles in each direction, and add 2 reps per week until you are doing 20 reps in each direction.

Correct Your Form

- Keep the lower back on the ground while the hips move.
- Allow your head to rest comfortably on the ground.

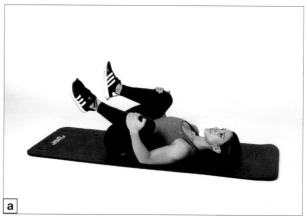

a

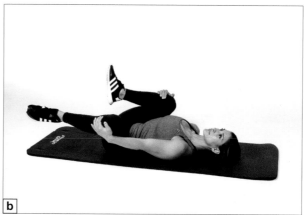

b

Hip Bridge

Benefits

This exercise strengthens the gluteal muscles responsible for extending the hips. Sitting all day can cause these muscles to be overlengthened, which reduces their ability to generate force. In addition, sitting can cause the hip flexor muscles (in the front of the hips) to become short, which restricts the ability of the hip to go through a full ROM. This exercise helps reduce tension in the hip flexors, allowing them to lengthen so the hips can move all the way through their designed path of motion.

Instructions

1. Lie flat on the floor with your palms facing the ceiling, knees bent, your feet slightly away from your tailbone, and your feet flexed so that your toes are pulled upwards toward your shins.
2. Squeeze your gluteal muscles to lift your hips toward the ceiling as you push your heels into the floor.
3. Pause slightly at the top, then lower slowly to the ground. The movement should be 1 to 2 seconds up, pause for 1 to 2 seconds, and lower for 3 to 4 seconds. Complete 8 to 12 reps, rest for 30 to 45 seconds, and perform a second set. Start with 2 sets of 8 to 12 hip bridges, and as you feel your mobility improve, add 2 reps per week until you are doing sets of 20.

Correct Your Form

- If you feel the backs of your upper legs tighten up, move your feet away from you.
- Lift your hips high enough so you reach full extension—a straight line from your thighs to your shoulders.

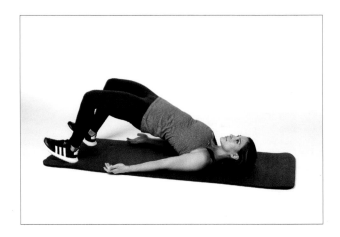

Offset Quadruped Rocking

Benefits

Placing the hands and knees in an offset position creates minor rotation in the lower back when rocking forward and back. This subtle motion can be important for reducing tightness and improving hip mobility. The position of the arms also creates pressure in the joint capsules of the shoulders, helping improve their mobility.

Instructions

1. Start in a quadruped position with your hands under your shoulders and knees under your hips.
2. Move your left hand and left knee forward just a few inches so your hands and knees are not aligned.
3. Keep your spine long while slowly rocking forward and back 10 to 12 times, then switch so your right hand and right knee are forward; rest for 30 to 45 seconds, and do a second set. As you feel your mobility improve, add 2 reps per week until you are performing 20 reps in each position.

Correct Your Form

- The right hand and knee only need to be a few inches in front of the left hand and knee.
- Let the hips move back while keeping the spine straight.

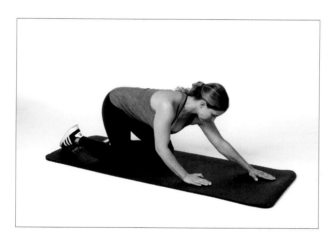

Spider-Man Stretch

Benefits

Hip mobility and strength of the deep core muscles are responsible for stabilizing the lumbar spine. This exercise strengthens the chest, shoulder, and triceps muscles of the upper body.

Instructions

1. Start in a high plank position with the hands directly under the shoulders and feet in line with the hips.
2. Bring your right knee forward to the outside of the right elbow while pushing back through the left heel to straighten the left leg. (This helps increase the stretch in the right hip.) Pause for 3 to 4 seconds, then place the right foot back to the starting position.
3. Bring your left knee to the outside of the left elbow, pause for 3 to 4 seconds, then bring the left foot back to the start position.
4. Keep your spine straight by bracing the core muscles and pressing the hands into the floor while slowly moving each leg forward and back.
5. Perform 5 to 6 reps with each leg; rest for 30 to 45 seconds and complete 2 sets. As you feel your mobility improve, add 2 reps to each leg until you can do 20 reps with each leg before taking a rest.

Correct Your Form

- Push back through the heel of the stabilizing leg while the knee of the opposite leg moves toward the elbow; this significantly increases the stretch in the stabilizing leg.
- Keep the spine straight by pressing your hands into the ground and flattening across your back.

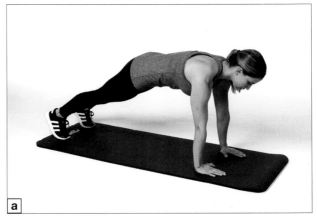

a

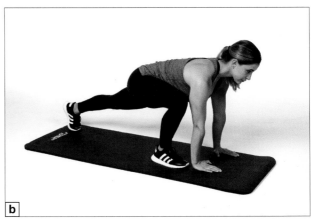

b

Slow-Motion Burpee

Benefits

This exercise increases hip mobility and upper-body strength, and elevates heart rate for metabolic conditioning. Additionally, using the different appendages can create a feedback loop that improves coordination in the entire body.

Instructions

1. Start in a standing position with your feet about shoulder-width apart. Sink into your hips and bend down to place your hands on the floor.
2. Slowly walk your hands forward to move into a high plank, and pause for 2 to 3 seconds.
3. Walk your hands back toward your feet as you sink into your hips so you end up in a squatting position.
4. In the low part of the squat, press your feet into the ground to stand up.
5. Start with 5 to 6 reps, and rest for 30 to 45 seconds before completing a second set. As you feel yourself get stronger, add 2 reps per week until you can complete 20 reps without stopping.

Correct Your Form

- Stand with the feet wide enough apart so that you can sink into the low squat position and place your hands on the floor.
- The pace of this exercise should be steady and controlled, not quick.

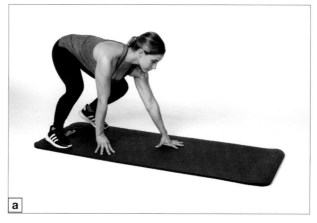

a

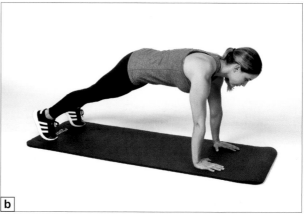

b

Multiplanar Kneeling to Standing

Benefits

Kneeling to standing can be an effective way to increase hip mobility, strengthen the hip extensors, and improve stability of the core muscles around the lumbar spine. Moving in multiple directions strengthens the tissues, allowing them to tolerate a variety of forces.

Instructions

1. Start in a kneeling position with the knees directly under the hips and the tops of your feet resting on the floor.
2. From the kneeling position, lift your left leg and place it directly to your left. Press the left foot into the ground and extend your left hip to move into a standing position with both feet next to each other.
3. Slowly lower back down to the kneeling position. Repeat, leading with the right leg.
4. Finally, from the kneeling position, take your left foot and rotate it to the left so your toes are pointing away from you in the 9 o'clock direction.
5. Press your left foot into the ground and extend your hip to bring yourself to a standing position with both feet next to each other. Rotate the right hip to the right, place your right knee on the floor, and slowly lower back to a kneeling position.
6. Repeat, leading with the right leg. Do the pattern in the following order: left (lateral and rotational) then right (lateral and rotational), completing 4 to 6 reps in each direction. Rest for 60 seconds after completing both legs and perform 2 sets. As you feel yourself get stronger and your hip mobility improve, add 2 reps to each direction until you are able to easily complete 10 reps on each leg, in both the forward and rotational directions, for a total of 20 reps on each leg in each direction without rest.

Correct Your Form

- Take your time; this is not a speed drill. Focus on planting your feet into the ground and using the hips to move from the kneeling to standing position.
- Keep your spine long and tall with chest lifted as you move from kneeling to standing.

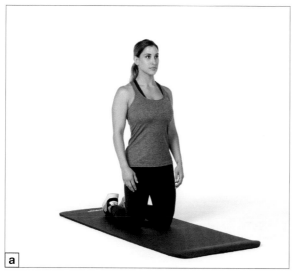

a

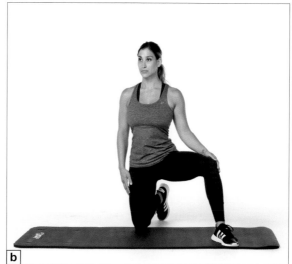

b

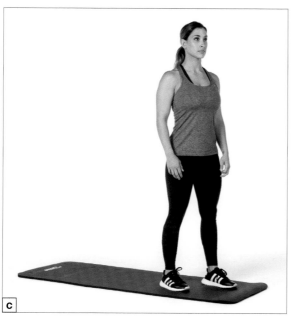

c

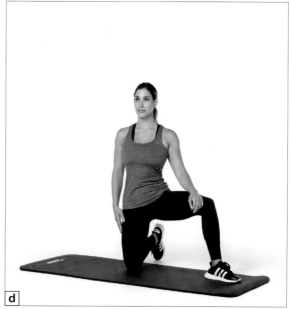

d

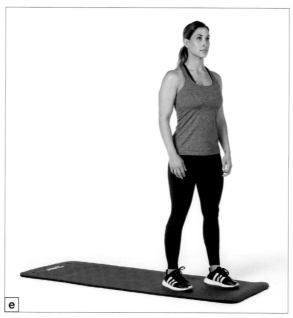

e

Quadruped Shoulder Rotation

Benefits

This exercise improves mobility of the thoracic spine and strength of the shoulder joints.

Instructions

1. Start in a quadruped position with your hands under your shoulders and knees under your hips.
2. Place your right hand on the back of your head. Keep your spine straight as you slowly lower your right elbow toward your left wrist.
3. Rotate the right elbow toward the ceiling as you pull your right shoulder back while pushing your left hand into the ground. (This increases the stretch in the chest.)
4. Do 8 to 12 reps with the right shoulder, then switch to the right hand on the ground and the left hand behind the head; rest for 30 to 45 seconds and complete a second set. As your thoracic mobility and core strength improve, add 2 reps per week until you are able to complete 20 reps on each arm.

Correct Your Form

- Keep the spine in a straight, neutral position during the exercise.
- When the right hand is behind the head, pushing the left hand into the ground while pulling the right shoulder back can increase the ROM from the thoracic spine while strengthening the shoulder.

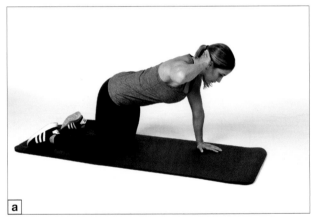

a

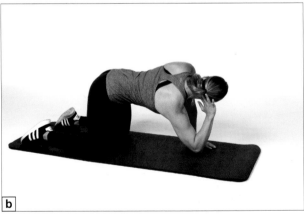

b

Kneeling Thoracic Spine Mobility

Benefits

This exercise improves mobility of the intervertebral joints of the thoracic spine and reduces tension in the lumbar spine while strengthening the muscles of the hip extensors, which is important for improving hip mobility.

Instructions

1. Kneel on both knees with your spine fully extended and your hands up on the back of your head.
2. Rotate to your left and slowly lower your left elbow toward your hips while keeping your spine straight. Slowly return to an upright position and rotate back to face forward.
3. Perform 4 to 5 rotations in each direction for a total of 8 to 10 reps; rest for 30 to 45 seconds, and complete a second set. As you feel your thoracic mobility improve, add 2 reps per week (1 to each side) until you can do 20 reps in each direction.

Correct Your Form

- It's important to start with a tall, straight spine for optimal mobility through the spine.
- As you rotate your body and reach down with your elbow, maintain stability by squeezing both glutes to keep your hips pressed forward.

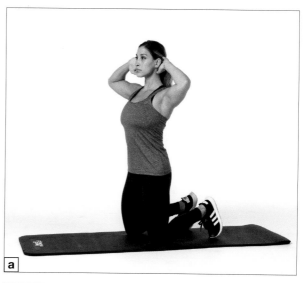

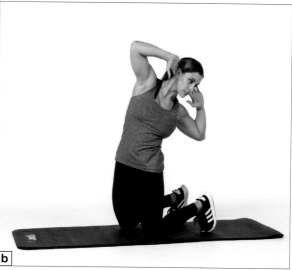

STABILITY BALL EXERCISES FOR MOBILITY

Mobility exercises with fitness equipment can provide more leverage to take a limb through a greater ROM while also increasing muscle fiber activation to help improve muscle contraction patterns. The stability ball creates two unique challenges for the body: 1) The unstable nature of the ball can cause muscle contraction, which is an important part of mobility training. As one set of muscles contract to maintain stability, the muscles on the other side of the joint will have to lengthen to allow the muscles to contract. 2) The shape of the ball creates a unique lever that can help move the body into positions that lengthen muscle and connective tissue while enhancing joint motion. For best results, use a fully inflated stability ball, as this will create the instability for enhanced muscle activation while providing a stiff surface to optimize leverage into a joint position. Once you reach 20 reps per each side, work up to doing 4 sets of each exercise; for the stretches, keep the length of time the same, but feel free to add additional sets.

When selecting a stability ball, use a 55-centimeter ball if you're 5' 7" or shorter. Select a 65-centimeter ball if you're between 5' 7" and 6' 4". Select a 75-centimeter ball if you're taller than 6' 4". The ball should be inflated until it's firm and you can sit on it so your knees and hips can comfortably hold a 90-degree bend.

Exercise	Sets	Repetitions	Rest interval
Child's pose	2	30-45 sec hold	30-45 sec
Kneeling cross-body reaching	2	30-45 sec hold	30-45 sec
Kneeling chest stretch	2	30-45 sec hold each arm	30-45 sec
Seated hip opener	2	30-45 sec hold each leg	30-45 sec
Seated adductor stretch	2	30-45 sec hold each leg	30-45 sec
Full body extension	2	30-45 sec hold	30-45 sec
Supine lateral roll	2	Slowly roll for 30-45 sec	30-45 sec

To increase the level of difficulty, complete all of the exercises in a row with no rest; allow 2 minutes of rest after the entire circuit. Work up to 4 circuits, and then add reps until you can do 20 of each exercise (10 on each arm or leg).

Child's Pose

Benefits

This exercise stretches the latissimus dorsi and upper-back muscles to reduce shoulder and back tightness.

Instructions

1. Kneel down facing the stability ball, place both hands on top of the ball as you lean back with your tailbone over your heels, breathe in, and as you exhale, allow your body to sink back deeper.
2. To increase length in the upper-back muscles, slowly roll the ball side to side, holding for 2 to 3 seconds at the end range of each motion.
3. To take the stretch deeper, rotate your palms up to face the ceiling as you roll your hands side to side. Hold for 30 to 45 seconds. Repeat for a total of 2 sets.

Correct Your Form

- Sit back as far as possible.
- For best results, hands should be placed right on top (at the twelve o'clock position).

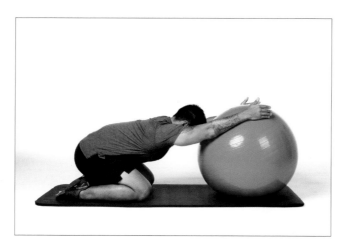

Kneeling Cross-Body Reaching

Benefits

This exercise reduces tightness in the back by increasing the length and stretching the muscles of the upper back and shoulders.

Instructions

1. Kneel down facing the ball, reach your left arm across your body, and allow the back of your left hand to rest on top of the ball.
2. Place your right hand on the floor and look to the right as you reach your left arm across your body. Hold for 30 to 45 seconds and repeat with the right arm. Repeat each stretch 2 times.

Correct Your Form

- To increase the stretch, the hand should be facing up to the ceiling, and you should reach with your arm as far as possible. If using the left arm, try to reach it across your body to the right side while leaning to your left.
- Turn your head to look in the direction of your arm in order to increase the stretch.

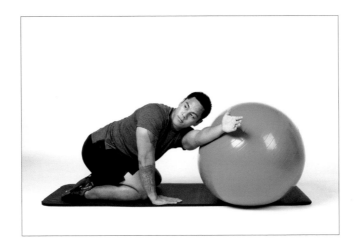

Kneeling Chest Stretch

Benefits

This exercise reduces tightness in the chest and shoulder muscles. *Note*: If these muscles become too tight (often from spending hours using a computer or phone), they will pull your shoulders forward, which increases tension on your upper back; stretching the muscles in your chest and along the front of your body can reduce stress through your spine and back.

Instructions

1. Kneel down to the right side of a stability ball, bend your left elbow to approximately 90 degrees, and place your entire left arm on the top of the ball. Your right hand should be on the ground directly under your right shoulder. Place your weight into your left arm as you rotate to look to your right.
2. To increase the intensity of the stretch, press down with your left arm for 3 to 5 seconds, then relax and lean deeper into the stretch. Repeat 3 to 5 times for a total of 30 to 45 seconds, then alternate arms. Repeat 2 times on each side.

Correct Your Form

Stretch only to a point of mild tension; attempt to go a little further into the ROM with each stretch.

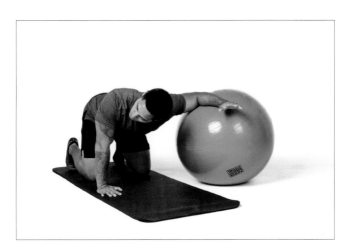

Seated Hip Opener

Benefits

This exercise stretches the hip flexor muscles to improve hip mobility and reduce tightness in the low back. (If the hip flexors become too tight, they will pull on the lower lumbar spine, which could be a potential cause of injury.)

Instructions

1. Sit on top of the stability ball so your right glute is on top of the ball, your right leg is directly in front of you, and your left leg is extended behind you.
2. Extend your left leg as straight as possible as you raise your left arm into the air, take a deep breath in, exhale slowly as you lean back to straighten your spine, and lean to your right as you rotate your left shoulder back (away from the front of your body) to increase the stretch.
3. Hold for 30 to 45 seconds, then repeat on the other side. Complete 2 stretches on each side.

Correct Your Form

- Lengthen the trail leg as far as possible.
- Maintain excellent posture; keep your spine tall and long to increase the stretch.

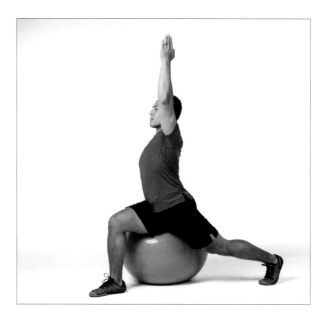

Seated Adductor Stretch

Benefits

This exercise lengthens the adductor muscles of the inner thigh to improve hip mobility.

Instructions

1. Sit on top of the stability ball so your tailbone is not directly on the top but forward (if the top is twelve o'clock, your tailbone should rest on the one- to two o'clock position).
2. Extend your left leg directly out to your left so your entire left foot is flat on the ground, shift your hips to the right as you keep your spine long, breathe deeply, and exhale as you rotate to look to your left. Hold for 30 to 45 seconds, then repeat on each side for 2 sets.

Correct Your Form

- Try to place your tailbone at the eleven o'clock position on the ball, and extend the leg as far as possible to the side while keeping your foot completely flat on the ground.
- Keep your spine long and straight as you rotate away from the extended leg.

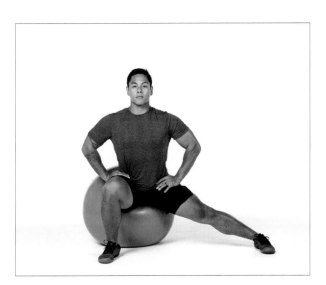

Full Body Extension

Benefits

This exercise lengthens all of the muscles in the front of your body. Sitting all day can make these muscles tight; if they become too tight they can pull your body forward, placing tension along the muscles of your back.

Instructions

1. Sit on top of the stability ball. Slowly drop your hips down to the front of the ball as you straighten your legs and raise your arms over your head. Lean back over the top of the ball so that you are fully extended.
2. Once you are fully extended over the ball, rotate the palms of your hands so they are facing up toward the ceiling.
3. Breathe deeply, and as you exhale, try to extend your body further. Hold for 30 to 45 seconds, sit tall for 30 seconds, then repeat for a total of 2 times.

Correct Your Form

- Allow your body to rest on the ball while fully extending.
- To increase the stretch, reach both arms directly overhead and exhale to increase the depth of the stretch.

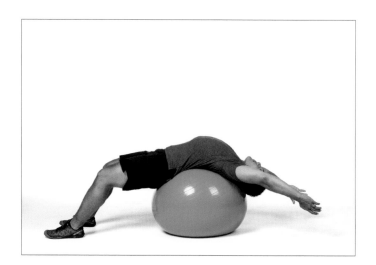

Supine Lateral Roll

Benefits

This exercise lengthens the muscles in the front of the body to reduce tightness in your upper back, and it improves strength of the hips and muscles of the lumbar spine to reduce overall tension in the lower back.

Instructions

1. Sit on top of the stability ball. Roll forward and stop when your upper back, shoulders, and back of your head are resting on the top of the ball as you hold both arms straight out to the side with your palms up in the air. (Imagine holding one plate in each hand.)
2. Keep your hips pressed up high (so your body is completely level) as you roll from side to side. Move slowly for a total of 30 to 45 seconds, rest for 30 to 45 seconds, then repeat for a total of 2 sets.

Correct Your Form

- Keep your hips pushed up toward the ceiling while pressing your feet into the ground.
- When rolling to each side, roll to your right until your entire left shoulder is on top of the ball, pause, then roll to your left until your right shoulder is resting on top of the ball.

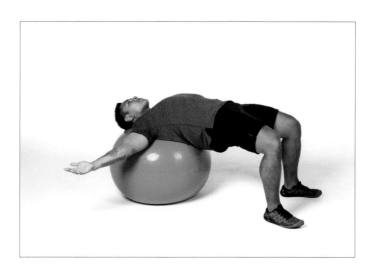

MEDICINE BALL EXERCISES FOR MOBILITY

Mobility exercises with fitness equipment can provide more leverage to take a limb through a greater ROM while also increasing muscle fiber activation to help improve muscle contraction patterns. The medicine ball can provide leverage to lengthen muscle and connective tissue while enhancing motion from a joint. The medicine ball can also provide a weight to help the body move into a complete range of motion. For best results, use a smaller medicine ball that can easily be supported by one hand while also providing enough weight so that it can be challenging to hold for more than 20 or 30 seconds with both arms fully extended. Using a medicine ball that is too light or too small may not provide the weight to properly lengthen the tissue or the leverage to completely optimize joint position. An additional benefit of using a medicine ball for mobility exercises is that you will be strengthening your muscle and connective tissue while also enhancing joint ROM. Once you reach 20 reps per each side, work up to doing 4 sets of each exercise; for the stretches, keep the length of time the same, but feel free to add additional sets.

Exercise	Sets	Repetitions	Rest interval
Child's pose cross-body reach	2	30-45 sec hold per arm	30-45 sec
Kneeling with overhead reach	2	30-45 sec hold per leg	30-45 sec
Offset kneeling with trunk rotation	2	3-5 each leg	30-45 sec
Trunk rotation with overhead reach	2	4-6 each arm	30-45 sec
Lateral lunge with trunk rotation and reach	2	6-8 each leg	30-45 sec
Rotational lunge with reach to ground	2	6-8 each leg	30-45 sec

To increase the level of difficulty, complete all of the exercises in a row with no rest; allow 2 minutes of rest after the entire circuit. Work up to 4 circuits, and then add reps until you can do 20 of each exercise (10 on each arm or leg).

Child's Pose Cross-Body Reach

Benefits

This exercise increases length and reduces tension in the upper-back muscles.

Instructions

1. Kneel down facing a basketball-sized or larger medicine ball, reach your left arm across your body, and rest your left hand on top of the ball.
2. Look to the right and pull your right shoulder back as you reach with your left arm across your body. Hold for 30 to 45 seconds.
3. Repeat with the right arm reaching across your body to the left side. Perform 2 times on each side.

Correct Your Form

Use a proper-size medicine ball; a basketball-sized or larger ball will allow better leverage into the shoulder joint.

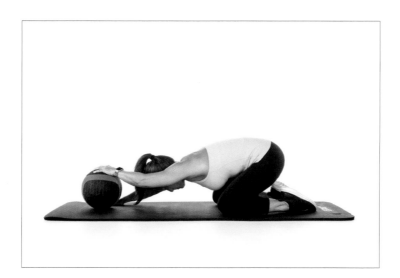

Kneeling With Overhead Reach

Benefits

This exercise releases tension in the hip flexors. If these muscles become overly tight, it can cause discomfort in the lumbar spine (low back). Additionally, this exercise improves mobility of the hip joints and reduces tightness in the upper back and shoulders.

Instructions

1. Place your right knee directly under your right hip with your left foot directly in front of your body. Keep your spine long and pelvis level as you raise both arms directly overhead, holding the medicine ball between both hands.

2. Squeeze your right glute and push your right hip forward as you keep your spine straight and rotate your right shoulder slightly to the right to increase the length in the muscles along the front of your body. The weight from the medicine ball should help increase the stretch in the hip flexors and increase ROM in the hip joint.

3. Hold for 30 to 45 seconds and switch legs. When the left knee is on the ground, rotate to your left while holding the medicine ball directly overhead. Repeat 2 times on each hip.

Correct Your Form

- Keep the pelvis level while leaning forward.
- Keep the spine tall to increase the stretch through the front of the hip.

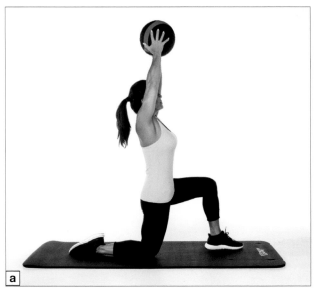

a

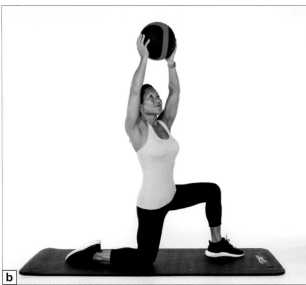

b

Offset Kneeling With Trunk Rotation

Benefits

This exercise reduces tension and increases length in the hip flexor and adductor muscles of the hips. Stretching these muscles can improve hip mobility and reduce low-back discomfort.

Instructions

1. Keep your left knee directly under your left hip. Turn your right leg so that it is 90 degrees relative to the front of your body. (If the left hip is at twelve o'clock, the right knee should be pointing toward three o'clock.) Hold the medicine ball in both hands so that it is directly in front of your chest.

2. Press your left knee into the ground as you lean your weight into your right leg. Think about trying to create distance between both knees. Hold the end ROM as you are looking toward the end of your right knee.

3. From this position, rotate your trunk to your right, keeping the medicine ball straight in front of your body. Once you hit the end of the motion to your right, slowly rotate back to your left so you end up where you started.

4. Repeat for 3 to 5 repetitions rotating to your right before switching legs and repeating to the left side. Complete 2 sets of 3 to 5 repetitions in each direction. As you feel your strength and mobility improve, add 2 reps (1 to each side) every week until you can do 10 reps on each leg (20 total) for 2 sets.

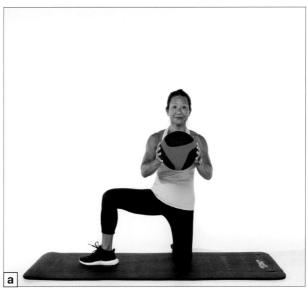

Correct Your Form

- The right thigh should be approximately 90 degrees relative to the left to ensure proper space between the hips.
- Pressing the down knee into the ground increases the stretch on the muscles of the left hip.
- Keep the spine straight and long while rotating, and keep your chest lifted and shoulders back to maintain proper length in your spine.

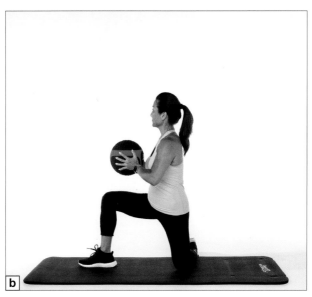

Trunk Rotation With Overhead Reach

Benefits

Stretch the shoulder and chest muscles while increasing motion in the intervertebral segments of the thoracic spine.

Instructions

1. Stand tall with both feet approximately hip-width apart, and extend the right arm directly overhead while resting the medicine ball in the palm of the right hand.
2. Keep your spine long and rotate to the right while reaching the right arm straight to lengthen the muscles through the front of the right shoulder and chest.
3. Move slowly, rotating to the right and reaching the arm to full extension. Pause at the end of the movement, then rotate back to the front.
4. Perform 4 to 6 repetitions to the right side before switching sides and repeating with the left arm while rotating to the left. Complete 2 sets of 4 to 6 repetitions to each side. As you feel your mobility improve, add 2 reps (1 to each side) until you can complete 10 reps on each side (20 total) without stopping.

Correct Your Form

- Keep the spine long during the movement to allow it to rotate properly.
- Extend the arm to increase the stretch into the right chest and shoulder muscles.

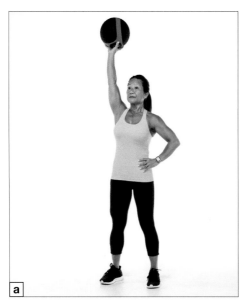
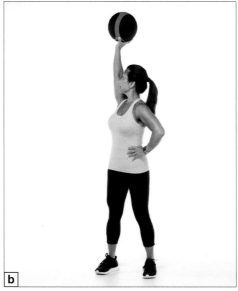

Lateral Lunge With Trunk Rotation and Reach

Benefits

This exercise increases ROM in the thoracic spine, improves mobility and strength of the hip muscles, and increases the strength of the obliques, which help control trunk rotation.

Instructions

1. Stand with your feet hip- to shoulder-width apart, holding a medicine ball with both hands directly in front of your chest. Step directly to your right. As your right foot hits the ground, make sure it is parallel to the left.

2. With your right foot on the ground, push the right hip back while keeping the left foot pressed into the ground, and rotate to your right as far as possible.

3. Pause at the end ROM and extend the medicine ball straight forward at chest height. Pull the medicine ball back, then rotate your trunk back to face the front.

4. Once you are facing forward again, push off with your right foot as you press your left foot into the floor to pull your body back to the starting position.

5. Perform 6 to 8 repetitions to the right, then perform the same number of repetitions to your left. Perform 2 sets on each side of the body. As you feel your strength and mobility improve, add 2 reps per week (1 on each side) until you can complete 10 reps on each leg (20 total) without stopping.

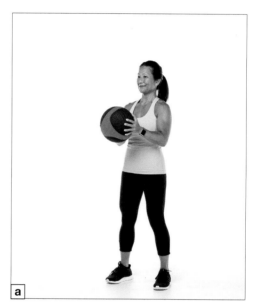

a

Correct Your Form

- Keep both feet parallel to one another during the lateral lunge. The right foot should be pointed straight ahead, and as the right foot hits the ground, it should remain parallel to the left.

- Maintain length through the spine. The straighter the spine, the easier it will be to rotate. (If you try to rotate while slouching, it could cause back discomfort.)

- Keep your planted foot pressed into the floor. When stepping to your left, pressing your right foot into the floor will help improve mobility of the right hip.

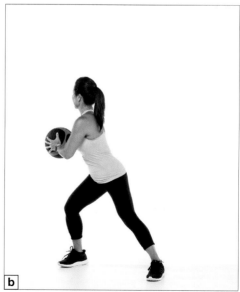

b

Rotational Lunge With Reach to Ground

Benefits

This exercise improves ROM of the hips, strengthens the muscles of the inner and outer thigh in a way that helps improve resiliency while reducing the risk of a strain, and increases strength of the muscles in the lower back.

Instructions

1. Stand with your feet hip- to shoulder-width apart, holding a medicine ball with both hands directly in front of your body.

2. With your right foot, step back and away from the left foot (toward the four o'clock position on a clock dial). Keep your left foot pressed into the ground as you step to the right and place weight into your right hip.

3. As your right foot hits the ground, push the right hip back into a hinge position and bend forward to reach for the ground directly in front of your right foot. (If you can't reach all the way to the ground, reach as low as possible; once your hip is in a flexed position, you can allow your spine to bend and round as you reach for the ground.)

4. Bring your trunk back to an upright position, push off with your right foot, and press your left foot into the ground as you bring both feet back to the original starting position.

5. Complete 6 to 8 reps on the right side before switching sides. Rest for 30 to 45 seconds and complete 2 sets. As you feel your strength and mobility improve, add 2 reps (1 to each side of the body) per week until you can complete 10 reps on each leg (20 total) without stopping.

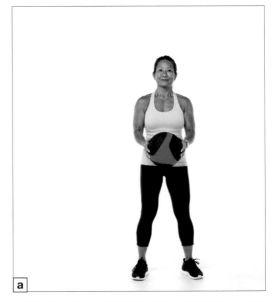

a

Correct Your Form

- Keep the front foot (the left foot in the example here) pressed into the ground so that it continues to point forward as you shift your weight into the foot you are stepping to (the right foot in the example above).

- As you reach for the ground, you should move from the hips by pushing them back before allowing your spine to bend.

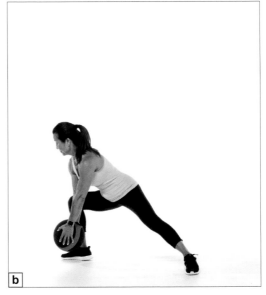

b

SANDBAG EXERCISES FOR MOBILITY

Mobility exercises with fitness equipment can provide more leverage to take a limb through a greater ROM while also increasing muscle fiber activation to help improve muscle contraction patterns. Like a medicine ball, the weight from a sandbag can provide leverage to lengthen muscle and connective tissue but, unlike a medicine ball, it can be used as a cushion to provide support in certain positions. For best results, use a smaller sandbag that can easily be supported by one hand while also providing enough weight so that it can be challenging to hold for more than 20 or 30 seconds with both arms fully extended. A sandbag that is too light may not help lengthen muscle and connective tissue while a sandbag that is too heavy could be too difficult to hold or move through a safe ROM. An additional benefit of using a weighted sandbag for mobility exercises is that you will be strengthening muscle and connective tissue while enhancing joint ROM. Once you reach 20 reps per each side, work up to doing 4 sets of each exercise; for the stretches, keep the length of time the same, but feel free to add additional sets.

Exercise	Sets	Repetitions	Rest interval
Pullover	2	5-8	30-45 sec.
Lying spinal rotation	2	30-45 sec hold each side	30-45 sec
Hip thruster	2	10-12	30-45 sec
Kneeling hip flexor stretch with overhead reach	2	30-45 sec hold each side	30-45 sec
Hip hinge with offset stance	2	5-6 each leg	30-45 sec
Lateral lunge with shoulder carry	2	6-8 each leg	30-45 sec
Forward lunge with reach to ground	2	6-8 each leg	30-45 sec

To increase the level of difficulty, complete all of the exercises in a row with no rest; allow 2 minutes of rest after the entire circuit. Work up to 4 circuits, and then add reps until you can do 20 of each exercise (10 on each arm or leg).

Pullover

Benefits

This exercise reduces tension in the upper chest and lengthens the muscles of the upper back.

Instructions

1. Lie on your back so you are face-up with your knees bent and feet flat on the floor.
2. Hold the sandbag in both hands so your arms are straight up with the palms facing each other. Reach overhead until your hands are resting on the floor. Hold for three to five seconds, allowing the weight of the sandbag to lengthen your muscles.
3. With your arms resting on the floor, pull your shoulder blades down toward your back pockets while pressing them into the floor, and lift your arms up until they are completely vertical (relative to the ground).
4. Move slowly and repeat for 5 to 8 repetitions. Rest for 30 seconds; complete 2 sets. As your strength improves, add 2 reps per week until you can complete 20 reps without stopping.

Correct Your Form

- Your feet should be about 18 inches (46 cm) from your tailbone. If your feet are too close, your hamstrings might cramp. Too far, and your back will be working instead of your glutes.
- Keep elbows straight while reaching overhead.

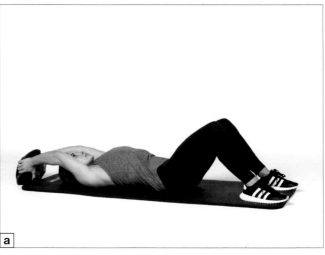

a

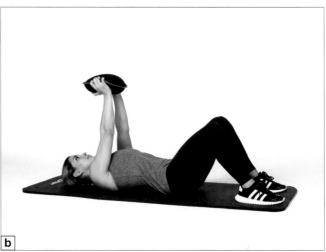

b

Lying Spinal Rotation

Benefits

This exercise improves mobility and ROM of the thoracic spine and oblique muscles that control trunk rotation. It also stretches the muscles of the shoulder and chest.

Instructions

1. Lie on your back so that you are face-up with your left arm extended straight out to the left side. The sandbag should be on the right side of your body, about 12 to 18 inches (30-46 cm) to the right of your hips, resting on your right hand to help increase the stretch in the right side of your chest and shoulder.
2. Keep your right leg straight as you bend the hip and knee of your left leg and cross it over your right. Your left knee should point toward the right side of your body in the three o'clock position and rest on the top of the sandbag.
3. Place your right hand on your left knee and press it into the sandbag while looking down your left arm.
4. Hold the stretch for 30 to 45 seconds before switching sides and holding for the same amount of time. Rest briefly, 30 seconds or less, after both stretches and repeat for 2 sets. As you feel your mobility improve, increase the number of sets until you are doing 4 on each side.

Correct Your Form

- Keep the right leg straight as your cross your left leg over it.
- Press your extended arm (the left arm in the instructions) into the floor to increase the stretch.
- Breathe normally. On the exhale, press your right hand harder on your left knee to increase the stretch.
- For best results, keep looking down your extended arm while pressing on the top of the bent knee.

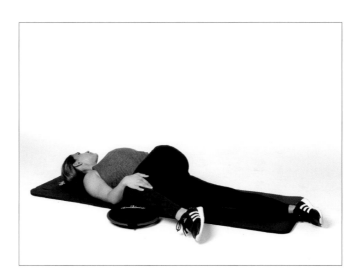

Hip Thruster

Benefits

This exercise activates and strengthens the hip extensor muscles of the gluteal complex while increasing the ROM of the hip flexor muscles. It also improves mobility of the hip joints to reduce stress on the lumbar spine.

Instructions

1. Lie flat on your back with both feet flat on the floor and your knees pointed up to the ceiling. (Your heels should be about 18 inches [46 cm] in front of your hips.) Place your arms along the side of your body so that your palms are rotated up to face the ceiling.
2. Place the sandbag across the front of your hips. If necessary, use both hands to hold it in place during the movement.
3. Push your heels into the ground while pulling your toes up toward your shins. Press your heels into the ground while squeezing your glutes and pushing your hips up toward the ceiling. Pause at the top and lower your hips slowly.
4. Push up for a count of 2, and lower for a count of 4. Perform 10 to 12 reps. Rest for 30 to 45 seconds and complete 2 sets. As your strength and mobility improve, add 2 reps each week until you can complete 20 reps without stopping.

Correct Your Form

- If you feel your hamstrings (the back of your legs) cramp and tighten, move your heels forward away from your tailbone.
- Pull your toes up toward your shins to strengthen the muscles along the front of the shins while stretching the muscles along the back of the calves, both of which can help improve ankle flexibility.
- Move at a slow and steady pace. Lowering the hips slowly keeps the muscles under tension longer, allowing them to develop strength while reducing tension in the muscles along the front of the hips.

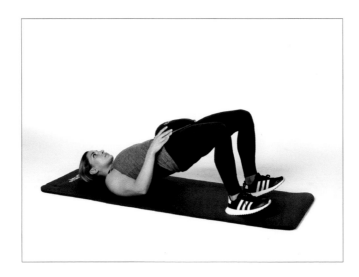

Kneeling Hip Flexor Stretch With Overhead Reach

Benefits

This exercise reduces tightness in the muscles along the front of the hip, which can reduce tightness and discomfort in the lumbar spine of the lower back. It also improves hip mobility and ROM of the hip flexor muscles and lengthens muscles of the upper back to improve shoulder ROM.

Instructions

1. Place your right knee directly under your right hip with your left foot directly in front of your body.
2. Keep your spine long and pelvis level as you raise both arms directly overhead, holding the sandbag between both hands.
3. Squeeze your right glute and push your right hip forward as you straighten your spine and lean back slightly to increase the length in the muscles along the front of your body. The weight from the sandbag should help increase the stretch in the flexor muscles along the front of the hip and increase ROM in the hip joint.
4. Hold for 30 to 45 seconds and switch legs. Perform 2 times on each hip.

Correct Your Form

- The pelvis should remain level. The motion should come from the hip joint, not from the pelvis tilting forward toward the front of the body.
- Keep the spine long and maintain length through the entire torso. This will allow more motion through the thoracic spine (mid-back).

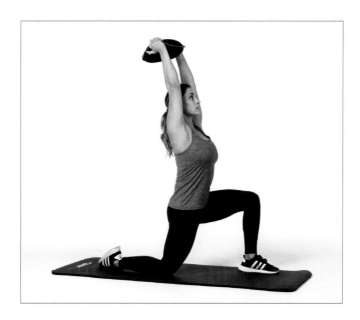

Hip Hinge With Offset Stance

Benefits

This exercise strengthens the extensor muscles of the gluteal complex while improving hip ROM, and it strengthens the muscles of the deep core responsible for maintaining stability in the lumbar spine.

Instructions

1. Stand with your feet hip-width apart. Move your right foot forward so that the toes of your left foot are even with the heel of your right. Keep your knees slightly bent and hold the sandbag in front of your chest, keeping it close to your chest through the entire ROM.
2. Keep your spine long as you push your hips back while hinging forward. The motion should come from the hip joints; the spine should remain straight through the entire movement.
3. Go to a comfortable end ROM. If your spine starts bending, that is too far to return to the top. Press your feet into the ground while driving the hips forward and squeezing your glute muscles.
4. Complete 5 to 6 reps with the right foot forward, then do the same number of reps with the left foot forward before resting for 30 to 45 seconds. Complete 2 sets. As your strength and mobility improve, add 2 reps each week (1 each side) until you are able to complete 20 reps (10 with each foot forward) in a row without stopping.

Correct Your Form

- The most common mistake in this and any hip hinge exercise is moving from the spine as opposed to the hips. During this movement, the spine should remain long. Motion should come from the pelvis rotating over the tops of the thigh bones. Anytime your spine starts rounding, you have gone too far.
- An offset stance where the toes of the back foot are even with the heel of the front creates different forces in the hips, allowing the muscles to become strong. Many times when you bend forward to lift something off the ground, your feet are in an offset position; this exercise can help strengthen your hip muscles relative to the way your feet are often placed during the movement patterns you perform on a regular basis. (The gym is the only place where movement happens symmetrically; most regular movements occur in a slightly offset position. Placing your feet and hands in asymmetrical positions allows the muscles to adapt to those forces.)

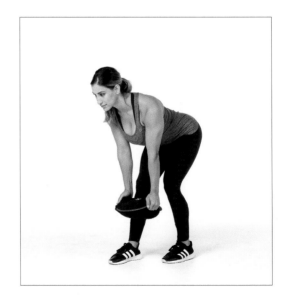

Lateral Lunge With Shoulder Carry

Benefits

This exercise strengthens the muscles of the hips while strengthening the muscles responsible for maintaining lumbar stability. It also strengthens the upper-back muscles to maintain stability when carrying an offset, unbalanced load.

Instructions

1. Hold the sandbag on the left shoulder with the left hand, and stand with feet about hip-width apart.
2. Step directly to your left, making sure your feet are parallel. As your left foot hits the ground, push your weight back into your left hip while keeping your spine long.
3. As you sink into your left hip, press your right foot into the ground and squeeze your right thigh to help maintain stability of the right knee.
4. To return to standing, push off with your left foot as you press your right foot into the ground and use your right inner thigh muscles to bring yourself back to standing.
5. Perform 6 to 8 reps moving to your right, then switch legs. Place the sandbag on your left shoulder and perform the same number of reps. Rest for approximately 1 minute and complete 2 sets. As your strength improves, add 2 reps per week (1 to each side) until you can complete 20 reps on each side without stopping.

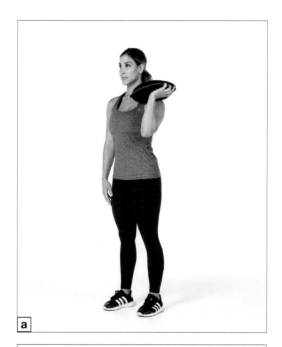

Correct Your Form

- Keep your spine long and straight as you step into the lunge. Rounding the back could cause discomfort or an injury.
- When stepping into the right leg, keep your left foot planted. It's important to try to keep both feet parallel during the lateral lunge movements.
- When stepping into the lunge, the hip should perform a hinging movement, with your weight going back into the hip, as opposed to the knee moving forward.

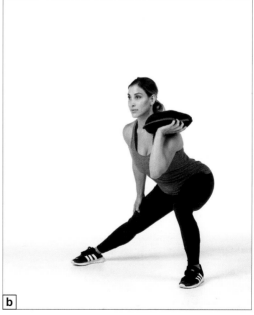

Forward Lunge With Reach to Ground

Benefits

This exercise strengthens the muscles of the posterior chain, specifically the hamstrings, glutes, and spinal erectors while improving mobility of the hips and lower back. It also increases the strength of the deep core muscles responsible for stabilizing the spine.

Instructions

1. Stand with feet hip-width apart and hold the sandbag with both hands in front of your waist.
2. Step forward with the left leg while keeping your right foot planted into the ground.
3. As your left foot hits the ground, hinge at the hip and lean forward while reaching with the sandbag as low as possible, trying to reach in front of the left foot. As you're leaning forward, make sure to keep your right heel pressed into the ground to lengthen the muscles along the back of the right leg.
4. As you return your spine to a tall, upright position, push off with your left leg and pull yourself back with your right leg.
5. Alternate legs. Step forward with the right leg while keeping the heel of the left foot flat on the ground. Reach the sandbag toward the ground in front of your right foot. Alternate legs for a total of 6 to 8 reps on each leg. Rest for 30 to 45 seconds and complete 2 sets. As you feel yourself get stronger, add 2 reps per week (1 to each leg) until you can perform 20 reps (10 on each leg) without stopping.

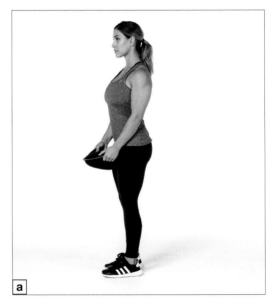
a

Correct Your Form

- Keep the heel flat on the ground to lengthen the muscles of the hamstrings and calves, allowing them to strengthen while stretching. Do not let the heel of your back foot come up as you perform this exercise.
- When your front foot hits the ground, the initial movement should be back into the hip before bending forward with the spine. When the hip moves first, it can reduce strain on the spine.

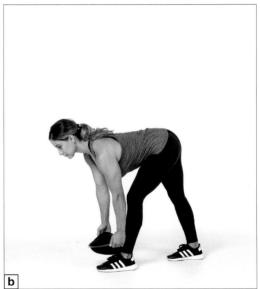
b

TWO-ARM RESISTANCE TUBING EXERCISES FOR MOBILITY

Mobility exercises with fitness equipment can provide more leverage to take a limb through a greater ROM while also increasing muscle fiber activation to help improve muscle contraction patterns. Resistance tubing can be used to create leverage for certain stretches as well as provide a little resistance to help enhance muscle activation during a movement pattern or static stretch. One way to increase the stretch of a muscle is to contract it while it is in a lengthened position then increase the stretch once the contraction is released. For example, when holding a straight leg stretch, contract the hamstring muscles in the back of the leg for 5 to 7 seconds; when you release the contraction, you can move into a deeper stretch taking the joint into a greater ROM. As you use the resistance tubing for mobility exercises, make sure to relax and breathe normally. If you hold your breath or contract muscles, it can reduce the effectiveness of the exercise. Once you reach 20 reps per each side, work up to doing 4 sets of each exercise; for the stretches, keep the length of time the same, but feel free to add additional sets.

Exercise	Sets	Repetitions	Rest interval
Leg-raise hamstring stretch	2	20-40 sec each leg	30-45 sec
Lying hip stretch	2	30-40 sec hold each leg	30-45 sec
Standing chest opener	2	30-50 sec hold each arm	30-45 sec
Standing pull and punch	2	6-8 each side	30-45 sec
Kneeling lift	2	6-8 each leg	30-45 sec
Overhead squat	2	8-10	30-45 sec

To increase the level of difficulty, complete all of the exercises in a row with no rest; allow 2 minutes of rest after the entire circuit. Work up to 4 circuits, and then add reps until you can do 20 of each exercise (10 on each arm or leg).

Leg-Raise Hamstring Stretch

Benefits

This exercise reduces tightness in the hamstring muscles along the back of the up leg (right in the photo) while stretching the hip flexors along the front of the down leg (left leg in the photo). It also improves flexibility and hip mobility to reduce discomfort or mild pain in the lower back.

Instructions

1. Lie flat on your back with both legs next to one another. Hold the ends of the band in both hands and loop the band around the bottom of the right foot.
2. Keep the left leg flat along the floor while picking the right leg straight up in the air.
3. With the band around the bottom of the right foot, gently pull your right leg up in the air until the point where you feel mild tension along the back of the thigh or the knee starts to bend.
4. To increase the stretch in both legs, push the back of the left leg into the floor while keeping the right leg straight. Contract the thigh of the right leg. As you relax the thigh of the right leg, use the band to pull the right leg higher into the air. Hold the stretch for 8 to 10 seconds after each contraction.
5. Repeat 2 to 4 times, holding the stretch for a total of 20 to 40 seconds, then alternate legs. Repeat for a total of 2 times on each leg.

Correct Your Form

- Keep the leg straight. (In the instructions, as soon as the right knee bends, the stretch is lost in the right hamstring.) Contract the thigh muscles to help keep the leg straight; the contraction of the muscles in the front of the thigh will help reduce tension in the muscles along the back of the thigh. If the knee starts to bend, lower the leg to reduce the stretch in the muscles.
- Keep the left leg flat and stable along the floor while lifting the right leg. This can help stretch the muscles along the front of the left thigh while the muscles in the back of the right thigh are being stretched.

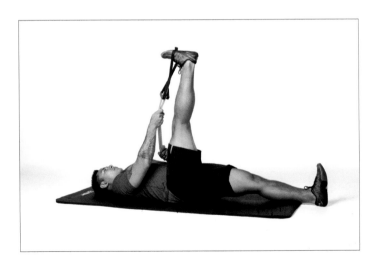

Lying Hip Stretch

Benefits

This exercise improves hip mobility and reduces tension in the hip rotators and improves extensibility of muscles in the lower back.

Instructions

1. Lie flat on your back with both legs next to one another. Hold the ends of the band in both hands and loop the band around the bottom and side of the left foot.
2. Bend your left knee to bring your left foot closer to the midline of your body. Use the band to create leverage on the left foot in order to increase the pressure in the muscles of the left hip. Hold the ends of the band with the right hand and place your left hand on the outside of your left knee so you are bringing your entire lower leg closer to your body. Keep your right leg straight along the ground as you bring your left foot up toward your midsection.
3. To increase the stretch, try to move your right foot away from you and press into the band and your right hand for 3 to 5 seconds. As you relax the right hip, move your leg into a new ROM and hold for 8 to 10 seconds.
4. Repeat the contract-and-relax cycle 2 to 4 times for a total of 30 to 40 seconds, then alternate legs. Complete 2 sets on each hip.

Correct Your Form

- This stretch works on the muscles that control hip mobility. For best results, keep the pressure on both the knee and foot. In the instructions above, keep the right leg flat on the ground. This creates more stability for the pelvis, allowing for a deeper stretch into the right hip capsule.
- Only move the limb to a point of mild tension; never force it to a point that is uncomfortable or painful.

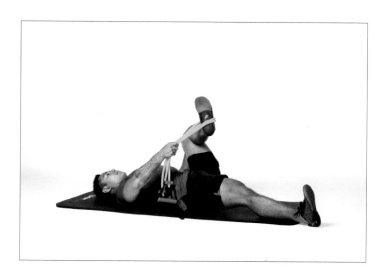

Standing Chest Opener

Benefits

This exercise stretches the muscles of the upper chest and shoulders, which often become tight as a result of typing on a cell phone or standard keyboard for an extended period of time. Stretching the muscles in the front of the torso can relieve tightness and tension in the muscles of the upper back and shoulders.

Instructions

1. Place the band in a doorframe at shoulder height to create a stable and secure base.
2. With your feet shoulder-width apart for stability, stand facing away from the doorframe so there is mild tension on the resistance bands. Place your right hand through both handles. Keep your right arm extended to your right side so that your right hand is at the same height as your right shoulder.
3. Press your right hand forward to contract the chest and shoulder muscles to place tension on the band. After contracting the muscles for 3 to 5 seconds, relax to release the muscles. Take a small step forward to increase the stretch on the right chest and shoulder, and hold for 8 to 10 seconds.
4. Repeat 3 to 5 times for a total of 30 to 50 seconds, then alternate sides. Complete 2 times on each arm.

Correct Your Form

- Make sure the anchor point for the band is at the same height as your shoulder.
- Keep the tension on your chest and shoulder muscles consistent without placing too much force on the shoulder.

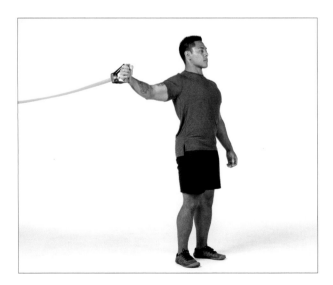

Standing Pull and Punch

Benefits

A combination of opposing movement patterns—pushing and pulling—along with rotation through the trunk can improve thoracic mobility and reduce tightness or tension in the muscles of the mid- to upper back.

Instructions

1. Place the anchor end of the band at a high point on a doorframe. With your feet wider than shoulder-width apart, stand facing the anchor point while holding one handle in each hand.

2. Pull your left arm back over your left shoulder while rotating your trunk to your left as you press your right hand across your body. Rotate your right foot towards your left foot as you turn over your left hip.

3. Pull your right hand back and rotate to your right, allowing your left foot to rotate to the right as you extend your right hand back over your right shoulder while reaching your left hand across your body.

4. Focus on leaning back to keep tension on the band, and rotate from the hips. Perform 6 to 8 reps on each side. Rest for 30 to 45 seconds and complete 2 sets. As you feel your strength and mobility improve, add 2 reps (1 to each side) each week until you can perform 10 reps on each side (20 total) without stopping.

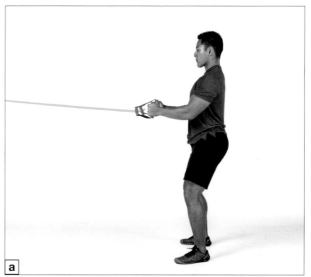
a

Correct Your Form

- Keep tension on the band during the entire movement. Leaning back to place tension on the back activates the posterior muscles, allowing more ROM to come from the front of the body.

- Allow your feet to rotate; they should rotate in the same direction as the hand reaching across your body.

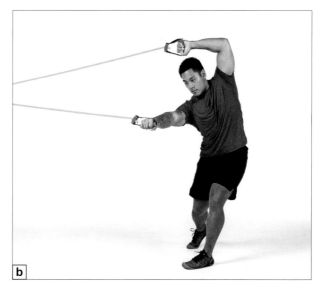
b

Kneeling Lift

Benefits

This exercise stretches the muscles and improves mobility in the hips, which can reduce tension on the lower back, thereby reducing pain. It also improves strength of the deep core muscles responsible for stabilizing the spine.

Instructions

1. Place the attachment end of the band at a low position (by the lower hinge if using a door-frame). Grip the ends of the band so that your palms are facing each other and your thumbs are pointed up to the ceiling. Kneel down on a pad or cushion, and place your right foot forward with your left knee directly under your left hip so that the left side of your body is facing the anchor point of the band. You should be far enough away from the anchor point so that there is slight tension in the band as you grip it.

2. Maintain a long spine as you pull the band up to your chest and then push it over your right shoulder as you keep your hands next to each other. Do not allow your upper body to move as you bring the resistance across your body. To increase stability and allow more motion from the spine, press your right foot into the ground.

3. At the top of the movement, pause before slowly reversing the motion to return the band to its original starting position.

4. Perform 6 to 8 reps, then alternate sides. Turn around so that your right knee is on the ground with your right side facing the anchor point and your left foot is planted on the floor. Perform 6 to 8 reps, rest for 30 to 45 seconds after both sides, complete 2 sets. Add 2 reps (1 to each side) per week until you are able to complete 10 reps on each side (20 total) without stopping.

Correct Your Form

- The spine should be long and tall to allow for optimal ROM.
- Push the forward foot down into the ground to create stability in the hips, which allows for more motion from the upper spine.

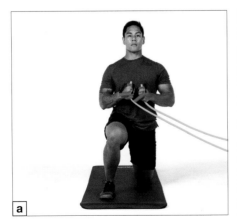
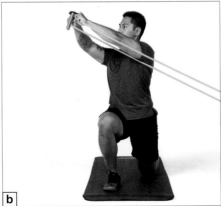

Overhead Squat

Benefits

This exercise improves hip mobility while strengthening the muscles of the shoulders and upper back. Using a band to help support your weight can allow you to sink lower into the bottom of the squat.

Instructions

1. Place the anchor point of the band in a doorframe at shoulder to head height.

2. Stand back facing the anchor point with your feet shoulder-width apart. Place your hands in the handles so the backs of your hands are pressing into the handles, with the palms facing the anchor point. As you raise your arms overhead, keep your arms extended overhead during the entire exercise. You should be far enough away from the anchor point that there is slight tension on the band.

3. Keep your spine long and push your hips back to lower into the squat position. As you lean back, the band will help support your weight allowing you to sink lower into your hips.

4. At the bottom of the movement, press both feet into the ground and think about pushing the floor away from you as you return to standing.

5. Lower yourself slowly for 3 to 4 seconds, then move more quickly to return to standing in 1 to 2 seconds. Perform 8 to 10 repetitions, rest for 30 to 45 seconds, and complete 2 sets.

Correct Your Form

- Keep your arms extended overhead during the entire movement, and keep the shoulders pulled down to help hold the shoulders stable.

- Stand back from the anchor point. You should be far enough so the tension on the band is pulling you forward; this allows you to sink deeper into your hips during the squat.

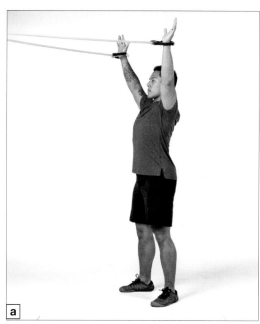

a

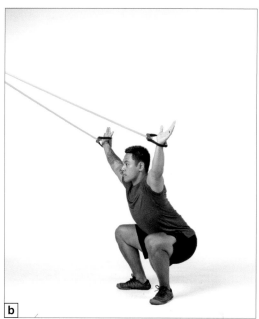

b

DUMBBELL EXERCISES FOR MOBILITY

Dumbbells can help improve muscle strength, and they can also be an effective tool for enhancing mobility because the weight can lengthen muscle and connective tissue while taking a limb through a complete ROM, helping to increase muscle fiber activation. In addition, using dumbbells requires coordination between the right and left sides of the body, which can help improve overall movement skill. Start with light dumbbells that can easily be controlled for the recommended number of repetitions; a weight that is too heavy could cause too much length in the muscle and be a potential cause of injury. Once you reach 20 reps per each side, work up to doing 4 sets of each exercise; for the stretches, keep the length of time the same, but feel free to add additional sets.

Exercise	Sets	Repetitions	Rest interval
Supine pullover	2	8-10	30-45 sec
Lateral lunge with reach to ground	2	6-8 each leg	30-45 sec
Split squat with single-arm overhead press	2-3	6-8 each leg	30-45 sec
Rotating shoulder press	2-3	6-8 each arm	30-45 sec
Sword draw	2-3	8-10 each arm	30-45 sec
Transverse plane lunge with reach to ground	2-3	6-8 each leg	30-45 sec
To increase the level of difficulty, complete all of the exercises in a row with no rest; allow 2 minutes of rest after the entire circuit. Work up to 4 circuits, and then add reps until you can do 20 of each exercise (10 on each arm or leg).			

Supine Pullover

Benefits

This exercise improves extensibility of the chest and shoulder muscles in the front of the body, and it increases ROM of the shoulder joints.

Instructions

1. Lie down on your back with your feet flat on the floor so your knees are pointed up to the ceiling. Hold one dumbbell in each hand, and extend your arms straight above your chest with your palms facing each other.
2. Slowly lower your arms overhead while keeping them straight. Once your arms are overhead, pause for 1 to 2 seconds before slowly pulling the weights back up to the original starting position.
3. Allow the weights to lower slowly, then bring them up quickly. Repeat for 8 to 10 repetitions, rest for 30 to 45 seconds, and repeat for a second set. Add 2 reps per week until you are able to complete 20 reps without stopping.

Correct Your Form

- Keep both knees bent so the feet are flat on the floor. This helps keep the pelvis in a neutral position to reduce tension in the low back.
- Keep the elbows straight during the entire movement. If the elbows bend, the triceps will do most of the work. Keeping your arms straight will ensure the latissimus dorsi muscles of the upper back receive the greatest stretch benefit.

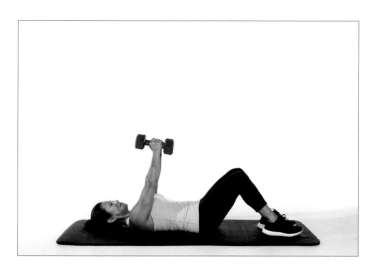

Lateral Lunge With Reach to Ground

Benefits

This exercise improves mobility of the hips and ankle complex while stretching the muscles that stabilize the deep core.

Instructions

1. Stand with your feet hip-width apart and hold one dumbbell in each hand.
2. Step directly to your right. As your right foot hits the ground, keep it parallel to your left and push your right hip back as you reach for the right foot with both hands.
3. As you lower yourself to reach for your foot, push your hips back before allowing your spine to bend as you reach for the floor.
4. To return to standing, pull your arms up to your waist and push your right foot into the floor while pressing your left foot into the ground and using your left inner-thigh muscles.
5. Perform 6 to 8 repetitions on the right leg before alternating legs. Rest for 30 to 45 seconds after completing the same number of reps on each leg; perform 2 sets. Add 2 reps per week (1 to each side) until you can complete 10 reps on each side (20 total) without stopping.

Correct Your Form

- Mobile hips protect the spine. Moving the hips first when reaching for the ground will help protect the back as it starts to round. If the hips don't flex properly, unnecessary stress and strain are placed on the muscles of the lumbar spine.
- To develop optimal movement in the hips, make sure both feet are parallel, pressed firmly into the floor, and facing the same direction as you perform the lunges.

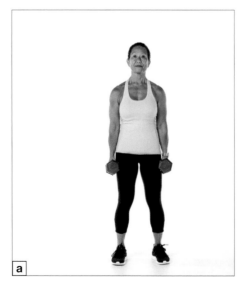

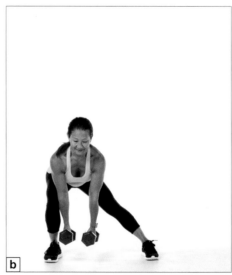

Split Squat With Single-Arm Overhead Press

Benefits

This exercise reduces tightness of the muscles in the front of the hip while improving hip mobility and increasing core stability. You walk and run on one leg at a time; this move replicates that action to allow for better strength development for how you actually use your legs.

Instructions

1. Start in a split stance with your feet hip-width apart so that your right foot is forward and your left foot is back behind your body with your toes on the ground.
2. Hold a dumbbell in your left hand in front of your left shoulder with your elbow tucked in to your rib cage.
3. Maintain a long spine as you sink back into your right hip, and extend your left arm directly overhead so that your palm faces the midline of your body. Lower yourself to a comfortable depth while keeping your pelvis in a relatively neutral position. At the bottom of the split squat your left arm should be extended directly overhead.
4. To return to standing, press your right foot into the ground as you lower your left arm. Repeat for 6 to 8 repetitions with the left arm, then switch to place your left leg forward, right leg back, and weight in your right hand. Perform the same number of repetitions with each arm. Rest for 30 to 45 seconds between sets. Complete 2 sets. As your strength and mobility improve, add 2 reps (1 to each side) each week until you can complete 10 reps on each side.

Correct Your Form

- The knee of your back leg should be almost directly under the hip. Placing your back leg (the left leg in the instructions) too far back increases the stretch and reduces your stability.
- To help increase the stretch when you extend your arm overhead, keep your spine long and straight.

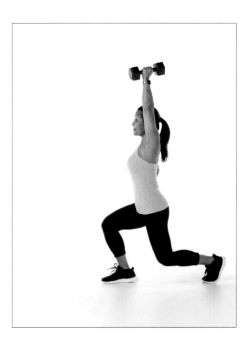

Rotating Shoulder Press

Benefits

This exercise improves mobility of the hip and thoracic spine while increasing strength of the deep core and shoulder muscles.

Instructions

1. Stand with your feet hip-width apart and knees slightly bent. Hold one dumbbell in each hand so they are directly in front of your shoulders.
2. Keep your spine long as you rotate to your right. At the end of the rotation, extend your right arm straight up while pressing your feet into the ground. (Creating force in opposite directions helps increase the stretch effect while also improving strength of the connective tissue.)
3. Pull the right arm back down and rotate to your left before extending your left arm overhead.
4. Move slowly as you rotate from side to side. Perform 6 to 8 repetitions with each arm. Rest for 30 to 45 seconds after each set. Complete 2 sets. As your mobility and strength improve, add 2 reps (1 to each side) until you can perform 10 reps to each side without stopping.

Correct Your Form

- Keep your spine long and straight to allow for optimal motion as you rotate. Do not allow spine to bend or slouch.
- Pressing your feet into the ground increases stability, which helps improve mobility and motion in the thoracic spine.

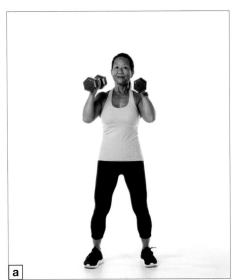
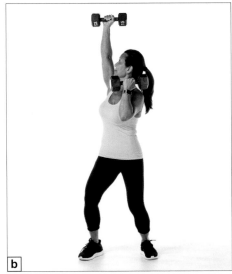

Sword Draw

Benefits

This exercise stretches the muscles in the front of the chest and shoulder while increasing the strength of the upper-back and shoulder muscles, which can help promote good posture.

Instructions

1. Stand with your feet hip-width apart. Hold one dumbbell in your right hand so that your right arm is straight and your right palm is resting in front of your left thigh.
2. Press both feet into the ground to increase stability. Maintain a level pelvis and a long, tall spine as you raise your right arm across your body and out to your right side so that the weight ends up at approximately shoulder height. Your right hand should move across the front of your body like you are drawing a sword from your left hip.
3. Perform 6 to 8 repetitions with the right arm, then switch arms. Rest for 30 to 45 seconds between sets and complete 2 sets. Once you can easily perform 8 reps, add 1 rep per week until you can complete 20 reps on each side.

Correct Your Form

- Keep the weight at or below shoulder height.
- Keep the spine long and straight to improve ROM of the shoulder joint and avoid possible injury.

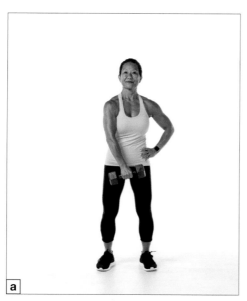
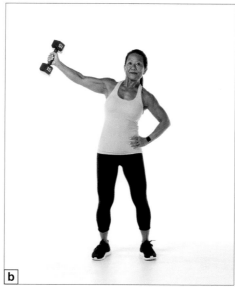

Transverse Plane Lunge
With Reach to Ground

Benefits

This exercise improves hip mobility and stretches the muscles of the upper thighs.

Instructions

1. Stand with your feet hip-width apart. Hold one dumbbell in each hand. Keep your left foot pointed straight ahead at the twelve o'clock direction as you step back with your right foot and place it facing in the four o'clock direction.
2. As your right foot hits the ground, push your weight back into your right hip while reaching for your foot with both hands.
3. To return to standing, push off the ground with your right foot as you press your left foot into the ground and use the inner-thigh muscles of your left leg.
4. Perform 6 to 8 repetitions with your right leg, then alternate legs, performing the same number of repetitions. Rest for 30 to 45 seconds between sets. Perform 2 sets. Once you can comfortably perform 8 reps on each leg, add 2 reps (1 on each leg) every week until you can complete a total of 20 reps (10 on each leg) without stopping.

Correct Your Form

- Keep the foot of the forward, planted leg (in the instructions, the left leg) pressed into the ground to allow the hip to rotate as you step back and reach for the foot.
- Pressing the forward foot into the ground while squeezing the thigh muscles can help protect the knee while allowing greater mobility in the hip joint.

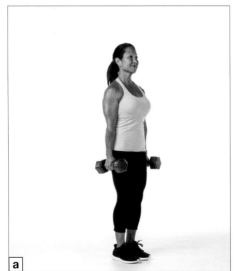
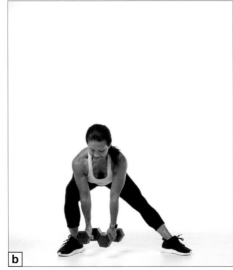

KETTLEBELL EXERCISES FOR MOBILITY

The unique design of the kettlebell with the handle outside of the center of mass makes it a great tool for improving tissue length and joint range of motion. Asymmetrical exercises where a kettlebell is held on just one side of the body can be an extremely effective way to enhance mobility one side of the body at a time. It's important to use a kettlebell that is not too heavy or too light; if it's too heavy it could over stretch the muscle causing a strain, and if it's too light it may not provide enough load to properly lengthen a muscle. If you can easily hold a kettlebell in a bottom-up position (holding the kettlebell by the handle so that the bottom is facing upwards toward the ceiling) for more than 20 seconds, then it is probably too light to provide any mobility (or strength or metabolic) benefits. A kettlebell that is the proper weight for mobility training should be difficult to hold in a bottom-up position for more than 10 or 15 seconds.

Exercise	Sets	Repetitions	Rest interval
Supine rollover with single-arm press	2	5-8 each side	45-60 sec
Reverse lunge in racked position	2	6-8 each leg	45-60 sec
Halo	2	6-10 each direction	45-60 sec
Reverse lunge with trunk rotation	2	5-8 each leg	45-60 sec
Trunk rotation with single-arm press	2	5-8 each arm	45-60 sec
Windmill low hold	2	4-6 each side	45-60 sec
To increase the level of difficulty, complete all of the exercises in a row with no rest; allow 2 minutes of rest after the entire circuit. Work up to 4 circuits, and then add reps until you can do 20 of each exercise (10 on each arm or leg).			

Supine Rollover With Single-Arm Press

Benefits

The weight and position of the kettlebell can help add leverage to improve mobility of the shoulder and spine, specifically, the intervertebral segments of the thoracic spine and the glenohumeral and scapulothoracic joints of the shoulder.

Instructions

1. Lie flat on your back with your left leg straight and your right leg bent so the right foot is flat on the ground. Hold the kettlebell straight up with the right arm and place your left arm directly overhead with the palm up facing the ceiling.
2. Press your right foot into the ground and press your right arm up as you roll over to the left side of your body. Pause for 1 to 3 seconds, then lower back to the initial lying position.
3. Perform 5 to 6 repetitions, then switch sides. Rest for 45 to 60 seconds after both sides. Complete 2 sets. As your mobility improves, add 2 reps (1 to each side) per week until you can complete 10 reps on each side without stopping.

Correct Your Form

- Keep constant tension in the arm holding the kettlebell (the right arm in the instructions). Allowing the elbow to bend could change the position of the weight and lead to a loss of control.
- Use the bent leg (the right leg in the instructions) to initiate the rolling movement. This will help integrate motion between the hips and shoulders.

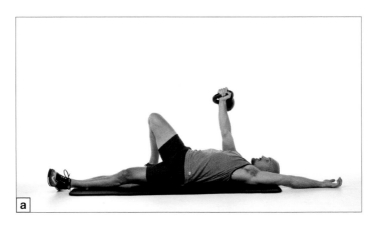

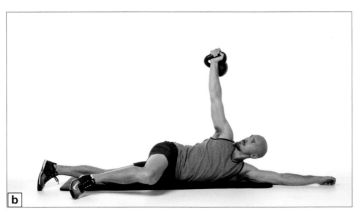

Reverse Lunge in Racked Position

Benefits

This exercise improves mobility in the hip while increasing strength of the muscles responsible for creating stability in the spine. Holding a weight in an offset, asymmetrical position (that is, on only one side of the body) can help strengthen the core muscles while enhancing mobility of the hips.

Instructions

1. Stand tall with feet about hip-width apart. With your right hand, hold a kettlebell in a racked position so that the knuckles of your right hand are resting against your collarbone while your right elbow is pressed into your rib cage. (The kettlebell should be resting on the right forearm.)

2. Keep your left foot pressed into the ground as you step back with the right leg. Place the top of your right toes on the ground. Lean forward slightly as you lower into the lunge to increase the activation of the left hip while stretching your back.

3. Lower yourself but do not let your right knee hit the ground. Pause at the bottom for 1 to 2 seconds, then press your left foot into the ground to pull yourself forward back to the starting position. Perform 6 to 8 reps, then switch sides. Rest for 45 to 60 seconds between sets. Perform 2 sets total. Once you can complete 8 reps on each leg, add 2 reps per week (1 on each leg) until you can complete 10 reps on each leg.

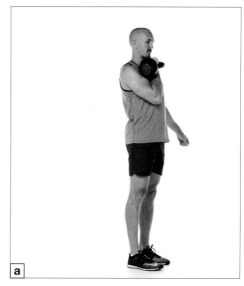

a

Correct Your Form

- Keep your spine long and straight during the lowering phase of the movement. A slight lean forward can increase strength of the hip extensor muscles, but the motion should come from the hip, not the spine.

- Move at a steady, slow pace. The focus of this movement is to improve mobility. Move slowly when stepping back to emphasize stretching the muscles of that hip (the right leg in the instructions).

- Pressing the forward foot into the ground (the left foot in the instructions) helps create and maintain stability of the forward hip joint.

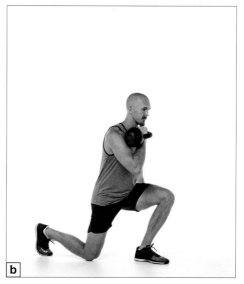

b

Halo

Benefits

This exercise improves mobility in the glenohumeral and scapulothoracic joints of the shoulders and the intervertebral joints of the thoracic spine. It reduces tightness of the chest and shoulder muscles. Tightness in the muscles in the front of the body could cause back pain.

Instructions

1. Stand with your feet approximately shoulder-width apart as you hold a kettlebell by the horns (the sides of the kettlebell handle) directly in front of your chest.

2. Maintain a tall, long spine as you move the kettlebell from in front of your chest to over your left shoulder as you reach across your body with your right arm. Continue moving the kettlebell behind your head to bring it back to your chest by passing it over your right shoulder.

3. Perform 6 to 8 repetitions moving over the left shoulder first before switching directions. Rest for 45 to 60 seconds between sets. Complete 2 sets. As your mobility improves, add 2 reps per week (1 in each direction) until you can complete a total of 20 reps (10 in each direction) without stopping.

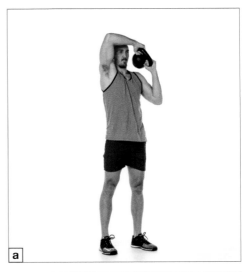

a

Correct Your Form

- Maintain excellent posture with a long, straight spine to ensure optimal mobility of the shoulders.
- Try to keep the head and neck stable with minimal movement. Move the weight around your head and shoulders as opposed to moving your neck and head to make room for the kettlebell.

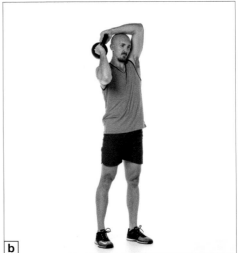

b

Reverse Lunge With Trunk Rotation

Benefits

This exercise improves mobility of the hips and intervertebral segments of the thoracic spine, and it increases stabilization strength of the deep core muscles.

Instructions

1. Stand with your feet about hip-width apart and with a tall spine. Hold a kettlebell in both hands by the bell so the bottom is up and the handle is between your forearms. The kettlebell should be in front of your chest so your upper arms are pressed against the front of your rib cage.

2. Step back with the left leg and lower yourself into your right hip until your right knee is almost 90 degrees and your left knee is almost touching the floor. Keep a tall spine and rotate to your right. To increase rotation, think about turning your left shoulder over your right thigh. Rotate back to face the front. Press your right foot into the ground to help pull yourself forward as you return to standing.

3. Perform 6 to 8 repetitions stepping back with the left leg before alternating legs and completing the same number of reps on that leg. Rest for 45 to 60 seconds between reps. Complete 2 sets. Once you feel your strength and mobility improve, add 2 reps per week (1 to each side) until you can complete 20 reps (10 on each side) without stopping.

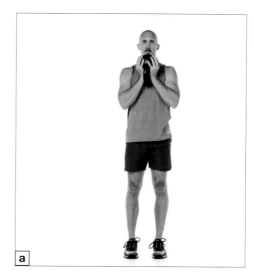

a

Correct Your Form

- For optimal rotation, keep the spine tall and straight; do not allow it to round or bend.
- Maintain stability in the front leg by pressing the foot into the floor (the left leg in the instructions).

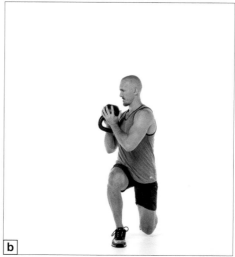

b

Trunk Rotation With Single-Arm Press

Benefits

This exercise stretches the chest and shoulder muscles while improving mobility of the intervertebral segments of the thoracic spine.

Instructions

1. Stand with your feet hip-width apart. Hold a kettlebell in the racked position with your right hand so that your knuckles are along your collarbone and your upper arm and elbow are against your rib cage.
2. Keep your spine tall and long, and rotate to your right. As you reach about 90 degrees (facing toward three o'clock), stop and press your right arm straight into the air. Lower your arm by pulling your elbow down to your right rib cage and then rotate back to face directly forward.
3. Perform 5 to 8 reps with the right arm, then switch to the left and perform the same number of reps. Rest for 45 to 60 seconds between sets. Complete 2 sets. As your strength and mobility improve, add 2 reps (1 to each side) until you can complete 12 reps on each side.

Correct Your Form

- Have a tall, straight spine to allow for optimal rotation.
- When rotating to your right, think about turning your left shoulder to face the two o'clock position.
- Keep your feet pressed into the ground and squeeze your glute muscles to create a solid base of support to allow the spine to rotate.

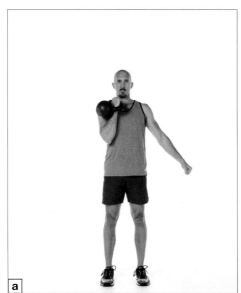
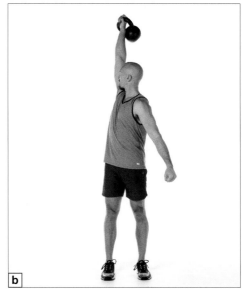

Windmill Low Hold

Benefits

This exercise enhances spinal stability while improving hip mobility, and it develops integrated strength between the muscles of the hips and shoulders.

Instructions

1. Stand with your feet wider than shoulder-width, with your right foot pointing straight ahead in the twelve o'clock position and your left foot in a staggered position in the three o'clock position. Even though they are in staggered positions, the toes of both feet should be pointed relatively in the same direction (forward).
2. Hold a kettlebell in the left hand so that it is hanging down along the front of the left thigh. Hold your right arm straight overhead and lower your left arm by your side while maintaining a long spine as you push your weight back into the right hip and turn to look at your right hand. Allow your left hand to slowly lower the kettlebell along the inside of your left (front) leg.
3. To return to standing, push your left leg into the floor and slide your hips forward as you bring your back up straight and tall.
4. Perform 4 to 6 reps, then alternate sides, completing the same number of reps on each side. After using both sides, rest for 45 to 60 seconds. Complete 2 sets. Once you can complete 6 reps, add 1 rep to each side every week until you can complete 12 reps with each side.

Correct Your Form

- For this exercise the movement should come from the hips. Keep the spine long and fully extended. Focus on pushing back into the hips and lower yourself only as far as you can while maintaining control of your spine. Stop before you feel your spine start to bend or round.
- Keeping your eyes on your raised hand helps position the spine to allow the motion to come from your hips.
- When returning to standing, push the back hip forward (the right hip in the instructions) to initiate the movement.

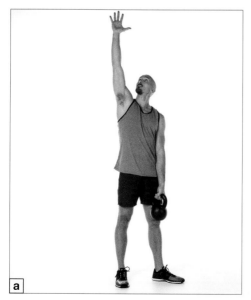 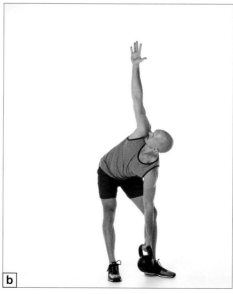

4

Core Strength Training

From video-based workouts to infomercials to group fitness classes at the local gym, it seems as if you can't hear any fitness instructor teach an exercise without using the words *contract*, *squeeze*, or *engage* in reference to your core. The rectus abdominis muscle provides the shape of the proverbial six-pack on the front of the abdomen. That's not the only muscle that's important, though. The area comprised of your upper legs, spine, and chest, often referred to as the body's core, is made up of a number of muscles that work together to create the necessary stability and mobility for efficient movement. Effective exercise strategies for the muscles often referred to as the core require more than merely squeezing or contracting. This chapter will provide effective strategies, along with a number of fun and challenging workouts, to help you develop true core strength.

Because they often require you to lie down on the floor, many traditional core exercises do not harness the inherent mechanical energy created when the body is in a vertical, upright position. Momentum occurs as the result of a mass moving at any rate of speed; the greater the mass or faster the speed, the higher the momentum. The muscles that attach your shoulders and pelvis to the spine can harness the momentum created by the competing forces of gravity and ground reaction to generate the mechanical energy for many of the movements you perform on a regular basis. When any part of your body starts moving, it generates momentum, and one of the primary functions of muscle, fascia, and elastic connective tissue is to control this momentum.

When it comes to core training, the abdominals can be controlled by the brain to flex the spine when you're lying on the ground, but this is not how they actually work during upright movement. During the gait cycle, which is the default pattern of human movement, the multiple layers of the abdominals are lengthened in all three planes as the rib cage and pelvis rotate opposite one another; these lengthening motions engage the muscles in their natural way of functioning. Therefore, it is easy to see how the crunch is really *not* the most effective exercise for strengthening core muscles.

All You Ever Needed to Know About Your Core You Learned Before You Could Walk

Every time your foot makes contact with the ground, your body is accelerated downward by the force of gravity. At the same time, the ground exerts an equal and opposite force upwards into your lower leg, called ground reaction force (GRF); these two competing forces intersect around the body's center of gravity. How we learn to control our bodies as we grow from newborns to infants to children provides important insights into how our muscles are designed to function. Humans are one of the only mammals born not knowing how to walk; when a four-legged mammal is born, it only takes a few minutes for it to learn how to stand on its feet. Quadrupeds have four legs to support the mass of the body, with a spine parallel to the ground, while humans are bipeds with a spine that is perpendicular to the ground and only two legs to support the weight of the body. This means that it can take a human approximately ten to fourteen months or longer to learn how to sequence and coordinate the muscle actions responsible for walking because the muscles and skeletal structures have to become strong enough to maintain a vertical position that resists the downward pull of gravity (Enoka 2002).

The natural stages of human motor skill development are extending the spine, rolling over, sitting up, belly crawling, crawling, cruising (which is standing and walking while holding on to stable objects), and, finally, walking. During the stages of development, the muscles are developing the timing, strength, and coordination to integrate movements of the hips, pelvis, spine, and shoulders. At no point during the natural progression of walking does a baby lie on its back and flex his or her spine to perform a crunch (Abernathy 2005).

Lying on your back to do abdominal and oblique crunches could actually be working against the way your muscles function. Attempting to isolate specific muscles with traditional core exercises will not train the tissues and skeletal structures to accommodate the multiplanar forces you could experience when performing a number of ADLs such as lifting a young child from a crib or carrying a big bag of groceries.

Functional Anatomy: Understanding Your Core Muscles

Core is commonly used to describe the muscles that control motion of the pelvis, femurs, rib cage, and spine, specifically, the lumbar and thoracic segments. However, any muscle that can influence motion of the upper legs, pelvis, or spine could be considered part of your body's core region as well. This means that a number of muscles not traditionally classified as part of the core could be considered core muscles because they can indeed influence motion at these segments. For example, both the long and short heads of the biceps (your upper-arm muscle) attach to the shoulder blade (at the supraglenoid tubercle and coracoid process, respectively), which sits on the thoracic rib cage. If the biceps remain in a state of contraction, the muscle could pull the scapula forward, creating a rounded shoulder, which then changes the position of the thoracic spine, causing it to flex and bend toward the front of the body. If the thoracic spine remains in a flexed position, it will affect the muscles responsible for controlling both position and motion of the entire spine, ultimately changing your center of gravity.

One group of researchers describes the core as the pelvic girdle, spine, shoulders, and all soft tissues (ligaments, tendons, fascia, and muscle) with proximal attachments originating on the axial skeleton formed by the skull, spine, and rib cage (Martuscello et al. 2013). This definition includes the numerous muscles that attach to the pelvis, abdominals, and spine (figure 4.1).

Dr. Stuart McGill describes the core as being "composed of the lumbar spine, the muscles of the abdominal wall, the back extensors and quadratus lomborum. Also included are the multi-joint muscles, namely, latissimus dorsi and psoas that pass through the core linking it to the pelvis, legs, shoulders and arms" (McGill 2010, 33). A separate model describes the abdominal muscles as being organized into layers—superficial, intermediate, and deep—based on their relation to the superficial surface of the skin and the deep, internal structures of the skeleton (Neumann 2010).

McGill is not alone in his thoughts that ground-based strength training can be effective for enhancing the strength of core muscles. According to researchers Bret Contreras and Brad Schoenfeld, "Most training can be considered 'core training' . . . With respect to program design, basic core strength and endurance will be realized through performance of most non-machine-based exercises such as during squats, deadlifts, chin-ups and push-ups" (Contreras and Schoenfeld 2011, 14). The human body is designed to move most efficiently when walking or running across the ground. The muscles, fascia, elastic connective tissues, and skeletal structures function most effectively when standing upright on the ground, not lying on the floor. Exercises to develop core strength, therefore, should enhance the ability of the muscles to function as a single, integrated system.

Regardless of the specific model referenced, the muscles that connect the hips, pelvis, spine, shoulders, and rib cage function as the transmission of the body because they are responsible for transferring forces generated from the ground through the legs and trunk and ultimately out through the upper extremities. If you want to improve your core strength, you need to perform exercises for a wide range of muscle groups, including the gluteal complex (gluteus maximus, medius,

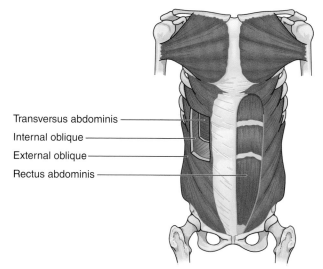

Transversus abdominis

Internal oblique

External oblique

Rectus abdominis

Figure 4.1 The core muscles are organized in layers and work together to create stability.

and minimus), hamstrings, quadriceps, adductors, spinal erectors, internal obliques, external obliques, hip flexors, latissimus dorsi (which attaches to the lower back, so it is considered a core muscle), and, finally, the rectus abdominis (otherwise known as the six-pack muscle). These muscles all attach to the core of the body.

Dr. McGill has found that using ground-based, vertical exercises to strengthen the core is extremely effective because muscles can develop the ability to produce force in the multiple directions necessary to support various positions and handle unexpected loads (McGill 2010). The external and internal obliques, rectus abdominis (RA), and transverse abdominis (TVA) are considered part of the deep layer in Neumann's model and make up the abdominal wall as described by McGill. The deep muscles create stability around the lumbar spine in order to allow motion of the thoracic spine, shoulders, and hips. The muscles of the abdominal wall are layered against one another like the individual layers of a sheet of plywood; as these layers contract, they create stiffness around the lumbar spine and pelvis to establish core stability. Because of the way these layers of muscles work as a single unit, they are only capable of working in isolation when you are in various positions lying on the floor or in an exercise machine with a specific ROM. A stationary posture is both the beginning and end point for all movement; as the deep muscles of the core get stronger, they will help you maintain a straighter posture, which in turn, can help you to move better. Plus, as the deep core muscles become stronger, they will act like a weight belt or girdle and actually help to flatten your stomach by holding the contents of your abdominal cavity in behind the walls of muscle.

The Role of Core Muscles in Movement

Exercise is a function of movement created by many muscles working together simultaneously, not a series of discrete actions. Nowhere is this more apparent than the core region. Exercises for core muscles are often performed in an inefficient manner that may not actually improve their ability to control movement when you are standing on your feet. Instead, exercises for your core muscles should be based on how the body is designed to move or, more specifically, how your muscles produce various movements when you're standing upright (see tables 4.1 and 4.2 and figure 4.2). For example, a common misunderstanding is that countless crunches are the best way to sculpt a six-pack. However, the *only* time the RA flexes the spine is when the body is lying on the ground, which begs the question, Is the crunch the most efficient use of your time during a workout?

A strength-training program for core muscles should feature exercises in a standing position to properly prepare the body to produce and control forces experienced in ADLs. Movements should integrate the hips, trunk, and shoulders to efficiently distribute the downward force created by gravity as well as the upward forces generated by GRF. Exercises in the prone (face-down) or supine (face-up) positions can help establish strength specifically through activating the motor units responsible for contracting the muscle fibers that stabilize the spine and pelvis. For example, the plank exercise requires minimal movement while contracting all layers of the abdominal fascia and is an excellent way to establish the muscle recruitment patterns required to stabilize the spine. When done properly, the plank not only uses the deep abdominal muscles but it also recruits hip, shoulder, and upper-back muscles (Hibbs et al. 2008). However, once you establish the ability to properly brace the spine, it becomes necessary to integrate movement at the hips before progressing to exercises performed in standing positions. As Dr. McGill's work has demonstrated, movement-based strength training exercises that involve your upper- and lower-body limbs working together from a standing position can be extremely effective for developing core strength (McGill 2010).

Understanding and Controlling Movement

When walking or running, the body has to move in all three different directions to create forward movement. Your chest and rib cage will counterrotate relative to the pelvis in reaction to the momentum created by the arms and legs moving opposite of one another. During gait, as the right leg swings forward, the left arm swings forward. This counterrotation of the torso and hips lengthens all layers of your core muscles, which are designed to facilitate this multiplanar action to make it smooth and efficient. That's right; the actual purpose of our core muscles is to work effectively and efficiently while the body is in an upright, vertical position (Earls 2014).

To store the elastic energy used for many upright movements, exercise strategies for core muscles should include movements that first lengthen the tissue before it shortens. For sustainable, long-term results, an exercise program should first enhance mobility and tissue extensibility in individual movement patterns before progressing to complex, dynamic movements that involve multiple planes of motion. Mobility exercises allow the CNS to develop efficient timing of muscle contractions before progressing to the more complex movement patterns that can improve strength and allow muscles to generate force in multiple directions.

Table 4.1 **Attachments and Actions of Deep Core Muscles**

Muscle	Superior attachments	Inferior attachments	Integrated function
External oblique	Lateral side of ribs 4-12	Iliac crest, linea alba, and fascial sheath of RA	Control motion at the trunk by producing flexion in the sagittal plane, lateral flexion in the frontal plane, and rotation in the transverse plane
Internal oblique*+	Iliac crest, inguinal ligament, and thoracolumbar fascia	Ribs 9-12, linea alba, and fascial sheath of RA	Control motion at the trunk by producing flexion in the sagittal plane, lateral flexion in the frontal plane, and rotation in the transverse plane
Rectus abdominis	Xiphoid process of the sternum	Pubic symphysis of the pelvis	Decelerate anterior tilting of the pelvis, control rotation of the trunk, co-contract with other layers to stabilize the spine
Transverse abdominis	Iliac crest, thoracolumbar fascia, inner surface of cartilage of ribs 6-12, and inguinal ligament	Linea alba and fascial sheath of RA	Compression of abdominal cavity, create stability by increasing tension on thoracolumbar fascia, provide attachment sites for other abdominal muscles

*The contralateral (opposite side) external oblique (EO) and internal oblique (IO) work together to create rotation; for example, the right EO works with the left IO to create rotation to the left.

Superior is an anatomical term and means "toward the head"; conversely, *inferior* means "away from the head."

+The ipsilateral (same side) EO and IO work together to create lateral flexion; for example, the right EO works with the right IO to create right lateral flexion of the spine.

Table 4.2   **Attachments and Actions of Superficial and Intermediate Core Muscles**

Muscle	Superior attachments	Inferior attachments	Integrated function
Hamstrings: biceps femoris (BF), semitendinosus (ST), semimembranosus (SM)	BF: ischial tuberosity (bottom of pelvis) ST: ischial tuberosity SM: ischial tuberosity	BF: top of fibula and lateral tibial condyle (lower leg) ST: inferior to medial condyle of tibia (top of lower leg) SM: medial condyle of tibia (top of lower leg)	Extend hip, extend knee (when foot is on the ground), control internal and external rotation
Adductor complex: brevis, longus, magnus	Brevis: pubic bone Longus: pubic bone Magnus: pubic bone and ischial tuberosity	Brevis: middle 1/3 of back of femur Longus: middle 1/3 of back of femur Magnus: linea aspera and adductor tubercle (back of femur)	Extend the hip when the leg is in front of the body and flex the hip when the leg is behind the body
Quadriceps: rectus femoris (RF), vastus medialis (VM), vastus intermedius (VI), vastus lateralis (VL)	RF: bottom front of pelvis VM: front of thigh bone (femur) VI: top 2/3 of thigh bone (femur) VL: top of thigh bone (greater trochanter—femur) front of thigh bone (femur)	RF: patella (kneecap) and tibial tuberosity VM: medial tibial condyle, medial patella, and medial aspect of RF tendon VI: inferior aspect of patella, tendons of VL and VM VL: lower patella, front of lateral tibial condyle (top of lower leg)	Flex hip, extend (straighten) lower leg, control stability of knee
Gluteal complex: maximus, medius, and minimus	Sacrum and coccyx (lower back), posterior gluteal line, and iliac crest (top of pelvis)	Gluteal line of thigh bone (femur), inferior and anterior to lateral condyle of tibia (top of lower leg)	Extend hip, create external rotation of hip (resist internal rotation of hip), adduct hip
Latissimus dorsi	Intertubercular groove of humerus (upper arm)	Spinous processes of lower 6 thoracic and all lumbar vertebrae, ilium and lower 3 ribs, inferior angle of scapula	Extend upper arm, pull arm closer to body (adduct), control rotation of the shoulder; the inferior segments can create forward tilt of pelvis
Spinal erectors	External occipital protuberance (bottom of skull)	Lumbar and sacral vertebrae	Extend (straighten) spine, decelerate forward flexion of spine, maintain lengthened position

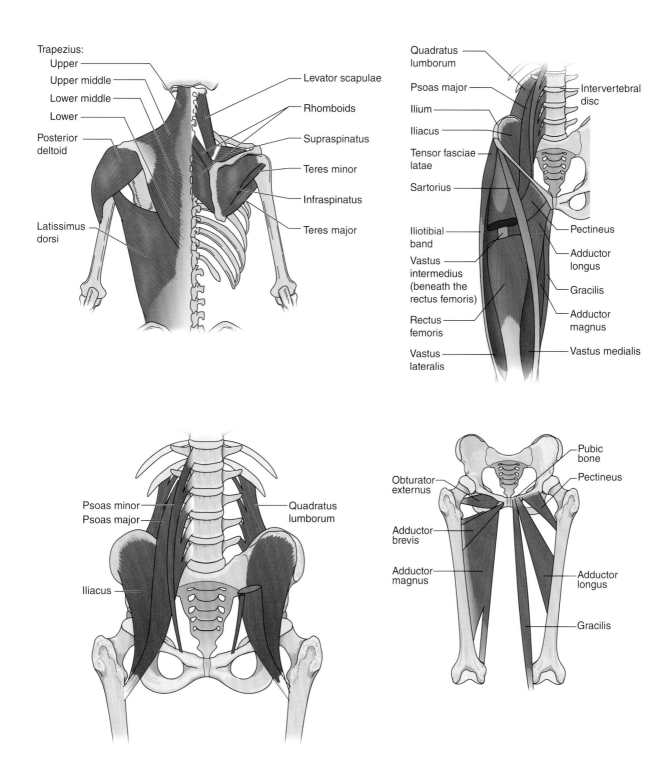

Figure 4.2 The muscles that work together to control movement of the spine, hip, thigh, and knee.

What the Science Says:
Benefits of Strength Training Throughout the Aging Process

Age-related reductions in muscle mass as well as the concurrent loss of force output can significantly impair the functional strength required for essential ADLs. Strength training exercises performed to a point of momentary fatigue can activate type II muscle motor units; if they are not regularly engaged through progressively challenging strength training exercises, it could result in a loss of muscle mass. In addition, age-related changes in hormone levels resulting in an imbalance between the anabolic hormones necessary for growth and the catabolic hormones used for energy production has been associated with muscle atrophy and reduced force production (Taylor and Johnson 2008).

Atrophy is the loss of muscle size, which can happen to adults who do not perform any strength training exercises during the aging process; without regular strength training, adults can lose an average of 5 pounds (2.3 kg) of lean muscle per decade (Taylor and Johnson 2008). Strength training can provide numerous benefits, including an increase in lean muscle mass, increased production of the hormones that promote muscle growth, improved cardiovascular efficiency, elevated resting metabolism (meaning you'll burn more calories throughout the day even when not exercising), and the ability to participate in your favorite activities. Whether you are male or female, if you are interested in maintaining a healthy, active lifestyle with the ability to enjoy your favorite activities as you age, you should make strength training a key component of your exercise program. Strength training provides the necessary stimulus to engage and activate the type II motor units and fibers related to increasing muscle force production as well as increasing the production of the hormones required for muscle growth.

Exercises in Your Core Strength Workout

Core exercises don't need to be overly complicated; however, they do need to be based on the foundational movement patterns and use a number of different muscles, especially if your goals include the ability to do an efficient and effective workout in a limited amount of time. The more muscles and whole-body movements you use during a workout, the higher your oxygen consumption and the greater your caloric expenditure. Strength training exercises like kettlebell swings, dumbbell Romanian deadlifts, or kettlebell Turkish get-ups can be extremely effective for enhancing strength in all layers of abdominal muscles. Core muscles contain a combination of type I and type II fibers. Low-intensity, long-duration stabilization exercises activate type I fibers, while heavy resistance strength or power exercises stimulate the type II fibers.

McGill's work studying strongman competitors provides important insights into how core muscles and the spine adapt to three-dimensional forces and the need to reflexively maintain spinal stability under many different loads (McGill, Karpowicz, and Fenwick 2009). Strongman competitions feature individual events requiring competitors to carry heavy loads, which can help develop the strength necessary to move the body and maintain dynamic balance while handling a variety of external forces. Because they compete in standing positions to move, lift, carry, and throw heavy weights, strongman athletes develop substantial core strength because the multiple layers of muscle reflexively co-contract to create the stiffness necessary to prevent the spine from buckling (McGill, Karpowicz, and Fenwick 2009b). McGill's work suggests that a successful core conditioning program can include exercises adapted from strongman competitions such as the one-arm overhead press, windmill, and carries to generate three-dimensional strength around the spine and pelvis (McGill and Marshall 2012).

The examples below demonstrate how movement patterns can become the foundation of an exercise program to enhance core strength while improving overall coordination and skill.

Hip-Dominant Movements

There is one thing that most top athletes and dancers have in common: a well-shaped behind. The reason is that the hips are one of the most mobile joints in the body, and the gluteus maximus muscles that control that mobility are responsible for generating strength and power, which is then used by all other segments in the body. Exercises that engage the muscle mass around the hip will develop functional strength of, shape, and sculpt this highly visible muscle and help burn more calories during the workout. Examples include glute bridges, squats, deadlifts, Romanian deadlifts, and swings.

Single-Leg Movements

Single-leg balance exercises can be important for helping integrate abdominal function with the lower extremities because your core muscles play an important role in controlling the position of your body any time you balance on a single leg. Walking or running is the process of transitioning from one leg to the other; therefore, being strong and stable while balanced on a single leg is an important part of improving human movement performance. Examples include single-leg glute bridges, single-leg balance exercises, lunges, or split squats.

Plank, Push-Up, or One of the Many Variations

The body is organized into two primary segments, upper and lower, which are connected via the spine and trunk muscles. Planks and their many variations are an important exercise for creating stability in the muscles around the spine that link the upper and lower body. The fascinating thing is that the core muscles that connect the upper and lower bodies act as a corset. If they get stronger, they can actually help your stomach become flatter. When doing a plank, it's important to keep the hips and shoulders at the same height so the spine is in a relatively neutral position. Once you master the basic plank (holding it for 45 seconds or longer without dropping your hips), you can progress to one of the more challenging variations, which can involve movement of the hips or shoulders while maintaining a stable spine. *Note*: A push-up can be considered a progressed version of the plank. When it comes to developing core strength, it is more important to do a good plank than a bad push-up.

Pulling Movements

If you're in the modern workforce, there is a good chance that you spend a portion of your day using a computer or mobile device. Whether we are sitting at a desk or using a tablet, we have a habit of slouching forward (cue: changing your posture to sit upright right now), which can cause our shoulders to internally rotate. Try this: Sit up nice and tall, and raise your right hand in front of your body as high as you can. Now slouch and try the same thing. When we slouch, we limit the space in our shoulder joint that allows easy, efficient overhead movements. Doing pulling exercises with a tall spine and a neutral (palms facing each other) or supinated (palms up) grip places the glenohumeral joint of the shoulder in an externally rotated position, helping alleviate pressure in the joint that occurs as a result of typing at a computer while sitting all day. Make sure to add one or two pulling movements to each workout. They're even better if they are in a standing position (e.g., bent-over dumbbell rows, or alternating arm resistance tubing pulls). Examples include bent-over rows, one-arm rows, pullovers, stability ball roll-outs, and band pulls.

Overhead Lifting and Pushing While Standing

Other than certain weight machines or seated dumbbell presses, how many times do you find yourself having to lift something over your head while in a seated position? Here's another question: How many times do you lift something overhead with your elbows out to the side (in the three and nine o'clock positions)? The shoulders are most effective during overhead movements when the elbows are pointed toward the front of the body (the eleven and one o'clock positions). This allows the cup of the shoulder blade to properly move and stabilize the ball of the humerus (upper arm bone) when your arm is moving overhead. Doing an overhead press while standing allows you to engage and use the muscles that connect your hips to your trunk. If you're seated, these muscles are not involved, and you lose the opportunity to burn a few extra calories. Whether it's a sandbag, dumbbells, kettlebells, or medicine balls, lifting something heavy overhead can help you develop strength from ground through hips and trunk and out through the upper extremities. Think of it as a standing plank using your shoulders and arms. Examples include standing dumbbell presses, standing kettlebell presses, windmills, and medicine ball lifts.

Rotational Movements

When walking or running, your shoulders rotate over your hips. Rotation is one of the foundational patterns of human movement, yet it is often overlooked in many traditional exercise programs. When you are in a standing position, your hip, abdominal, and upper-back muscles work together to create rotational movement. In fact, a rotational movement is part pulling and part pushing, making it a pattern that supports strength development in the other patterns. Examples include medicine ball chops, medicine ball twists, kettlebell windmills, and rotations with resistance tubing.

These six movement types should be the foundation of any effective exercise program to enhance the function and strength of core muscles. An additional benefit is that because they use a number of muscles at the same time, these movement-based exercises can be an effective way to burn calories while increasing strength. It may be tempting to change exercises frequently in an effort to avoid becoming bored. However, it is important to remain consistent with the exercises for a number of workouts so that the different systems of the body, specifically the CNS and muscular, learn how to execute the pattern as a reflex without any conscious effort.

The following workouts provide examples of how to organize these movement patterns into time-efficient exercise programs that can help you improve coordination, movement skill, and, most importantly, strength of the muscles responsible for stabilizing and moving your body.

Core Strength Training Workouts

The primary purpose of core strength training is to improve your muscles' ability to produce and distribute force throughout the entire body. As mentioned, gait is the default pattern of human movement. During the gait cycle, your shoulders and hips counterrotate to generate the force and momentum to move you forward. Therefore, the most effective strength training for core muscles involves working in a standing position where you use both your hips and shoulders at the same time. Many of these core exercises are essentially traditional strength training exercises, but when done with the right intention from a standing position they can help develop the integrated strength of all of the muscles that both stabilize and move the core.

To increase the overall energy expenditure (the amount of calories burned), these workouts are designed to be performed as circuits, where you move from one exercise to the next with minimal rest time between each exercise. Rest for 90 seconds to 2 minutes once all exercises are completed. The exercises should be performed at a steady tempo of one to three seconds in each direction. Going slower during the muscle lengthening phase (when muscles are stretching) is a technique that can increase the number of motor units activated.

When starting a new workout program, the exercises should seem challenging but not cause any pain or discomfort. The starting range of repetitions is a total of 8 to 10, 4 to 5 on each arm or leg. As you feel yourself getting stronger, add 2 reps every week until you are doing a total of 20 reps for each exercise (10 on each arm). *Note*: if 20 reps becomes easy, then you will be developing endurance, the ability to maintain a consistent amount of force, as opposed to strength, which is the ability to generate a greater amount of force, and it will be time to use heavier weights or change the piece of equipment to place a new challenge on the body. Start with two complete circuits of each workout. Once you can complete the two circuits relatively easily, add a third circuit. Once three circuits feels relatively easy, or if you have the time, add a fourth, then possibly a fifth circuit. The goal is to get to a point where you are doing each exercise for at least 10 reps for each arm or leg (20 total for the exercise) 4 times through the circuit. It should take about 10 to 12 weeks to progress from starting a workout to reaching the point where you are completing multiple circuits of at least 20 reps (total) for each exercise. Once that has occurred, it will be time to either change the equipment or the workout, for example, switching from bodyweight to a sandbag or transition from doing core training to metabolic conditioning. See chapter 5 for more discussion of how circuits can work in metabolic conditioning. For easier reference, flip to the blue-colored tabs on the sides of the pages to help you quickly identify the core-strength exercises in this book.

BODYWEIGHT EXERCISES FOR CORE STRENGTH

Using only your body weight can be an extremely effective strategy for strengthening your core muscles. The movement-based exercises should be performed at a steady pace under control in order to keep the muscles under tension; the isometric exercises should be held for the designated period of time to keep the muscles under tension. The great thing about bodyweight workouts is that they can be done anywhere, which makes them an excellent option if you travel a lot for work or your time is extremely limited and you need exercise solutions that fit a tight schedule.

Exercise	Sets	Repetitions
High plank	2	20 sec hold
Side plank	2	20 sec hold each side
Glute bridge	2	8-10
Single-leg balance with arm reaches	2	8-10 each side
Lateral lunge with trunk rotation	2	4-5 each side
Reverse lunge with overhead reach	2	4-5 each leg
Squats with forward reach	2	8-10
Perform this workout as a circuit with little-to-no rest between each exercise, rest for 90 seconds to 2 minutes after completing all exercises.		

High Plank

Benefits

Because the high plank position uses the arms in an extended position, both the shoulders and hips are integrated, making this exercise effective for strengthening many of the muscles that help stabilize the pelvis and spine.

Instructions

1. Start in a prone high plank (top of the push-up) position with your hands directly under your shoulders and your legs extended behind you, approximately hip-width apart.
2. Press your hands into the ground as you press your back up into your shoulder blades (this opposing motion will create the tension to activate more muscles) while squeezing the muscles in your thighs and glutes to maintain stability.
3. Breathe normally as you hold this position for at least 20 seconds; add 5 seconds per week until you reach 50 to 60 seconds.
4. Once you can hold a high plank for at least 50 seconds, you can increase the level of difficulty by raising a leg and pointing your toes. Hold for 3 to 4 seconds, alternating legs.

Correct Your Form

- If you notice your back or hips start to sag, it is time to end the exercise. It is much better to rest than to do a plank with poor form.
- As you get stronger, try to add 5 seconds every week; however, the longest you want to work up to is 50 to 60 seconds. Holding a plank any longer than that is not necessary.
- It's very important to relax and breathe normally during this exercise. If you hold your breath, your heart rate could unnecessarily increase.

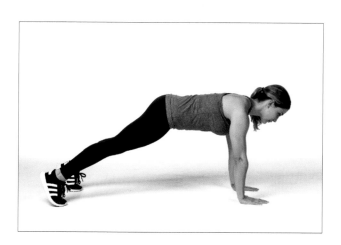

Side Plank

Benefits

This variation of the plank engages the muscles that provide lateral stability of your hips and spine, which is important for maintaining a tall posture and reducing the risk of injury in the lower back.

Instructions

1. Lie on your left side and place your left hand directly under the right shoulder so that your fingers are pointed up, away from your feet.
2. Stack your legs and feet on top of one another and squeeze your thighs together to help increase stability. Think about squeezing a coin between your legs.
3. While holding this position, push your left hand down and right hip up. This will create tension that activates the muscles that stabilize your pelvis and spine. Your trunk should be straight so that your right shoulder is stacked directly over your left.
4. Hold the position for at least 20 seconds or until you can no longer maintain a straight line between your hips and shoulder. Alternate sides before moving to the next exercise.
5. Add 5 seconds every week or so until you are able to hold this position for 50 to 60 seconds on each side.
6. Once you can hold this position for 50 seconds, you can increase the difficulty by lifting and holding the top leg for 2 to 3 seconds at a time.

Correct Your Form

- If fully extending your arm is uncomfortable, then bend your elbow and place it directly under your shoulder to reduce the leverage. Another option is to bend your knees so that your left elbow (directly under the left shoulder) and left knee (with both knees bent so your lower legs are behind you) are the points of contact with the ground.
- To increase stability, think about squeezing your hip and thigh muscles. This will help create stability through your entire core region.
- Having one side much stronger than the other could be a cause of low-back pain. If you notice that one side is stronger than the other, perform this exercise for the same amount of time on both sides to help correct the imbalance.

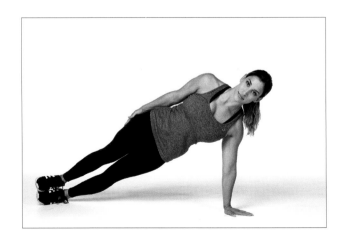

Glute Bridge

Benefits

Tight hip flexor muscles and weak glutes could be a cause of low-back pain. The gluteus maximus is the primary muscle responsible for extending the hips and moving the lower body; this exercise can help improve strength in the glute muscles while stretching the hip flexors. This exercise teaches the foundational movement pattern of hip flexion and extension in a position that is safe for the spine, allowing you to improve the strength of your glutes so you can perform other exercises like squats and lunges more effectively. If you spend a long time in a seated position, this exercise is an excellent dynamic stretch that can help reduce tightness and restore range of motion (ROM) in your hips. The more mobility you have in the hips, the better it is for your low back.

Instructions

1. Lie on your back so that your feet are flat on the floor with your knees pointed up to the ceiling. Your feet should be about 18 inches (46 cm) or so away from your glutes. Keep your arms along your side with your palms rotated up to face the ceiling, which helps stretch your shoulder muscles.
2. Pull your toes up toward your shins so that you are resting on the heels of both feet.
3. To perform the movement, press your heels down as you squeeze your glutes and lift your hips up toward the ceiling. (Think about squeezing a coin between your glute muscles to increase the muscle activation.). Push up for a count of 1 to 2 seconds and lower for a count of 3 to 4 seconds.
4. Start with 8 to 10 repetitions and add 2 reps per week until you are doing 20 reps at a time.

Correct Your Form

- If you notice your hamstring muscles (along the back of your thighs) cramping, simply move your feet forward a little bit.
- If you feel a little discomfort in your lower back, move your feet back toward your tailbone.
- Focus on squeezing your glutes to increase activity in those muscles and improve extensibility of the muscles along the front of your hips.

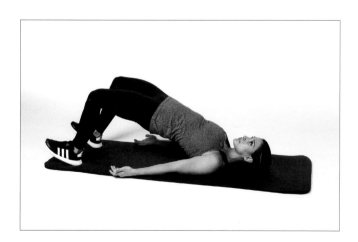

Single-Leg Balance With Arm Reach

Benefits

The muscles along the front of your core are designed to work best when standing in an upright position. This exercise stretches these muscles under resistance to help increase strength while your body is in the position in which it is designed to move. Lengthening muscle can help improve the strength by adding collagen fibers parallel to the muscle fibers, which could reduce the risk of injury from a strain or tear. If you've been stuck in a seated position for a long time, this exercise can also help strengthen the core muscles while stretching the hips to reduce lower-back tightness.

Instructions

1. Stand on your left foot and keep your right foot off the ground by bending your right knee. Hold your right arm directly overhead with your palm facing the midline of your body and your thumb pointing behind you. Hold your left arm directly out to your side at shoulder height.
2. Extend your right leg behind you. Think about pushing back through your heel, while moving both arms backwards; you should feel the pull along the front of your body.
3. Perform 8 to 10 reps, then switch sides. Add 2 reps per week until you are doing sets of 20 reps.

Correct Your Form

- If balancing on one leg is hard, place the toes of your lifted foot on the ground behind you like a kickstand. Keep most of the weight in your stance leg and focus on moving your arms for the exercise.
- To increase stability in the stance leg (the left leg in the instructions), press the foot into the ground while squeezing the glute muscle in the left leg.
- If you feel tightness in your lower back, work on keeping your spine straight while moving your arms and legs slowly in a limited ROM, moving your limbs too fast or too far could place strain on the lumbar spine, causing the soreness. As your arms and leg move behind you, they lengthen the fascia along the front of your core; and movements that lengthen the fascia can be an effective method of strengthening it.

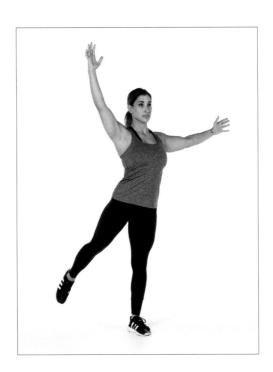

Lateral Lunge With Trunk Rotation

Benefits

Moving your shoulders over your hips is one of the most effective ways to lengthen and strengthen all of the muscles that connect the upper- and lower-body segments together.

Instructions

1. Begin in a standing position with your feet hip-width apart. Step your left foot directly to your left toward the three o'clock position. As your left foot hits the ground, make sure it is pointed straight ahead so that it is parallel to your right foot. As your left foot hits the ground, push your left hip back and maintain a long spine as you rotate to your left while keeping both arms extended in front of your body. (Think about turning your right shoulder to point toward the wall to your left.)

2. Rotate your trunk back to the center and push off the ground with the left foot to return to standing, then alternate to the right foot.

3. Perform a total of 8 to 10 lunges (4-5 on each leg). This places a lot of strain on the connective tissues between your hips and shoulders, so starting with a lower number of reps allows you to improve your strength without overstraining the muscles.

4. After the first 2 weeks, add 2 reps per week until you are doing 10 on each leg (20 total). At that point, if you want to gradually work up to doing 20 on each leg, go for it!

Correct Your Form

To reduce the strain on your knees, it is important that both feet are parallel when you plant your stepping foot on the ground. Keep the pressure on the outside foot (the left in the instructions); this will ensure the rotation comes from your thoracic spine and hips, the joints that are designed to rotate.

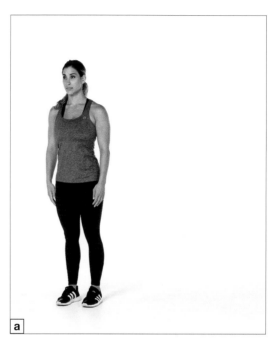

a

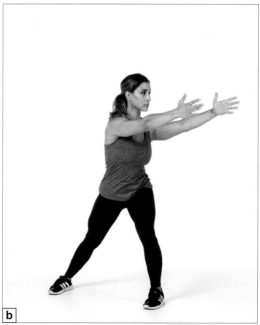

b

Reverse Lunge With Overhead Reach

Benefits

This exercise strengthens the abdominal and lower-body muscles from a standing position. Reaching overhead during a lunge lengthens the abdominal and hip muscles at the same time, which can help improve overall integration and coordination of how the muscles of the lower body and core work together.

Instructions

1. Stand with your feet hip-width apart and with both arms by your side. Step back with your left leg to lower yourself into a lunge while reaching overhead with both arms. Lower yourself to a comfortable depth while keeping your spine long.
2. Pause for a moment at the bottom, then press your right foot into the ground as you pull yourself back to standing while lowering both arms.
3. When you are back to the starting position, pause at the top, then repeat with the right leg.
4. Alternate legs for a total of 8 to 10 repetitions (4-5 on each leg). Once that becomes easy, add 2 reps every 2 weeks until you are doing 16 to 20 reps (8-10 on each leg). Once you can easily do 20 total, start adding more reps until you are able to do 15 to 20 repetitions on each leg.

Correct Your Form

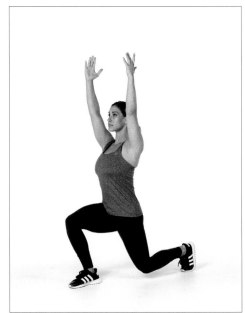

- If the knee of your planted leg (the right leg in the instructions) collapses toward the midline of your body, reduce the depth of the lunge and focus on pressing the front foot into the ground.
- The strength to return to standing should come from your front leg (the right leg in the instructions) as you press it into the ground.
- Like the previous exercise, this movement will use your muscles in ways they haven't worked before, which is why it is better to start with fewer reps and gradually add reps as you progress through the workout.

Squat With Forward Reach

Benefits

Squats can help strengthen all of the muscles in the lower body; reaching forward during a squat can increase hip flexion to enhance activation of the hip extensor muscles (the gluteus maximus).

Instructions

1. Start with your feet approximately hip- to shoulder-width apart and parallel, with your toes facing forward (pointed in the twelve o'clock position). Hang your hands along the sides of your body with the palms facing inwards.
2. Keep your spine long, and lower into the squat by pushing your hips back as though you are sitting in a chair. As you lower yourself, raise both arms in front of you to about chest height and reach in front of your body. This increases the length of the muscles along the entire backside of your body.
3. At the bottom of the squat, both arms should be reaching out front. As you return to standing, bring your hands back down by your side.
4. Start with 8 to 10 reps, and add 2 reps every 2 weeks until you can do 20 reps. Rest for 30 to 45 seconds after each set. Start with 2 sets, and once you feel comfortable, gradually progress to doing 4 sets.

Correct Your Form

- Emphasize pushing your hips back before your knees move forward to ensure that your hips are doing most of the work. If your knees move forward before your hips move backwards, it could create strain on the front of the knees and be a potential cause of pain.
- If you feel your heels coming off of the ground, don't go so low. Only lower your hips part way and keep your focus on pushing both feet into the ground.
- If you feel your knees collapsing inward, externally rotate your feet toward the outside of the body so your feet are pointed in the eleven and one o'clock positions).

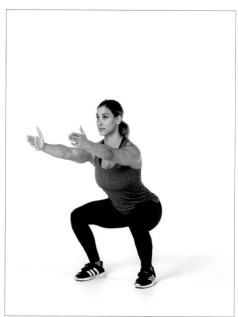

STABILITY BALL EXERCISES FOR CORE STRENGTH

Exercising on an unstable surface could help increase the number of muscles used for a particular movement because the body has to create the stability that the surface lacks. The stability ball creates an unstable surface so muscles have to work harder to maintain control of any specific exercise. In addition, in many exercises the ball creates a fulcrum for the body to move as a lever; changing the position of the ball can increase the challenge and level of difficulty of a particular exercise. Please note that for a number of years, fitness professionals have advocated using stability balls instead of a bench for certain weightlifting exercises such as chest presses or pullovers. However, now the manufacturers and distributors of stability balls warn users to not lift weights on the stability balls for safety reasons. Stability balls are still an extremely effective tool for bodyweight exercises because they can create a number of unique challenges that strengthen both the contractile and elastic components of muscle tissue.

When selecting a stability ball, use a 55-centimeter ball if you're 5' 7" or shorter. Select a 65-centimeter ball if you're between 5' 7" and 6' 4". Select a 75-centimeter ball if you're taller than 6' 4". The ball should be inflated until it's firm and you can sit on it so your knees and hips can comfortably hold a 90-degree bend.

Exercise	Sets	Repetitions
Hip bridge to hamstring curl	2	6-8
Stir-the-pot	2	5-6 each direction
Supine hip rotation	2	4-5 each side
Pike	2	6-8
Russian twist	2	3-4 each side
Hip roll to knee tuck	2	3-4 each side
One-leg squat	2	4-6 each side
Crunch	2	6-8
Perform this workout as a circuit with little-to-no rest between each exercise, rest for 90 seconds to 2 minutes after completing all exercises.		

Hip Bridge to Hamstring Curl

Benefits

This exercise strengthens the muscles along the back of the body responsible for extending the hips and controlling stability of the spine in a safe position that is not directly affected by the downward pull of gravity.

Instructions

1. Start by lying flat on your back with your arms by your side and your heels on top of the ball with your toes pulled up toward your shins. Squeeze your glutes and lift your hips in the air. Press both arms into the ground to create stability.

2. Once your body is in a straight line, pull your heels up to your tailbone, bringing the ball closer to your body. Slowly extend your legs back to a straight position before slowly lowering your hips to the ground.

3. As you learn the exercise it should be a single, fluid motion to raise the hips up as you bring your heels toward your tailbone. Start with 6 to 8 reps, and add 2 reps every 2 weeks until you reach a total of 16 to 20 reps.

Correct Your Form

- If you feel your calves tightening and cramping up, make sure you are pulling your toes up to your shins. This increases the length of your calf muscles, reducing the risk that they become overtight during the exercise.

- If you feel a strain in your lower back, move the starting position of the ball closer to your body so the backs of your calves, instead of the heels, are resting on the top of the ball.

- To increase stability with your hips off the ground, place your arms wider and keep them pressed into the ground.

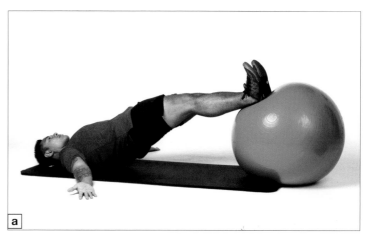

a

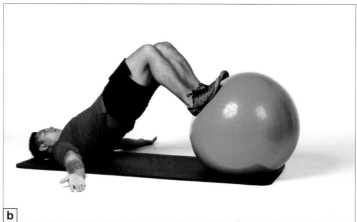

b

Stir-the-Pot

Benefits

This unique exercise is essentially a plank on an unstable surface; maintaining stability on the ball requires the deep abdominal and hip muscles to work together to create and control stability of the core region.

Instructions

1. Place your elbows on the top of the stability ball with both hands clasped together.
2. Keep your feet about shoulder-width apart and squeeze your glute and thigh muscles as you move into a position where your toes are on the ground and your elbows are on top of the ball. Keep your hip and thigh muscles squeezed to maintain stability throughout the exercise.
3. While holding this position use your elbows to move the ball counterclockwise for 5 to 6 circles, then create circles in the opposite direction for a total of 10 to 12 circles.
4. Add only 1 or 2 reps every 2 weeks until you can easily do 18 to 20 reps in each direction.

Correct Your Form

- If you have a hard time maintaining a straight body during the exercise, you can reduce the lever arm by dropping to your knees. Once you can do 12 to 14 circles in each direction, you can move back to the fully extended position.
- The wider you have your feet as you hold the plank, the more stability you will have. If you want to make the exercise harder, you can move your feet and legs closer together to create a narrower base of support.

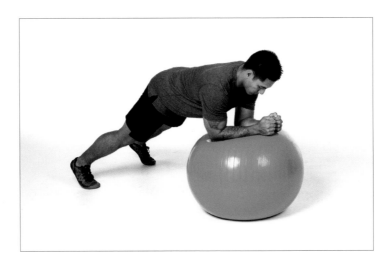

Supine Hip Rotation

Benefits

The obliques (both external and internal) work together to create rotation through the trunk and hips. The right-side external obliques work with the left-side internal obliques to rotate your trunk to your left, and the left-side external obliques work with the right-side internal obliques to rotate your trunk to the right. The ball creates a unique fulcrum for rotation that causes both sides of the obliques to work together like they do when you walk or run.

Instructions

1. Start by lying flat on your back with your arms out by your side and the backs of your lower legs on top of the ball with your toes pointed straight up into the air. Squeeze the ball into the back of your glutes and press both arms into the ground to create stability, keeping your hands wide.
2. Rotate your hips and drop both legs to your left while keeping your shoulders on the ground and your arms pressed down, allow your legs to drop as far as they can to your left before rolling your knees back over to your right side.
3. Perform 4 to 5 rotations in each direction for a total of 8 to 10 repetitions.
4. Once you can control movement during this exercise, add 2 reps every 2 weeks until you can perform 8 to 10 reps in each direction for a total of 16 to 20.

Correct Your Form

Keeping the ball closer to your tailbone so the backs of your calves are on top of the ball gives you more control of the movement. To ensure that the rotation comes from the thoracic spine, keep your shoulders, upper back, and arms pressed solidly into the ground.

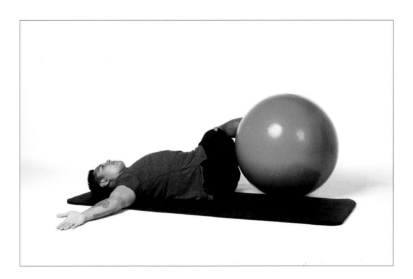

Pike

Benefits

This move strengthens all of the abdominal muscles along the front of the body in addition to your chest, shoulder, and upper-arm muscles, making it an excellent option for improving strength. Because you will be using so many muscles, you will also be burning more calories.

Instructions

1. Start facing the stability ball so that your chest is on the top of the ball. Walk forward with your hands until the tops of your thighs are on the ball.
2. Keep your hands directly under the shoulders, with your elbows rotated back toward your feet, and keep your hands pressed into the floor throughout the exercise for stability.
3. With your thighs on top of the ball, lift your tailbone up in the air so the ball rolls along the front of your legs. Pause for a moment at the top before allowing your legs to slowly lower back to the starting position.
4. To increase the level of difficulty, roll the ball all the way until the tips of your toes are on the top of the ball. Begin with 6 to 8 repetitions. Once you have control, add 2 repetitions a week until you are able to do 16 to 20 repetitions in a row.

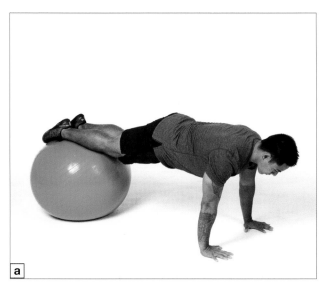

Correct Your Form

- At the start and end of this exercise, your body should be a straight line from the shoulders through the ankles. If your hips drop, start with the ball closer to your waist to shorten the lever arm.
- Throughout the movement, think about holding a coin between your thighs. This will help create stability in your legs through the entire ROM.
- If you find that the position bothers your wrists, you can use dumbbells to hold on to for handles, which can reduce the stress on your wrists.

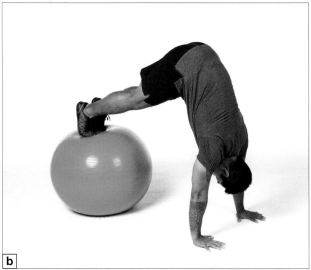

Russian Twist

Benefits

This rotational exercise strengthens the muscles between your trunk and hips, helping to improve strength and coordination between your upper and lower body.

Instructions

1. Start in a seated position on the top of the ball. Slowly walk forward, allowing your back to roll down on the top of the ball until the widest part of your back (between your shoulders) is directly on top of the ball.

2. Clasp the fingers of both hands directly over the top of your chest and press your hands together. Move your shoulders by dropping your hands to the left and lifting the right shoulder so that you roll on to your left shoulder. As you do this with your upper body, push your left foot into the ground and right hip into the air to create stability.

3. Pause on your left shoulder before roll-ing your back over the top of the ball to move over to your right shoulder. As you move to your right shoulder, pick up your left shoulder and allow the top of your right arm to roll on to the ball. Again, push your right foot into the ground and left hip into the air to enhance stability.

4. Start with 3 to 4 reps on each side, for a total of 6 to 8. Once you can do those with control, start adding 2 reps every week until you can do 8 to 10 reps on each side, for a total of 16 to 20.

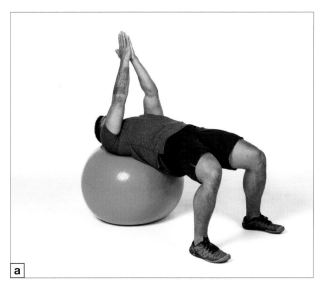

Correct Your Form

- This is a challenging exercise that requires a lot of control from your hips and lower body. Pressing your feet into the ground and squeezing your glute muscles throughout the entire move-ment will help create stability and allow you to rotate your upper body with more control.

- Keeping your arms straight with both hands pressed together will create more stability through your upper body, allow-ing it to roll over the top of the ball.

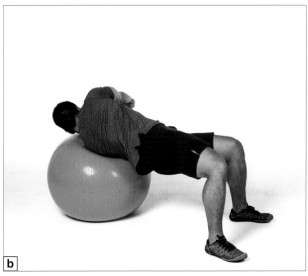

Hip Roll to Knee Tuck

Benefits

Pressing your hands into the ground while rotating your hips over the top of the ball helps enhance the strength of your shoulders and the muscles responsible for rotating your trunk, making it an effective exercise for strengthening both your internal and external obliques at the same time.

Instructions

1. Start by facing the stability ball so that your chest is on the top of the ball. Walk forward with your hands until the tops of your thighs are on the ball. Keep your hands directly under the shoulders, with your elbows rotated back toward your feet, and keep your hands pressed into the floor throughout the exercise for stability.

2. With your thighs on top of the ball, squeeze your legs together as though you are holding a coin in between them. To start the movement, press your hands into the ground while lifting your right hip so that the side of your left hip rolls on to the top of the ball.

3. Once the side of your left leg is on the ball, keep your legs squeezed together and pull both knees closer to your waist, pause for 2-4 seconds then extend the legs, and roll to the other side. Pick up your left hip as your right side rolls on to the top of the ball. When your right side is on top of the ball, bring both knees to your waist, then straighten the legs and return to the starting position with the tops of both legs on the ball.

4. Start by alternating between 3 to 4 reps on each side, for a total of 6 to 8. As you get stronger, add 2 reps per week until you are able to do 8 to 10 repetitions on each side, for a total of 16 to 20.

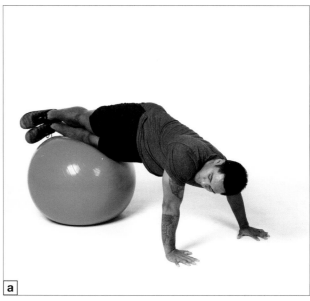

a

Correct Your Form

- This is a challenging exercise but one that is great for developing core strength. When on the side of your left leg, think about lifting your right hip into the air, and vice versa.

- Pressing your hands into the ground and squeezing your legs together can enhance stability, which is essential throughout this exercise.

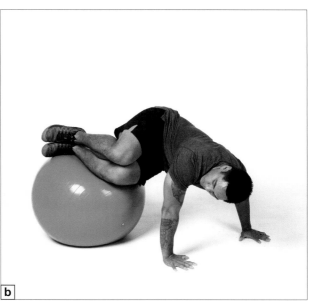

b

One-Leg Squat

Benefits

This balance-based move strengthens the muscles in the front leg while stretching the hip muscles of the leg that is on top of the ball. Balancing on one leg can help engage the muscles of the deep core to enhance stability of the pelvis and spine.

Instructions

1. Start standing with the ball directly behind you. Pick up your left leg and place the top of your left foot and lower leg directly on top of the ball. Press your left shin and foot into the top of the ball and lower yourself into your right hip while extending your left leg directly behind you to perform a lunge. Keep your right foot pressed into the ground to help create stability during the movement.
2. During the movement keep your spine long so that your hips are doing the work. Start with 4 to 6 reps on each leg. Once you can do that with control, add 2 reps every week until you can do 10 to 12 reps on each leg.

Correct Your Form

- If balancing with one leg on the ball is a challenge, do this exercise next to a wall so you can use it to help maintain balance. The side of your body with the leg on top of the ball should be next to the wall (the left side in the instructions).
- When learning the exercise, don't worry about going down too low. Instead, focus on maintaining balance while extending the leg on top of the ball. As your balance improves, slowly start lowering yourself into your right hip.

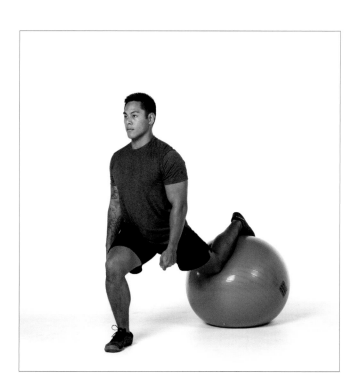

Crunch

Benefits

Even though the natural function of the abdominals is to control movement of the pelvis and rib cage when standing, doing crunches uses the ab muscles in a way that *can* help improve definition. Crunches on the top of the ball allow you to achieve full extension of the spine, which is not possible when lying on the floor. This helps strengthen the muscles *all* the way through the ROM.

Instructions

1. Sit on the top of the ball, then slowly walk both feet forward until your rear end is hanging off the ball and the curve of your low back is resting on the curve of the ball.

2. Press both feet into the ground and place the backs of the fingers of both hands on the front of your forehead (keeping the hands on the front of your head will reduce the temptation to pull your head forward, which could strain your neck). *Note*: as your ab muscles get stronger, you can move your arms further from your waist to increase the lever length, which can add resistance. The core muscles respond to resistance; therefore, increasing resistance could improve strength and definition of the ab muscles.

3. Exhale as you slowly roll your spine off the top of the ball. Think about pulling the bottom of your rib cage to the top of your pelvis. Pause at the top before slowly lowering back to the starting position.

4. Start with 6 to 8 reps. Once you can do them under control, add 2 reps per week. Once you can do 12 to 14 reps under control, change the position of your arms from the front of your chest to the top of the head, then to extended completely overhead.

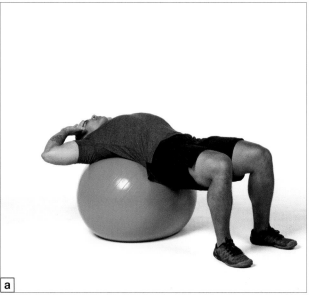

a

Correct Your Form

- It is not necessary to do a high number of repetitions. If you want to work harder, change the length of the lever by changing the position of your arms and hands.

- This exercise is for your ab muscles, *not* your neck. Your head should remain in a neutral, stable position throughout the ROM. Think about squeezing an egg between your chin and throat to maintain a stable position.

- If you feel your neck becoming sore, press your tongue into the roof of your mouth to activate the muscles that stabilize your neck.

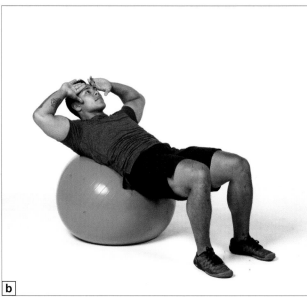

b

MEDICINE BALL EXERCISES FOR CORE STRENGTH

Moving a weight through gravity while standing in an upright position challenges a number of muscles to work together to generate the forces that create and control those movements; this is one of the greatest benefits of using a medicine ball for core strength training. You can use a medicine ball to perform pushing and pulling movement for upper-body muscles, rotational movements where your hips and shoulders counterrotate to involve a majority of your core muscles, and hinging, squatting, and lunging movements to strengthen lower-body muscles.

Exercise	Sets	Repetitions
Hip bridge with pullover	2	8-10
Romanian deadlift	2	6-8
Standing rotation	2	5-6 each direction
Vertical chop	2	8-10
Diagonal low-to-high lift	2	6-8 each side
Reverse lunge to chop	2	4-6 each leg
Transverse plane lunge with lift	2	4-6 each side
Perform this workout as a circuit with little-to-no rest between each exercise, rest for 90 seconds to 2 minutes after completing all exercises.		

Hip Bridge With Pullover

Benefits

This move will strengthen the muscles responsible for controlling extension of the hips and spine from the glutes to the upper back and shoulders.

Instructions

1. Lie face-up on the floor with your knees bent and feet flat on the floor. Hold a medicine ball between both hands with your arms extended directly over your head so they are resting on the ground.
2. Pull your toes up toward your shins, and push your heels into the floor. Squeeze your glutes and push your hips up toward the ceiling. As you hold your hips in the up position during the exercise, your upper back and shoulders should remain on the floor.
3. While holding your hips in the air, lift your arms up until the medicine ball is directly over your chest. Pause, then slowly lower the medicine ball back to the floor.
4. Start with 8 to 10 reps. Once 10 is relatively easy, add 2 reps a week until you can do 18 to 20 reps in a row.

Correct Your Form

If the hamstring muscles along the backs of your legs start tightening or cramping up, move your heels a little further away from your tailbone.

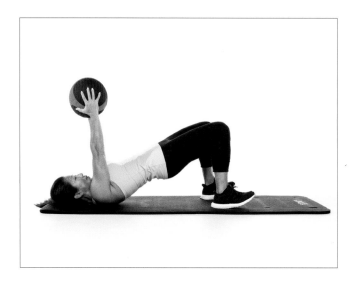

Romanian Deadlift

Benefits

This exercise strengthens the muscles responsible for extending the hips and spine. Doing so from a standing position helps the body become stronger against the downward pull of gravity.

Instructions

1. Stand with your feet hip-width apart and your knees slightly bent. Hold the medicine ball between both hands directly in front of your hips. Keep your spine long, and push your hips back in a hinging motion as you lower your upper body toward the floor.
2. Pause briefly at the end ROM. To return to standing, press your feet into the floor as you push your hips forward and lift your upper body back to a full standing position.
3. Begin with 6 to 8 reps. Once that becomes easy, add 2 reps a week until you can do a total of 18 to 20.

Correct Your Form

- Keep your spine long and straight during this movement and focus on moving from your hip; the motion for this exercise should come from your hips, not your lower back.
- Think about pushing your tailbone toward the wall behind you as you lower yourself. As you return to standing, focus on pressing your hips toward the wall in front of you.

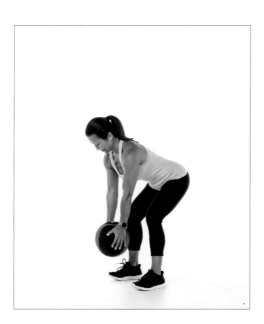

Standing Rotation

Benefits

This exercise strengthens the muscles of the hips, core, and upper shoulders by using all of them together during this movement.

Instructions

1. Stand with your feet hip-width apart and your knees slightly bent. Hold the medicine ball between both hands directly in front of your chest. Keep your spine long as you push your left foot into the floor to rotate to your right. As you turn your hips and shoulders to the right, keep your right foot pressed firmly into the ground as you rotate your left foot toward the midline of your body.
2. At the end ROM, quickly push your right foot into the floor and rotate to your left as you turn your shoulders and hips to face to your left. The goal is to move quickly from side to side by turning the feet and the hips.
3. Perform 5 to 6 rotations on each side, for a total of 10 to 12. Once you can do that under control, add 2 reps—one to each side—per week until you are doing a total of 9 to 10 on each side, for a total of 18 to 20.

Correct Your Form

- Rotation comes from your feet and hips, so to perform this movement correctly—and to protect your knees and spine—focus on turning your feet and hips quickly during this exercise.
- Your feet should rotate on the ground like you're putting out a cigarette (that someone else left burning).
- Your spine should remain long and straight as you move your feet, hips, and shoulders.

> **TIP** To increase the intensity of this exercise, extend your arms forward so the medicine ball is farther away from your center of gravity.

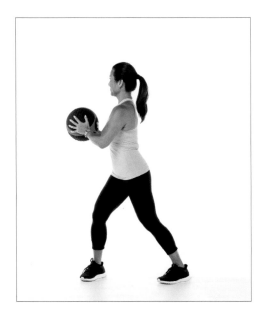

Vertical Chop

Benefits

This exercise uses the resistance of the medicine ball when the arms are fully extended to lengthen the abdominal muscles, which can be the most effective way to strengthen the muscles while improving coordination between the hips and shoulders. In addition, because you are doing a squat during the movement, you will be using the muscles of the thighs and glutes, which makes this effective for strengthening most of the muscles in your lower body.

Instructions

1. Stand with your feet shoulder-width apart and your knees slightly bent. Hold the medicine ball between both hands directly in front of your waist. Keep your spine long as you push your hips back to lower into a squat. Keep your arms straight so the medicine ball comes down between your knees; this should be the lowest part of the squat.

2. To return to standing, press your feet into the ground and your hips forward as you swing your arms directly overhead, keeping your elbows straight.

3. At the top position your arms should be directly overhead so you feel your abdominal muscles lengthened. Start with 8 to 10 repetitions. As you get stronger, add 2 repetitions per week until you can do 20 repetitions straight.

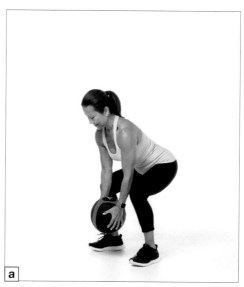

a

Correct Your Form

- When doing a squat, it is important that the first movement be from your hips as they move backward. It doesn't matter how deep you squat as long as you are moving from the hips first.

- When standing up from the bottom of the squat, pressing your feet into the ground activates most of the muscles in your legs and hips.

- Keep your spine long during the movement to ensure the hips can do their job.

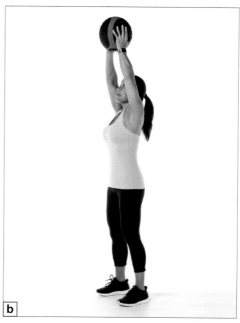

b

Diagonal Low-to-High Lift

Benefits

This exercise creates coordinated movement between your hips and shoulders, which is how they are designed to function during the gait cycle. The diagonal pattern of the medicine ball places a majority of the force from the exercise into the oblique muscles (both internal and external), which connect your pelvis to rib cage in a similar diagonal fashion.

Instructions

1. Stand with your feet shoulder-width apart, your knees slightly bent, and your right foot slightly in front of your left. The heel of the right foot should be even with the toes of the left.

2. Hold the medicine ball between both hands by your left hip. Keep your spine long and push your hips back so you sink into a quarter-squat with most of your weight in the left hip.

3. Push your left foot into the ground as you raise the medicine ball across the front of your body toward your right shoulder. As the medicine ball passes the midline of your body, allow your left foot to rotate (like putting out a cigarette someone left on the ground) and shift your weight into your right hip.

4. The medicine ball should end up over your right shoulder. As you bring it down in the same diagonal line, allow your left foot to rotate back so it points straight ahead, and sink back into both hips as the ball returns to your left hip.

5. Start with 6 to 8 reps moving from left hip to right shoulder, then switch sides for a total of 12 to 16 reps. As you get stronger add 2 reps per week until you can do 16 to 20 reps on each side.

Correct Your Form

- The rotation comes from your hips and feet, not your spine, which should stay long and straight through the duration of this movement.

- When rotating the foot as you lift the medicine ball (the left foot in the above example) think about pushing it into the ground as you shift your weight to the right—when the ball is at the end of the movement over your right shoulder, most of your weight should be on the right leg.

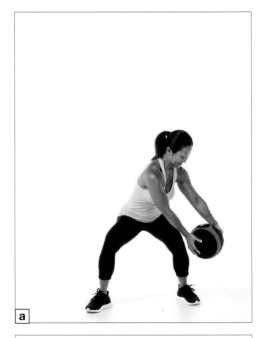

a

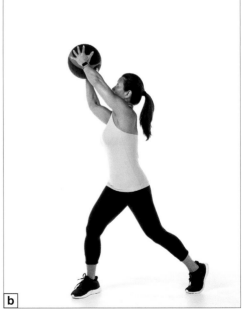

b

Reverse Lunge to Chop
(Over Forward Leg)

Benefits

This exercise strengthens the muscles that stabilize the spine while strengthening the muscles that control movement of the hips, shoulders, and upper back.

Instructions

1. Stand with your feet hip-width apart and hold a medicine ball in both hands directly in front of your chest. Keep your left foot planted on the ground as you step back with the right foot, placing the toes of the right foot on the ground.
2. Lower your right knee toward the ground (do not let it hit the ground) to sink into your left hip, and bring the medicine ball down to the left side of your left thigh, which should be almost parallel to the ground.
3. Press your left foot into the ground to pull yourself back to standing as you raise the medicine ball back to the front of your chest.
4. Perform 4 to 6 reps on the left hip, then switch legs for a total of 8 to 10 repetitions. As you get stronger, add 2 reps per week until you can do 16 to 20 reps on each side.

Correct Your Form

- Keep your spine long and straight during the lunge. As you bring the medicine ball across the front of your body, you can hinge forward at the hip, but do not allow the spine to bend.
- When returning to standing from the bottom of the lunge, press your foot into the ground to pull yourself forward using the muscles in the back of your leg.

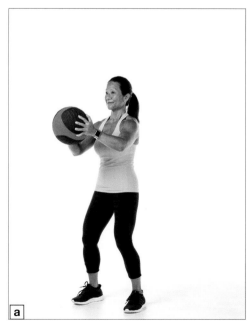

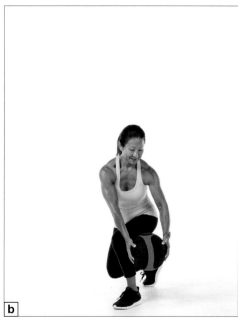

Transverse Plane Lunge With Lift

Benefits

Rotation is one of the most important movements the hips are designed to perform—specifically, the rotation of the pelvis over the thigh bone (femur) when the foot is fixed on the ground, and the rotation of the femur under the pelvis as the feet are rotating during a movement. Rotational lunges take a hip through a full ROM to strengthen the muscles that control the movement as well as the bones and joint capsule where the movement occurs. Lifting a weight overhead at the end range of the transverse plane lunge lengthens the tissues along the front of the body, helping strengthen these core muscles while at the same time improving strength and mobility of the hips. This exercise could be challenging to learn and could cause some soreness because the muscles will be working in new and different ways, but it is so effective that it will soon be one of the exercises you like to dislike.

Instructions

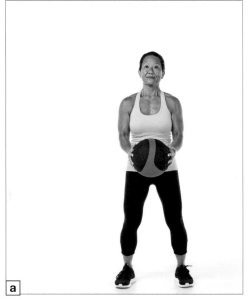

1. Stand with your feet hip-width apart and hold a medicine ball in front of your waist with both hands. Keep your left foot pressed into the ground as you step back with your right foot, and turn to your right so you place your foot on the ground, pointing in the three or four o'clock position.

2. When your right foot is planted on the ground, keep your spine long as you raise the medicine ball directly overhead. Pause for a moment at the top before lowering the medicine ball back to your waist.

3. To return to the starting position, push off with your right foot while pressing your left foot into the ground to use the inner thigh muscles to bring your body back to the starting position.

4. Perform 4 to 6 reps on the right hip, then switch legs for a total of 8 to 10 repetitions. As you get stronger, add 2 reps per week until you can do 16 to 20 repetitions on each side.

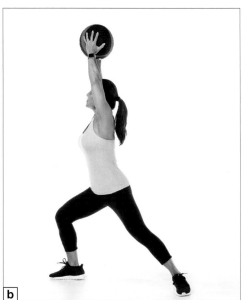

Correct Your Form

• While stepping back and to the right with the right leg, squeeze the muscles of your left thigh and keep your left foot pressed into the ground to help stabilize and protect the left knee. Most of the movement should come from your left hip joint.

• Keep your spine long so that as you step back and plant your foot on the ground (the right in the instructions) you have the ability to raise the medicine ball directly over your head without any restrictions.

SANDBAG EXERCISES FOR CORE STRENGTH

Controlling the movement of a weight through gravity while standing in an upright position challenges a number of muscles to work together to create and control the movements, which is one of the greatest benefits of using a small, handheld sandbag for core strength training. Like a medicine ball, you can use a sandbag to perform pushing and pulling movements, rotational movements, and hinging, squatting, and lunging movements. A significant difference between a medicine ball and a sandbag is that the softer, more pliable surface of a sandbag allows for an easier way to grip the weight because your hands can squeeze the surface while moving the weight, helping to improve grip strength.

Exercise	Sets	Repetitions
One-leg hip bridge	2	6-8 each leg
V-sit with press	2	6-8
Reverse lunge with rotation (over forward leg)	2	5-6 each leg
Single leg Romanian deadlift	2	5-6 each leg
One-arm bent-over row	2	6-8 each arm
Lateral lunge with forward press	2	5-6 each leg
Transverse plane lunge reach to ground with overhead press	2	5-6 each leg
Perform this workout as a circuit with little-to-no rest between each exercise, rest for 90 seconds to 2 minutes after completing all exercises.		

One-Leg Hip Bridge

Benefits

Strengthening the muscles responsible for extending the hip on one leg at a time in this position can help improve strength for standing one-leg exercises such as lunges, single-leg Romanian deadlifts, and single-leg squats. The cyclic action of one hip flexing while the other extends is also effective for improving ROM of the joint during extension exercises.

Instructions

1. Lie flat on your back with your left leg extended and right leg bent so the heel is on the floor. Pull the toes of the right foot up toward the shin.
2. Place the sandbag on top of the right hip, and keep your left leg along the floor. Keep your upper back flat along the floor as you push your right heel into the ground while pressing your right hip up toward the ceiling and pulling your left knee toward your chest (your left knee should be moving up toward your chest as you press your right foot down to extend the hip).
3. Pause at the top of the movement before lowering yourself back down with the right hip.
4. Perform 6 to 8 reps with the right hip, then switch legs, for a total of 12 to 16 reps. As you get stronger, add 2 reps per week until you can do 16 to 20 reps on each side.

Correct Your Form

- To increase activation of the glute muscles that extend the hip, focus on pushing your heel into the ground and hip up to the ceiling as you lift your hip off the ground.
- When placing your heel on the ground, it should be approximately 18 inches (46 cm) from your hip. Too far and you could use more of your back muscles; too close and it could cause cramping in the hamstrings.
- It may be necessary to hold the sandbag on your hip. For example, use your right hand when using the right hip.
- Keeping the toes pulled up toward the shin will help improve strength of the muscles along the front of the lower leg while stretching the muscles on the back of the lower leg.

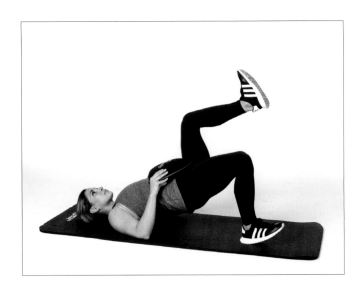

V-Sit With Press

Benefits

This exercise coordinates muscle actions between the shoulders and hips while strengthening the muscles responsible for stabilizing the spine to help improve posture.

Instructions

1. Start in a seated position with your feet in front of your hips so that your knees are bent. Keep your spine long and straight, and hold the sandbag in front of your chest.
2. Contract your abdominals by bracing your core muscles. (Think about getting punched in the stomach to contract all layers of muscle together.) Pick your feet up off the ground and balance on your tailbone while slowly pressing the sandbag away from the front of your body, hold at the end of the movement before slowly pulling it back to your chest—it should be 2-3 seconds in each direction.
3. Perform for 6 to 8 reps. As you get stronger, add 2 reps per week until you can do 16 to 20 reps.

Correct Your Form

- When starting, keep your feet close to your body. As you increase your strength and ability to hold the position, start straightening your legs away from your body.
- The purpose of pushing the sandbag in front of your body is to change the leverage and increase the workload on the muscles. If it is too challenging, keep the sandbag close to your body.

TIP To increase intensity, straighten your legs in front of your body to increase the lever arm, which adds resistance to strengthen the muscles while holding the position.

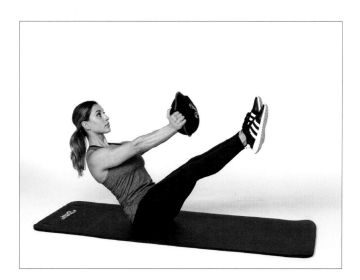

Reverse Lunge With Rotation
(Over Forward Leg)

Benefits

Your shoulders and hips counterrotate over one another as you walk and run. This exercise uses your muscles the same way to improve core strength in a standing position. This exercise helps improve the strength of the external and internal obliques as they work together to rotate the trunk. Lying on the ground to perform normal oblique crunches uses only the external obliques in the front of the body, creating a possible muscle imbalance.

Instructions

1. Stand with your feet approximately hip-width apart as you hold the sandbag directly in front of your chest with both hands.
2. Keep your elbows tucked next to your rib cage and your spine long as you step back with your right foot and sink into your left hip.
3. At the bottom of the movement, make sure not to let your right knee hit the ground, and keep your spine tall as you rotate to your left over your left leg. Return to center. To return to the starting position, press your left foot into the ground and swing your right leg forward.
4. Perform 5 to 6 reps with the left hip, stepping back with the right leg, then switch legs for a total of 10 to 12 reps. As you get stronger, add 2 reps per week until you can do 16 to 20 reps on each side.

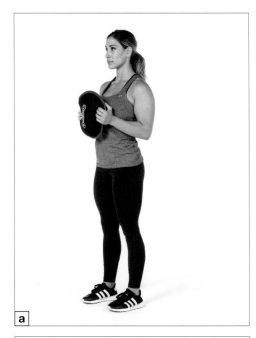

a

Correct Your Form

- Keep your front foot planted on the floor as you step back with your other leg. When stepping forward, press your foot into the ground and think about pulling from the back of your leg.
- Keep your spine long and straight as you rotate over the forward leg.

TIP To increase your strength, extend your arms in front of your body before making the rotation. The further the sandbag is from your body, the harder the muscles will have to work.

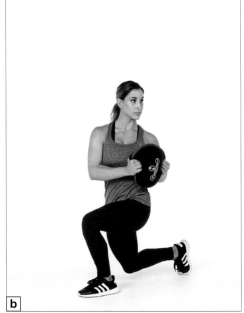

b

Single-Leg Romanian Deadlift

Benefits

Exercising on one leg can improve balance and coordination while also focusing all of the strength into the working muscles on the stance or balance leg. Exercising on one leg can engage a number of core muscles to maintain control of posture and balance during the movement.

Instructions

1. Stand with your feet hip-width apart, your spine lengthened, your right foot pressed firmly into the ground, and your left knee slightly bent so that the toes of your left foot are resting on the ground. Hold the sandbag in your left hand directly in front of your thigh.

2. Push your hips back as you begin to lift your left foot off the ground.

3. Keep your spine long as you straighten your left leg and point your left foot directly behind you.

4. Continue hinging forward from your hips to a comfortable distance. Allow the sandbag to lower to the floor in a straight line directly in front of your body. To return to standing, pull the bottom of your right pelvis down toward the back of your right thigh while swinging the left leg down toward the floor.

5. Perform 5 to 6 reps standing on the right leg, then switch legs for a total of 10 to 12 reps. As you get stronger, add 2 reps per week until you can do 16 to 20 reps on each side.

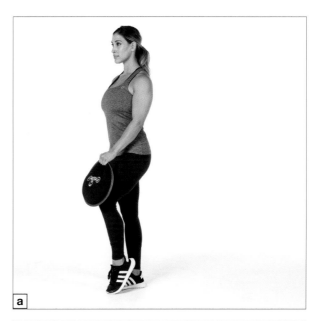

a

Correct Your Form

- When hinging forward on the right leg (as in the instructions), keep your left leg straight and point your toes. Straightening your left leg will help you control the hinge on your right.

- Keep your spine long and straight throughout the movement.

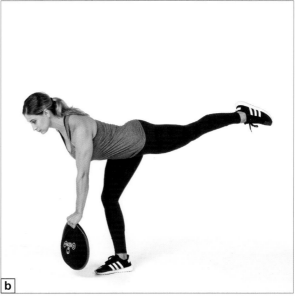

b

One-Arm Bent-Over Row

Benefits

Doing a one-arm row in a hinged position—without supporting yourself with the other arm—can recruit more of the deep stabilizer muscles that control your spine. This exercise will help integrate the strength of the muscles connecting the hips and upper back.

Instructions

1. Keep feet hip- to shoulder-width apart. Hold the sandbag in your left hand. Keep your spine long and straight as you hinge forward at your hips.
2. Stop at a point where you are leaning forward, and plant your feet into the ground for stability. Keep your right arm by your side; try not to use it to brace yourself.
3. Keep your left elbow close to your rib cage and pull the sandbag toward your waist, then slowly lower it to the starting position.
4. Perform 6 to 8 reps with the left arm, then switch arms for a total of 12 to 16 reps. As you get stronger, add 2 reps per week until you can do 16 to 20 repetitions on each side.

Correct Your Form

- Hold the sandbag with your hand, but as you pull it toward your body, think about pulling from your elbow. This will use more of your back muscles.
- Hinging forward without bracing yourself (the right arm in the instructions) will challenge you to use more deep muscles to help stabilize an unbalanced load in your spine.

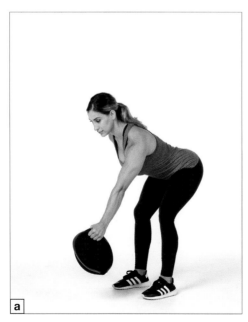
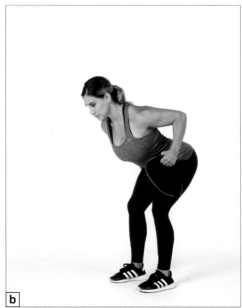

Lateral Lunge With Forward Press

Benefits

The sideways movement of this lunge variation strengthens the hip muscles to enhance control and stability. Adding the forward press increases leverage to activate more muscles of the posterior chain, including the spinal and hip extensors.

Instructions

1. Stand with both feet hip-width apart. Grip the sandbag in both hands and hold it in front of your chest so that your elbows are tucked in close to your body.
2. Maintain a long spine as you step directly to your left with your left leg. Keep your right foot planted on the floor and squeeze your right thigh to help stabilize your knee.
3. As your left foot hits the floor, push your left hip back to hinge into your left hip as you press the sandbag directly in front of your chest.
4. At the bottom of the lunge, pause and pull the sandbag back toward your chest while pressing your right foot into the floor and pushing off with your left foot.
5. Complete 5 to 6 reps on the left leg before switching to the right, for a total of 10 to 12 reps. As you get stronger, add 2 reps per week until you can do 16 to 20 reps on each side.

Correct Your Form

- When stepping to the side (to the left in the instructions), keep your right foot pressed into the ground and make sure that both feet are parallel as the left foot hits the ground.
- While lowering into the lunge, think about pushing your tailbone directly behind you to create the proper movement.
- If pushing the sandbag forward is too challenging, keep it close to your chest. As you become stronger (and you will), begin pushing it forward for only a couple reps at a time.

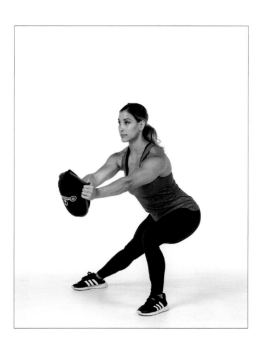

Transverse Plane Lunge Reach to Ground with Overhead Press

Benefits

The transverse plane lunge takes the hip through all three planes to help improve joint mobility as well as enhance strength of the muscles that control joint motion. The reach to ground with overhead press lift helps involve the extensor muscles of the posterior chain to improve postural strength as well as the coordination between the hips and shoulders.

Instructions

1. Stand with your feet hip-width apart, and hold the sandbag in front of your waist with both hands. Keep your left foot pointed straight ahead (the twelve o'clock direction).
2. Step back with your right foot and place it facing in the three or four o'clock direction.
3. As your right foot hits the ground, push your weight back into your right hip while reaching for the ground in front of your foot with the sandbag (keep your left foot pointed straight ahead).
4. To return to standing, push off the ground with your right foot as you press your left foot into the ground to pull yourself with the inner thigh muscles of your left leg. As you return to standing, push the sandbag directly overhead, then lower it and begin the next rep.
5. Complete 5 to 6 reps, including the overhead press, on the right leg before switching to the left, for a total of 10 to 12 reps. As you get stronger, add 2 reps per week until you can do 16 to 20 reps on each side.

Correct Your Form

- If you are not able to comfortably reach all of the way to the ground, reach to the level of your knee.
- When doing the overhead press, keep both elbows pointed to the front of your body.

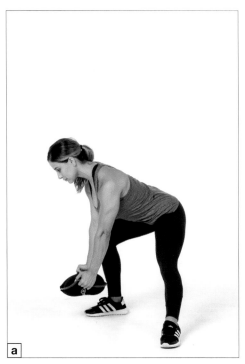
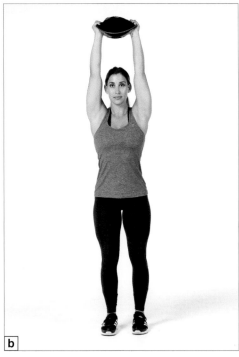

a

b

TWO-ARM RESISTANCE BAND EXERCISES FOR CORE STRENGTH

In a gym or health club, the adjustable cable machine is often one of the most underutilized pieces of equipment, and when it is used, it is not to the best of its ability. A two-arm resistance band allows for a number of cable machine–type exercises to be performed anywhere you can identify a secure anchor point for the band. The benefit of using either a two-arm resistance band or cable machine is that you can perform pushing, pulling, or rotating movements from a standing position, which will engage most of the muscles responsible for controlling both stability and mobility. These exercises can be some of the most effective movements for developing the core strength that can help you to enjoy all of your favorite activities.

Exercise	Sets	Repetitions
Standing crunch (facing away from anchor point)	2	8-10
High-to-low band chop	2	5-6 each side
Lunge to one-arm pull	2	5-6 each side
Split squat with trunk rotation	2	5-6 each side
Two-hand forward press	2	6-8 each side
Squat-to-row	2	6-8
One-arm press	2	6-8 each side
Perform this workout as a circuit with little-to-no rest between each exercise, rest for 90 seconds to 2 minutes after completing all exercises.		

Standing Crunch
(Facing Away From Anchor Point)

Benefits

The abdominal muscles help control movement between your rib cage, spine, and pelvis as you walk. This exercise strengthens your RA muscles the way they are designed to function.

Instructions

1. Place the end of the resistance band at head height or higher (up to 12 inches [30 cm]).
2. Stand facing away from the anchor point with both feet hip-width apart while keeping your pelvis level and your knees slightly bent so that you are pulling against the resistance.
3. Hold both ends of the band in both hands and keep them directly over the top of your head. Both of your elbows should be pointed forward.
4. To perform the movement, draw your belly button in to your spine and shift your rib cage down toward the top of your pelvis. Focus on rolling your rib cage down against the pull of the band, then slowly return to the top.
5. Perform 8 to 10 reps. As you get stronger, add 2 reps per week until you can do 18 to 20 reps. To increase the intensity, move farther away from the anchor point.

Correct Your Form

- The abdominals attach from the front of your rib cage to the bottom of your pelvis, so the movement should focus on pulling these two parts together as opposed to bending or rounding forward from the spine.
- Once you can do 18 to 20 reps, add some variety: Place your right foot approximately 18 inches (46 cm) in front of your left for 8 to 10 reps, then place your left foot forward for 8 to 10 reps.

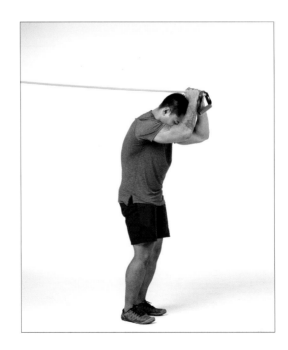

High-to-Low Band Chop

Benefits

The rotation of your trunk combined with the lateral shift of the hips uses the muscles responsible for controlling both stability and rotational mobility of your spine and hips, respectively.

Instructions

1. Anchor the resistance band at or slightly above (up to 18 inches [46 cm]) shoulder height. Step away from the anchor point until you have a minimal amount of tension when holding both handles in your hands.

2. Stand so that the right side of your body is facing the anchor point with your feet wider than shoulder-width apart. Grip both handles with your right hand first before placing your left hand on top; start with your hands in front of your right shoulder and your weight in your right leg. Push your right foot into the ground as you rotate your hands in front of your body while shifting your weight into your left leg.

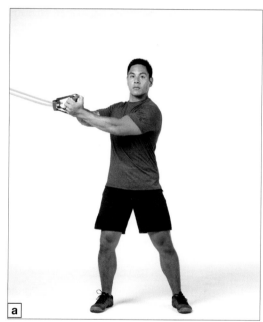
a

3. Keep both arms in front of your body and rotate your torso while lowering your hands from shoulder to hip height. Keep your spine straight the entire time.

4. At the bottom of the movement, your weight should be in your left hip and your hands in front of your left leg.

5. To return your hands to their initial position above your right shoulder, push your left foot into the floor as you slowly rotate both hands in front of your body.

6. Complete 5 to 6 reps moving from right to left, then switch directions. (When you switch, your left hand should hold the handles and your right hand should be on top.) Perform the same number of reps, for a total of 10 to 12 repetitions. As you get stronger, add 2 reps per week until you can do 16 to 20 reps on each side.

Correct Your Form

- If holding both handles is too challenging, use just one handle, but stand further from the anchor point for more resistance.

- Keep both feet parallel. Rotate from the trunk as you shift your weight from your right to left hip (in the instructions). Press your feet into the ground to create stability so that you rotate from both hip joints.

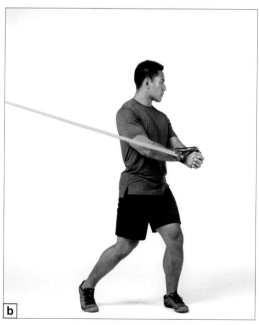
b

Lunge to One-Arm Pull

Benefits

Pulling from a single-leg balance requires using most of the muscles that control spinal stability as well as the muscles that control motion of the hip to hold the balanced position. Balancing on the one leg while pulling with the opposite arm strengthens your core muscles the way they function when walking or running, making this one of the most effective core exercises that you will love to dislike.

Instructions

1. Place the anchor point at or above head height. Stand facing the anchor so that your right foot is forward and your left leg is back, with the ball of your foot on the ground. Grip one (or both if the band's resistance is not that hard) of the handles in your left hand so that your palm is facing the midline of your body.

2. Stand far enough away from the anchor point so that there is tension on the band with no slack. Lower yourself into a static lunge so that your left knee moves closer to the floor while you continue to hold your left arm straight out in front of you.

3. At the bottom of the movement, push your right foot into the floor as you pull back with your left hand, keeping your left elbow close to your body while lifting your left leg off the ground to swing it forward as you balance on your right leg.

4. Hold the standing position balanced on your right leg with your left hand back by your chest. Pause for one second before slowly extending your left arm and lowering yourself back into a lunge position with your left leg behind you.

5. Perform 5 to 6 reps with your left hand and right leg, then switch to the other limbs for a total of 10 to 12 reps. As you get stronger, add 2 reps per week until you can do 16 to 20 reps on each side.

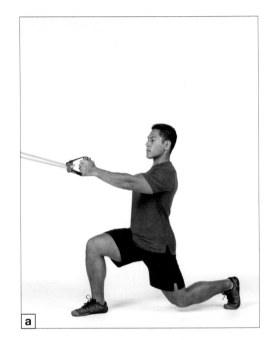

a

Correct Your Form

- Having more tension on the band helps you keep control of your body, so you want to start with the band already slightly stretched.

- If you need more resistance, hold both handles in one hand.

- When pulling back on the band, think about pulling from your elbow. This is the attachment point for your upper back muscles and will help increase the fluidity of the movement.

- As you lower yourself in to the lunge, stop before your knee hits the ground.

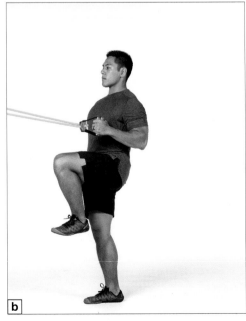

b

Split Squat With Trunk Rotation

Benefits

This exercise creates rotational strength of trunk muscles while maintaining a neutral, static position with your hips. It also improves coordination between your upper and lower body.

Instructions

1. Place the anchor point of the resistance band at approximately shoulder height. Stand so the right side of your body is facing the anchor point, and place your left leg forward and right leg back to hold yourself in a static lunge position. You should be far enough away so that there is a slight amount of tension on the band with no slack.

2. Hold one handle in both hands with the left hand down first and the right hand on top. Extend both arms straight in front of your body, and lower yourself so that you are sinking into your left hip. Hold the bottom position and rotate over your left leg. Pause for 1 to 2 seconds at the end of the rotation, then rotate back to the starting position and raise yourself up to the starting height.

3. Perform 5 to 6 reps with your left leg forward, then turn around and switch to your right leg forward so that you are rotating to the right. Complete a total of 10 to 12 reps. As you get stronger, add 2 reps per week until you can do 16 to 20 reps on each side.

Correct Your Form

- Stand far enough away so that there is tension on the band at the start of the movement. Keep your front leg pressed into the ground to increase stability, and maintain a tall, long spine during the entire movement.

- If you need more resistance, first move further away from the anchor point, then grab both handles in your hands.

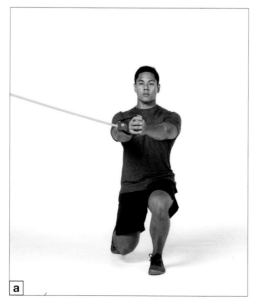
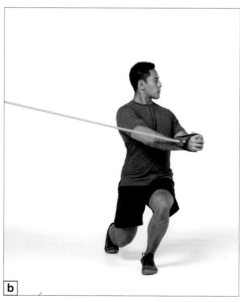

Two-Hand Forward Press

Benefits

This exercise is a progression from the front plank, which takes place in a face-down position, to increase the strength and coordination between your hips and shoulders. You will also strengthen the muscles that stabilize your spine. As they become stronger, they can give the appearance of a flatter stomach.

Instructions

1. Place the anchor point of the resistance band at approximately shoulder height, and stand with feet hip-width apart and with the left side of your body facing the anchor point. Keep your pelvis level, with your knees slightly bent during the exercise so that you are anchoring yourself with your hips and feet—the harder you press your feet into the ground, the more you engage and activate your core muscles.
2. Stand far enough away from the anchor point so that there is tension on the band. Grip a handle in both hands so that your fingers are laced together. Begin with your elbows in by your sides so they are touching your rib cage. Keep your spine tall and long as you press the handle forward. Pause at the end of the movement for 2 to 3 seconds before slowly pulling your elbows back to your sides.
3. Perform 6 to 8 reps with your right side facing the anchor point, then turn around and switch so that your right side is facing the anchor point, for a total of 12 to 16 reps. As you get stronger, add 2 reps per week until you can do 16 to 20 reps on each side.

Correct Your Form

- For optimal stability, keep both feet pressed into the ground while squeezing your thighs and glutes.
- To add more resistance, step further away from the anchor point to increase the tension, or hold both handles in your hands.

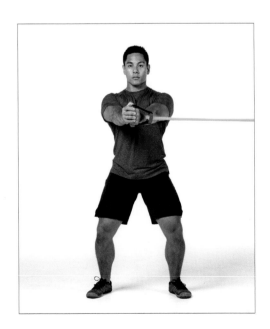

Squat-to-Row

Benefits

Pulling movements from a standing position can integrate both the large muscles of the upper back, with the larger muscles responsible for extending the hips and legs. Using more muscle mass can increase energy expenditure while improving strength.

Instructions

1. Place the anchor point of the band at approximately chest height, and stand facing the anchor point far enough away so that there is tension on the band. Hold one handle in each hand so that your thumbs are pointed up to the ceiling and your palms are facing each other. Keep both feet hip-width apart and your spine tall and long.
2. Lift your chest, hold your arms straight in front of you, and push your hips back to lower yourself into a squat.
3. At the bottom of the squat, continue to keep your arms extended, and hold your spine long as you push your feet into the ground to return to the standing position.
4. While you're standing up, pull the handles toward your body, keeping your arms parallel to the floor and elbows close to your side. Your hands should reach the front of your body as you reach the standing position. Pause and slowly extend your arms as you drop down into the next squat.
5. Perform 6 to 8 reps. As you get stronger, add 2 reps per week until you can do 18 to 20 reps.

Correct Your Form

- For optimal resistance, stand far enough away so there is tension on the band when you start the exercise.
- To increase stability, keep both feet pressed into the ground.
- Work on the timing so that your arms are moving forward as you lower yourself into the squat and so they are moving back toward your body as you return to the standing position.

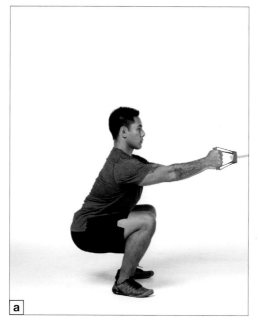
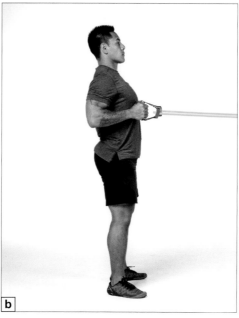

One-Arm Press

Benefits

Pushing from one side of your body can help recruit more muscles to generate and maintain stability through your hips and spine. Chest presses from a standing position allow more motion through the shoulder blade when compared to normal chest presses on a hard bench, which can restrict motion of the shoulder blade.

Instructions

1. Place the anchor point of the band at approximately chest height. Stand facing away from the anchor point far enough away so that there is tension on the band.
2. Hold one handle in the left hand (if the band is lower resistance, grip both handles to increase the level of difficulty). Keep your feet shoulder-width apart and with your right foot slightly forward. The heel of the right foot should be even with the toes on your left.
3. Hold your pelvis level and your spine tall and long, with your knees slightly bent. Press both feet into the floor as you press your left arm forward. Pause at the end for 1 second before slowly bringing your arm back to the starting position.
4. Perform 6 to 8 reps with your left arm, then switch to use your right, for a total of 12 to 16 reps. As you get stronger, add 2 reps per week until you can do 18 to 20 reps on each side.

Correct Your Form

- Keep your spine long, and lift your chest as you press your arm forward.
- To increase resistance, move further away from the anchor point or hold both handles so that you are using both arms of the resistance band.

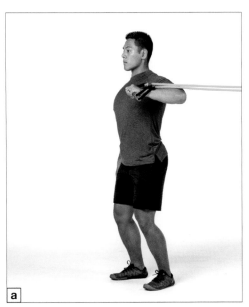
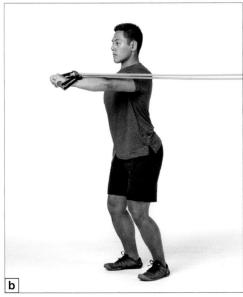

DUMBBELL EXERCISES FOR CORE STRENGTH

Dumbbells are an effective training tool for improving strength because they are easy to store out-of-the-way for home use and are almost always available in any fitness center, from hotel to apartment complex to commercial health club. When using dumbbells for core strength, the stabilizer muscles work harder to coordinate strength and create balance between both sides of the body. This is especially true if you use your dominant hand more than your non-dominant one; your brain will have to coordinate the muscles in both limbs to work together, which helps to improve overall coordination and strength. Use a weight heavy enough to make 4 to 5 reps with each relatively difficult. If the goal of the workout is to improve strength, then it should be challenging to extremely difficult to complete 10 reps. Once you can perform 10 reps without too much difficulty, it is time to increase the weight to ensure the muscles are properly engaged and challenged.

Exercise	Sets	Repetitions
Pullover to crunch	2	6-8
Hip press	2	6-8
Romanian deadlift to biceps curl	2	6-8
Lateral lunge reach-down to overhead press	2	5-6 each side
Alternating arm bent-over row	2	5-6 each side
Rotating uppercut	2	5-6 each side
Squat to overhead press	2	6-8
Single-leg sword draw	2	6-8 each arm
Perform this workout as a circuit with little-to-no rest between each exercise, rest for 90 seconds to 2 minutes after completing all exercises.		

Pullover to Crunch

Benefits

This exercise uses the large muscles of the upper back and abdominals along the front of the body to develop coordinated strength through both muscle groups.

Instructions

1. Lie on the ground flat on your back with your feet on the floor and knees pointed to the ceiling. Extend your arms straight up while holding one dumbbell in each hand so that your palms are facing each other.
2. Keep your feet pressed into the floor and your elbows fully extended as you slowly lower your arms to the floor. Pause for 1 to 2 seconds, then pull both arms back to the starting position. When the weights are directly over your chest, draw your belly button into your spine as you shift your rib cage toward your pelvis and lift your back off the ground to perform a curl. Slowly lower your back down to the floor and continue to the next repetition.
3. Perform 6 to 8 reps. As you get stronger, add 2 reps per week until you can do 18 to 20 reps.

Correct Your Form

- When performing the crunch, keep your chin tucked in to your neck and focus on moving from your rib cage.
- Keep your elbows straight throughout the entire movement to make sure you are using your back muscles instead of your upper arms.

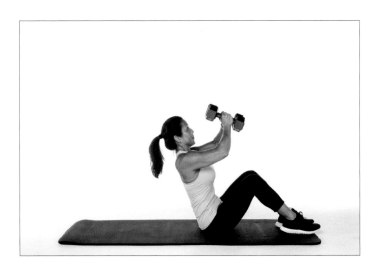

Hip Press

Benefits

This exercise increases strength from the glutes without putting any pressure on your back or knees.

Instructions

1. Lie on the ground flat on your back with your feet on the floor, knees pointed to the ceiling, and toes of both feet pulled up toward your shins so that your heels are resting on the floor.
2. Place the dumbbell in your right hand on your right hip and the one in your left hand on your left hip. Press your heels into the ground as you push your hips up toward the ceiling. Pause at the top and hold the position for 2 to 4 seconds.
3. Slowly lower your tailbone back toward the floor while keeping the weights on your hips.
4. Perform 6 to 8 reps. As you get stronger, add 2 reps per week until you can do 18 to 20 reps.

Correct Your Form

- Your heels should be about 18 inches (46 cm) away from your heels. Too close and you'll feel it in your hamstrings; too far and you'll feel it in your back.
- Raise your hips for a count of 2 to 3 seconds, pause for 2 to 4 seconds at the top, and lower your hips for 3 to 4 seconds to increase the amount of tension in the muscles. The greater the tension, the greater the strength.

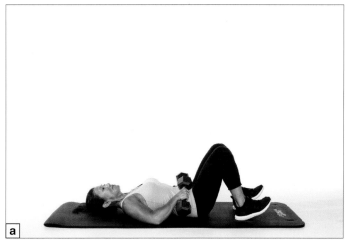

a

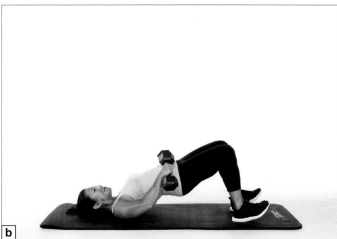

b

Romanian Deadlift to Biceps Curl

Benefits

Romanian deadlifts strengthen the hip extensors (glutes), spinal erectors, as well as the hamstring and adductor muscles of the legs; adding a biceps curl provides the opportunity to do more work during the movement.

Instructions

1. Stand with your feet hip-width apart and knees slightly bent. Hold one dumbbell in each hand so that your hands are resting along the front of your thighs.
2. To start the movement, push your hips back behind you as you hinge forward at the hips while keeping your spine straight during the entire movement. Lower yourself to the end of the movement, then push your feet into the ground as you press both hips forward to return to the standing position.
3. Once you are standing up tall, perform a biceps curl with both hand at the same time. Start with your palms resting along the sides of your thighs. As you bend your elbows, rotate your palms so they finish the movement facing up to the ceiling.
4. Perform 6 to 8 reps. As you get stronger, add 2 reps per week until you can do 18 to 20 reps without stopping.

Correct Your Form

- During the Romanian deadlift, keep the spine straight and push your tailbone behind you so that you are moving from the hips, not the spine.
- When hinging forward, focus on the exhale. Inhale as you return to the standing position.

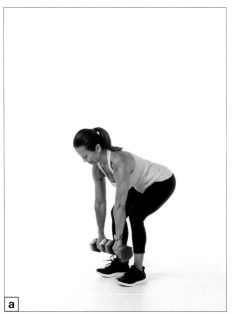
a

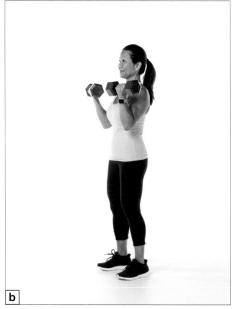
b

Lateral Lunge Reach-Down to Overhead Press

Benefits

The lateral lunge with reach-down uses the lateral hip, quadriceps, and glute, while the reach-down to overhead press uses your upper back, shoulder, and arms muscles. Because you are using your hips, legs, arms, back, and shoulders, you will be strengthening several muscles that work around your center of gravity while burning a number of calories.

Instructions

1. Stand with your feet hip-width apart and hold one dumbbell in each hand. Step directly to your right. As your right foot hits the ground, keep it parallel to the left and push your right hip back as you hinge forward to reach for the right foot with both hands.
2. To return to standing, pull your arms up to your waist. Push your right foot into the floor while pressing your left foot into the ground to pull yourself up with your left inner thigh muscles.
3. When you are back in the standing position, bend your elbows to bring each dumbbell to the front of your shoulders, then press both weights overhead into a shoulder press. Lower the weights and continue to the next lateral lunge.
4. Perform 5 to 6 reps with your right leg, then switch to the left leg, for a total of 10 to 12 reps. As you get stronger, add 2 reps per week until you can do 16 to 20 repetitions on each side.

Correct Your Form

- When stepping to the side, make sure both feet are parallel, and focus on pushing your hips back as you hinge forward to reach for the ground with both weights.
- To increase intensity, alternate from right to left instead of performing all reps on one side at a time.
- If the overhead press is challenging, focus on the lateral lunges, and add the overhead press later after becoming a little stronger.

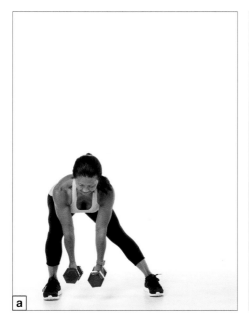

a

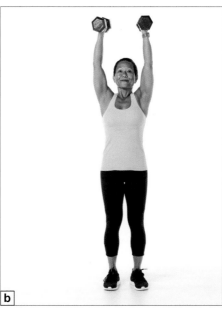

b

Alternating-Arm Bent-Over Row

Benefits

Holding the position of the bent-over row uses the deep muscles that stabilize the spine. Alternating from one arm to the other during the rowing movement challenges the muscles to work harder to maintain stability in the spine.

Instructions

1. Hold one dumbbell in each hand so that your arms are hanging along your side with your palms facing in toward your body. Stand with your feet approximately hip-width apart and with a slight bend in your knees.

2. Hinge at your hips by pushing your tailbone back and keeping a straight spine. Try to lower your trunk as low as possible, but stop before your spine starts to bend.

3. At the lowest position, allow both hands to hang toward the floor until the elbows are fully extended. Keep your spine long, chest lifted up, and palms facing each other as you pull the right hand back toward your body. As your right hand is moving, allow your left hand to hang toward the floor, and as your right arm returns to the starting position, rotate to your left as you pull back with the left elbow—there should be constant moving from right-to-left arms.

4. Perform 5 to 6 reps with each arm for a total of 10 to 12 repetitions. As you get stronger, add 2 reps per week until you can do 18 to 20 repetitions with both arms (9 to 10 each arm).

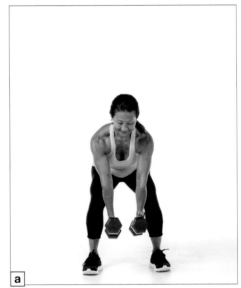

a

Correct Your Form

- To increase stability in your spine, press your feet into the floor while squeezing your hip and thigh muscles.

- Once you can maintain a totally straight spine during all reps, allow your shoulders and trunk to rotate each time you pull back an arm; for example, as you pull back with your right arm, rotate your trunk by pulling back on the right shoulder and turning your chest to the right side.

- Grip the dumbbell with your hand but focus on pulling the weight back from your elbow—this will use more of your upper-back muscles.

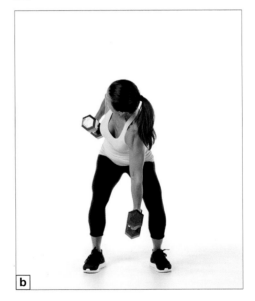

b

Rotating Uppercut

Benefits

The rotating movement helps strengthen the muscles around the hips, while lifting the arms in the uppercut movement strengthens the muscles in the upper arms and shoulders. Overall, the movement helps improve integrated strength and coordination between the shoulders and hips.

Instructions

1. Stand with your feet shoulder-width apart, and hold one dumbbell in each hand so that your palms are facing up. Keep your elbows tucked in by each side and place your weight back in your hips.
2. To start the movement, press your left foot into the ground to rotate to your right; keep your right foot pressed firmly into the ground so that you rotate around your right hip. Keep your left elbow bent as you lift your left arm to perform an uppercut to bring your left elbow to shoulder height.
3. Lower your left arm and rotate back to center, where you push your right foot into the ground to rotate around your left hip while swinging your right arm up in an uppercut.
4. Alternate sides and perform 5 to 6 reps on each side, for a total of 10 to 12 reps. As you get stronger, add 2 reps per week to each side until you can do 18 to 20 repetitions.

Correct Your Form

- The rotation comes from your hips, while the lifting movement of the arm should come from your shoulder.
- Keep your elbows bent at 90 degrees throughout the duration of the exercise.

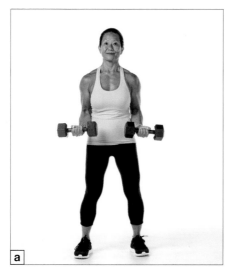 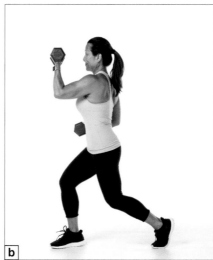

Squat to Overhead Press

Benefits

This movement uses the hip muscles to raise and lower your body, the deep core muscles to stabilize your spine, and the shoulder and arm muscles to raise the weight over your head, making this exercise effective for strengthening a number of muscles while increasing energy expenditure.

Instructions

1. Standing with your feet approximately hip- to shoulder-width apart, grip one dumbbell in each hand, and hold both hands in front of each shoulder with your elbows tucked close to your body.
2. Push your hips back and maintain length in your spine as you lower into a squat while holding the weights on the front of your shoulders.
3. From the bottom of the squat, press your feet into the ground to return to the top of the standing position. Once there keep both palms facing each other as you press the dumbbells overhead.
4. Slowly return the weight to your shoulders and move into the next rep.
5. Perform 6 to 8 reps. As you get stronger, add 2 reps per week until you can do 18 to 20 reps.

Correct Your Form

- To increase your leg strength, press both feet into the floor as though you are trying to push the floor away from you as you return to standing.
- For optimal movement through the shoulders, keep your palms facing the middle of your body as you press both arms overhead.

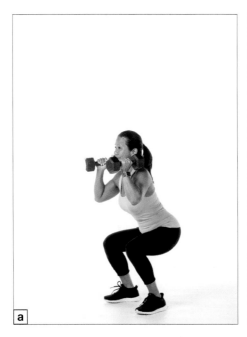
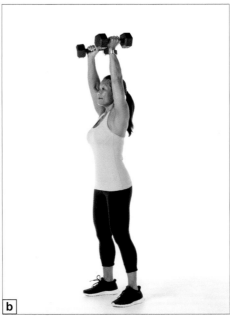

Single-Leg Sword Draw

Benefits

Remaining in a seated position for an extended period of time, whether at a desk or while driving a car, can cause weakness in the shoulder and upper-back muscles. This exercise strengthens the muscles that can help you maintain a tall posture. In addition, this movement can help improve overall strength and ROM of the shoulder joint.

Instructions

1. Stand balanced on your left leg, and keep your right knee bent so your pelvis is level during the movement. Hold one dumbbell in your right hand so that your right arm is straight and your right palm is resting in front of your left hip. Press both feet into the ground.
2. Maintain a long spine as you raise your right arm across your body and out to your right side so that the weight ends up at shoulder height.
3. Return the weight back to the front of your left hip.
4. Perform 5 to 6 reps with the right arm, then switch to the right leg and left arm for a total of 10 to 12 reps. As you get stronger, add 2 reps per week until you can do 18 to 20 reps.

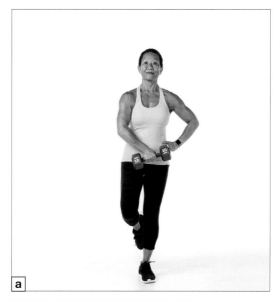

a

Correct Your Form

- Your right hand should move across the front of your body as though you are drawing a sword from your left hip out to your right side.
- If you need extra stability, keep your right foot resting lightly on the ground like a kickstand, with most of your weight in your left hip and leg.

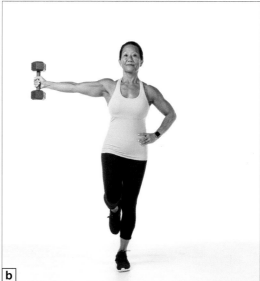

b

KETTLEBELL EXERCISES FOR CORE STRENGTH

Holding the kettlebell by the handle in an upside down position (called bottom-up) requires the forearm and grip muscles to work much harder to maintain control of the mass. Kettlebells can be used one at a time or one in each hand. When used in only one hand (as in the workout below), a kettlebell can create an asymmetrical, off-balanced load that requires the muscles of your body to work harder to maintain balance and control between both sides. Don't be intimidated by the fact that the kettlebell looks like a cannonball with a handle. Learning how to use this tool properly can help you perform a variety of effective exercises to improve core strength.

Exercise	Sets	Repetitions
Pullover to crunch	2	6-8
Reverse lunge to balance with offset weight	2	5-6 each side
Windmill	2	4-6 each side
Goblet squat	2	6-8
One-arm overhead press	2	5-6 each arm
One-arm bent-over row	2	6-8 each arm
Reverse lunge with one-arm overhead carry	2	5-6 each leg
Perform this workout as a circuit with little-to-no rest between each exercise, rest for 90 seconds to 2 minutes after completing all exercises.		

Pullover to Crunch

Benefits

The muscles responsible for moving the core have a large number of type II muscle fibers, which respond to heavier loads; this exercise can help improve your core strength without having to do a high volume of repetitions. In addition, this move can help improve the coordination and synergy between the abdominal muscles along the front of your body and the large latissimus dorsi muscle of your upper back.

Instructions

1. Lie flat on the ground with your feet flat on the floor and knees bent up in the air.
2. Hold a kettlebell in both hands so your hands are wrapped around the horns of the handle (the sides of the handle).
3. Keep your back resting on the ground and lower the weight overhead while keeping both arms straight. Once the kettlebell is resting on the floor, pull it from the overhead position to the top of your chest (so the kettlebell is right over the center of your chest).
4. As your arms pass over your chest, pull your belly button in toward your spine, which will help pull your rib cage toward your pelvis to lift your back off the ground and perform a crunch.
5. Lower yourself back to the floor. Once your back is flat on the ground, lower the kettlebell back overhead.
6. Perform 6 to 8 reps. As you get stronger, add 2 reps per week until you can do 18 to 20 reps.

Correct Your Form

- Keep your feet flat on the floor and push them into the ground to help increase stability. Allow your spine to rest along the floor. Do not curl up into the crunch until your hands (and the kettlebell) pass over the center of your chest.
- To reduce the strain in your neck, press your tongue into the roof of your mouth and keep your chin tucked into your neck.

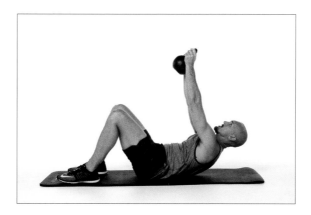

Reverse Lunge to Balance With Offset Weight

Benefits

Carries can be a very effective way to strengthen your core muscles from a standing position. This lunge to a balance can replicate the basic movement pattern of a carry without having to walk a long distance, which may not be possible at home. Balancing on one leg while holding the kettlebell in your opposite hand will recruit many core muscles to help you control your center of mass.

Instructions

1. Stand with your feet hip-width apart as you grip a kettlebell with your left hand and hold it along the left side of your body.
2. Maintain a long spine as you step back with your left leg. As your left knee lowers toward the floor, push your right hip back so that you hinge at the hip while lowering your body.
3. Keep your spine long as you descend to a comfortable ROM. To return to standing, push your right foot into the ground to pull yourself forward with your right leg as you swing your left leg forward to bring both legs next to one another, but keep your left foot off of the ground so that you balance on your right leg for 2-3 seconds. To increase the level of difficulty, try to step back with the left leg without placing it on the ground
4. Perform 5 to 6 reps with the right leg, then alternate to your left, for a total of 10 to 12 reps. As you get stronger, add 2 reps per week until you can do 9 to 10 lunges on each side, for a total of 18 to 20 reps.

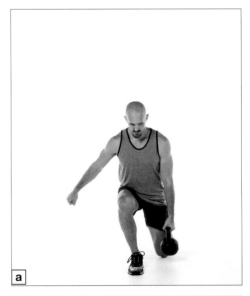

a

Correct Your Form

- Keep your spine long throughout the movement to reduce strain on the spine.
- Pressing your foot in to the ground to pull yourself forward can help recruit more of the muscles that help stabilize the knee, extend the hip, and control rotation.
- To increase the level of difficulty, hold the kettlebell in a "racked" position so that the knuckles of the hand holding the kettlebell are against your collarbone and the elbow is next to your rib cage.

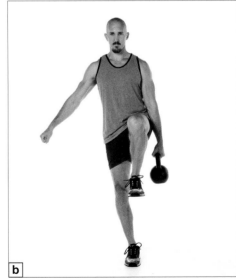

b

Windmill

Benefits

The shoulders and hips work together to provide the energy for walking or running, and this is one of the most effective exercises for strengthening the muscles that help the shoulders and hips function as a single, integrated structure.

Instructions

1. Stand with your feet wider than hip-width apart so that your right foot is pointing straight ahead in the twelve o'clock direction and your left foot is in a staggered position, pointing in the five o'clock direction.

2. Hold a kettlebell in the right hand in the racked position. The right wrist should be bent so the knuckles of your right hand are by your right collarbone and your right elbow is next to your rib cage, with the kettlebell resting on your forearm.

3. Press the kettlebell straight overhead and hold the right arm straight during the movement. Hold your left arm by your side and maintain a long spine as you push your weight back into the right hip and turn to look at your right hand while allowing your left arm to drop along the inside of your left (front) leg.

4. Lower yourself as far as you can while keeping a straight spine. To return to standing, push your right leg into the floor and slide your hips forward as you bring your back up straight and tall.

5. Perform 4 to 6 reps with the right arm, then switch arms and change feet position, for a total of 8 to 12 reps. As you become stronger, add 1 rep a week until you can do 8 to 10 reps on each side.

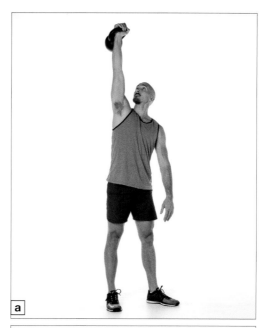

a

Correct Your Form

- This is a challenging exercise, so take your time to learn it properly.

- Your spine should remain straight throughout this movement. As soon as you feel it starting to bend or round, stop—that is your end ROM—and return to the starting position. As you do this exercise regularly, you will increase your hip mobility.

- You should feel this movement in your hips, not your spine. Specifically, you will feel it in your right hip when holding the kettlebell in your right arm and your left hip when holding the kettlebell in your left arm. If you feel this in your back or spine, hold the kettlebell in the hand by your leg (the left in the instructions) and work on your mobility before holding the kettlebell overhead.

- To increase stability, imagine pushing the kettlebell up toward the ceiling as you hinge forward into your hips. This increases the tension in the tissue, which can help improve overall stability.

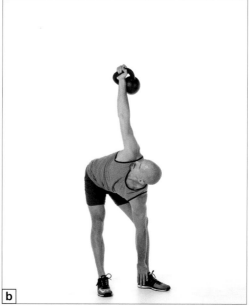

b

Goblet Squat

Benefits

Squats are a great exercise for strengthening the muscles that help control your center of gravity. The goblet variation allows you to hold a weight in front of your body as opposed to uncomfortably resting a barbell on your shoulders, which could cause discomfort in the upper back and neck. Using more muscles can help increase overall energy expenditure during a workout.

Instructions

1. Stand with your feet hip- to shoulder-width apart. Hold the kettlebell in between both hands so the bottom of the kettlebell faces up and the handle is between both of your forearms.
2. Keep both hands directly in front of your chest so that your elbows are right next to your rib cage.
3. Maintain a long spine as you push both hips back to lower yourself into a squatting position. From the bottom of the movement (as low as you can comfortably go before allowing your spine to bend or round), press both feet into the floor to return to the standing position.
4. Perform 6 to 8 reps. As you become stronger, add 2 reps per week until you can perform 18 to 20 reps continuously.

Correct Your Form

- The first movement should be your hips going back as you lower yourself into the seated or bottom portion of the squat.
- Maintain a long, straight spine to help give yourself more core stability and to allow a greater ROM from the hips.
- Lower yourself for a count of 3 to 5 seconds. When you return to standing, move quickly so that it only takes you 1 to 2 seconds.

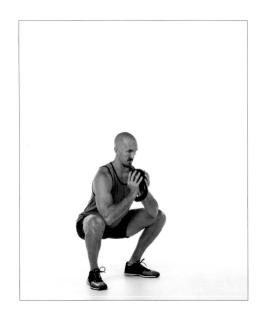

One-Arm Overhead Press

Benefits

The one-arm overhead press uses your hips, arm, shoulder, forearm, and grip muscles with one move that is a true test of strength. Using only one arm at a time for certain exercises gives you the ability to focus all of your energy into that muscle.

Instructions

1. Stand with your feet hip-width apart with your right foot slightly in front of your left. Grip a kettlebell with your right hand while holding it in the racked position. The right wrist should be bent so the knuckles of your right hand are by your right collarbone and your right elbow is next to your rib cage, with the kettlebell resting on your right forearm.

2. Start the move by pushing your left foot into the ground to shift your weight forward. As your weight moves into your right hip, press your right arm straight overhead, keeping the palm of your right hand facing the midline of your body. To lower the weight, think about pulling your right elbow back down to your rib cage.

3. Perform 5 to 6 reps with the right arm, then switch arms and foot position, to perform a total of 10 to 12 reps. As you become stronger, add 2 reps per week until you can do at least 16 reps with each arm.

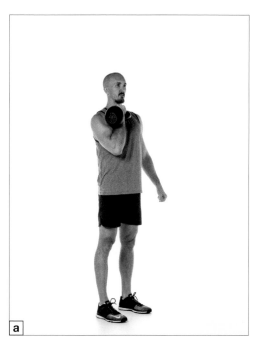

a

Correct Your Form

- Even though this is primarily a shoulder exercise, the feet and hips play an important role. You start the move with your feet by pressing into the ground and complete it once your arm is fully extended while holding the kettlebell.

- Keep your spine long and tall so that you have an optimal ROM from your shoulder joint.

TIP If you can easily do more than 16 repetitions in a row, it may be time to use (or invest in) a heavier kettlebell.

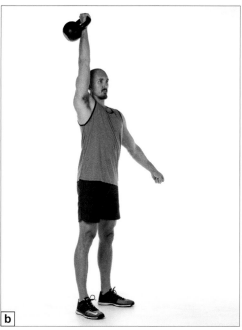

b

One-Arm Bent-Over Row

Benefits

The bent-over row combines the hip hinge with the plank to improve the strength of the hips and the stability of the spine in a standing position while using the large muscles of the upper back.

Instructions

1. Stand with your feet approximately shoulder-width apart. Hold a kettlebell in your right hand so that your right arm is hanging along the right side of your body with your palm facing in.

2. Keep a straight spine and a slight bend in both knees while hinging forward at your hips by pushing your tailbone straight back. Lower your right hand toward the floor until the elbow is fully extended. Keep your chest lifted up as you pull the kettlebell back toward your belly button, keeping your right elbow along the right side of your body. Pause at the top, then slowly lower the kettlebell back toward the floor.

3. To maximize core strength, keep your left arm hanging by your side. Use it to brace yourself by placing it on your left thigh *only* if you need the stability. Perform 6 to 8 reps with the right arm before switching to the left, for a total of 12 to 16 reps. As you become stronger, add 2 reps per week until you can do 18 to 20 reps with each arm.

Correct Your Form

- Hold the kettlebell tightly in your hand. When pulling it back toward your body, think about pulling from your elbow. This will help use the larger muscle of the upper back.

- To increase stability, keep your feet pressed firmly into the floor. Think about pushing the floor away from you to fully engage both legs.

- If you need additional stability, use a staggered stance by moving your left foot forward slightly when using your right arm, so that the heel of your left foot is even with the toes of your right.

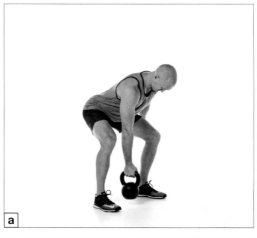

a

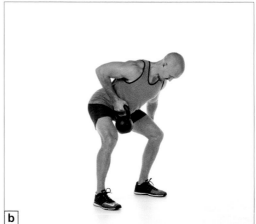

b

Reverse Lunge
With One-Arm Overhead Carry

Benefits

One-arm kettlebell overhead carries (walking while holding a single kettlebell with your arm extended directly overhead) are an effective exercise for developing core strength, especially in the muscles responsible for maintaining a tall, straight spine, stability of the shoulder, and lateral stability of the hips. This lunge replicates the overhead carry without having to walk, making it an effective solution when space is limited.

Instructions

1. Hold a kettlebell in your right hand with your right arm extended straight up overhead and your right palm facing the midline of your body.

2. Stand with your feet approximately hip-width apart. Step straight back with your right leg, and lower yourself into a lunge so that you are bending at the left hip.

3. Keep your chest raised and your spine long as you descend into the lowering phase, stopping before your right knee hits the floor. At the bottom of the movement, press your left foot into the floor and push off with the right leg to return to the standing position.

4. Perform 5 to 6 reps, then switch arms and legs to complete a total of 10 to 12 reps. As you become stronger, add 1 to 2 reps a week until you can perform 14 to 16 reps with each side of the body. (If you can easily do more than 16 reps, it may be time to invest in a heavier kettlebell.)

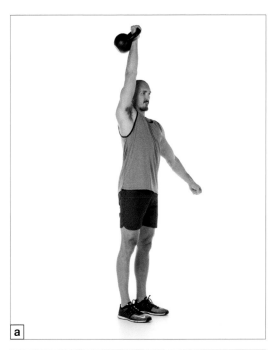

a

Correct Your Form

- To maintain proper stability of the shoulder while holding the kettlebell overhead and optimal mobility of the hip while stepping back, make sure to maintain a straight, fully extended spine with each rep.

- When returning to standing from the lowered position of the lunge, think about pulling the knee of the forward leg back (the left leg in the instructions) while pressing the foot firmly into the ground. This will help recruit and engage the extensor muscles along the back of the leg and hip.

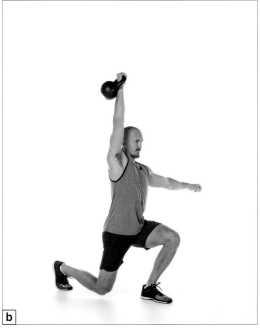

b

5

Metabolic Conditioning

Exercise is often used for the specific purpose of weight loss, with many people mistakenly believing that it is necessary to perform hours of cardio exercises such as cycling, swimming, walking, hiking, or using many of the machines you'll find in a health club (think: treadmills, elliptical runners, stationary bikes, and stair climbers) to achieve this goal. Admit it: When you first start thinking about the need to exercise you probably feel obligated to lace up your running shoes and go for a jog. Jogging *can* be an effective way to exercise, and it does deliver many health benefits. But many people—and you might be one of them—simply don't like to run. While running can be an efficient way to burn calories, the downside is that it involves moving over the ground at a fast pace, which sends impact forces into your body. The faster you move, the more force is placed into your body when your foot hits the ground. This could increase the risk of injury, especially if you have poor posture, poor running mechanics, or a previous injury. If you've ever started a running program because you wanted the health benefits but stopped because you found it to be uncomfortable or downright painful, there is good news: If you don't like to run, you don't have to!

The body stores excess energy from the food you eat as fat before your body uses it, along with oxygen, to fuel physical activity. Here's more good news: *Any* type of physical activity that elevates your heart rate and pumps more oxygenated blood to your working muscles can be considered a mode of cardiovascular exercise, and *any* exercise that increases oxygen consumption can help burn calories from fat. Oxygen is necessary to help convert fat into energy to fuel physical activity, and that oxygen is delivered via the cardiovascular system (your heart, lungs, and blood vessels). When performed on a regular basis, exercise that elevates the heart rate delivers a number of well-established health benefits, including enhanced cardiac efficiency (the ability to move blood around the body), increased mitochondrial density, a reduced risk of developing heart disease, lower cholesterol, and reduced excess body fat—all of which can help improve your overall quality of life (Haff and Triplett 2015; Taylor and Johnson 2008).

To help put this type of exercise into perspective, it's important to provide some clarification about terms. *Cardiovascular* refers to the heart pumping oxygenated blood to the working muscles as well as pumping deoxygenated blood back to the heart. *Cardiorespiratory* refers to how the lungs place oxygen in the bloodstream before the heart pumps the oxygenated blood to the working muscles. Whichever definition you choose, the term *cardio* usually refers to a mode of exercise where the main focus is to improve the function of the heart and lungs to do their job of placing oxygen in the blood (as well as the opposite function of removing carbon dioxide) and moving it around the body. While not incorrect, *cardio* is yet another incomplete way to describe what is happening in the body during exercise—delivering oxygen to the working muscles in your body. It's more appropriate to use the term *metabolic conditioning* to refer to exercise that's done for the purposes of burning calories or improving the ability to sustain physical work for longer periods of time. This conditioning helps your body become more efficient at the process of metabolizing energy from the macronutrients in your diet in order to fuel the muscle contractions required for physical activity.

Understanding Your Metabolism

Your body's metabolism is responsible for converting the food you eat into the fuel your body uses for functions such as tissue repair, digestion, and physical activity. The most important outcome of metabolic conditioning is that your body develops the ability to produce and use adenosine triphosphate (ATP), the chemical that fuels muscle contractions, more efficiently. Skeletal muscle is where fat and carbohydrates are converted into the ATP required to fuel muscle contractions. Fat requires oxygen to be turned into ATP, while carbohydrates, transported in blood as glucose or stored in muscle and the liver as glycogen, can be converted to ATP either with or without oxygen.

The amount of muscle you have is one component of the body's resting metabolic rate (RMR), which is the amount of energy your body uses to support the function of organs and physiological systems. The RMR accounts for approximately 60 to 75 percent of your total daily energy expenditure (TDEE). The thermic effect of physical activity (TEPA) is the amount of energy your body expends during both exercise and normal activity throughout your day, and is responsible for approximately 15 to 30 percent of your TDEE. After a workout, your muscles use energy to repair themselves; we commonly call this excess postexercise oxygen consumption (EPOC), and the process helps skeletal muscle remain active for up to 24 hours after a workout. If you don't use your muscles regularly, you will experience a gradual loss of muscle. It's a natural thing, but the bad news is that this muscle loss can lower the RMR and reduce your body's ability to use energy, and that energy could be stored as fat. That means that it becomes harder and harder to maintain a healthy weight or even to move comfortably as you get older because your muscles aren't using as much energy.

So, what can you do to combat age-related muscle loss? Circuits featuring resistance training exercises can increase lean muscle mass, decrease fat mass, and raise the RMR, creating an effective solution to sarcopenia, the loss of lean muscle mass during the aging process (Alcaraz et al. 2010). While you can't guarantee specific results from a resistance training program, research shows that individuals who regularly participate in resistance training for the purpose of increasing lean muscle mass can improve the body's ability to produce and use energy.

Whatever you call it, exercise for the purpose of weight loss can be unpleasant and arduous work. It is no fun to go to a health club only to wait in line for a piece of equipment so you can do an activity that you don't necessarily enjoy. There is a reason why fitness equipment manufacturers integrate TVs into their equipment: It's to distract you from what you're doing. Even if you like to run or bike outside, it can be difficult to make the time to get outside for exercise. Or, to save travel time and hassle, you may like the idea of having a piece of cardio equipment for use at home, but that may not be an option because of finances or space or a combination of the two. If spending an excessive amount of time on a machine literally running in place is not your idea of fun or if you live in an area with an extreme environment that makes outdoor exercise unpleasant, there is good news. You have another solution for doing metabolic conditioning: circuit training. It can be an effective strategy for metabolic conditioning because it can help increase the amount of lean muscle mass as well as helping your body become more effective at producing and using energy for exercise. Learning how to create exercise circuits using a single piece of fitness equipment can help you do metabolic conditioning workouts that save time and, because they are over relatively quick, are more bearable than lengthy bouts of traditional exercise (Alcaraz et al. 2010).

EPOC

Circuit training can be an effective means of elevating the EPOC, allowing the body to continue burning calories after the cessation of the training session. The body is most efficient at producing ATP through aerobic metabolism. At higher intensities, when energy is needed immediately, the anaerobic pathways can provide the necessary ATP much more quickly. This is why we can only sustain high-intensity activity for a brief period of time. We simply run out of energy! As the research on high-intensity interval training (HIIT) indicates, EPOC is also influenced by the intensity of exercise and not necessarily the duration. During EPOC, the body uses oxygen to restore muscle glycogen and help rebuild muscle proteins damaged during exercise. Even after a HIIT workout is over, the body will continue to use the aerobic energy pathway to replace the ATP consumed during the workout, enhancing the EPOC effect (Borsheim and Bahr 2003). Table 5.1 provides an illustration of how different metabolic pathways burn energy.

One way to get results from your workouts is to exercise at an intensity that can maximize the EPOC effect. Admittedly, there is some debate about the significance of the EPOC effect for the average exercise participant because the high-intensity exercise required for EPOC can be extremely challenging for many people. However, if you want results and are up for the challenge, increasing the intensity of your workouts by completing more repetitions, taking shorter rest intervals, or moving at a faster pace may be worth the effort. Remember that HIIT places a higher stress load on the body, meaning that it is extremely important to allow at least 48 hours of recovery time between high-intensity exercise sessions. Limit yourself to no more than three strenuous workouts like this per week.

Circuit Training and HIIT

In general, circuit training involves doing a series of exercises for specific body parts or executing a series of movement patterns with little to no rest between each one. For best results, an exercise circuit should alternate between upper- and lower-body muscles or between movement patterns like moving from push-ups to rows to step-ups or from squats to overhead presses to lateral lunges. Knowing how to use a single piece of equipment, such as a medicine ball, for circuit training can deliver the benefits of metabolic conditioning without having to perform a repetitive motion such as running that could lead to an overuse injury. Most importantly, performing exercise circuits with only one piece of fitness equipment can give you

Table 5.1 Descriptions of the Metabolic Pathways and How They Produce ATP

Exercise intensity(RPE)	Metabolic pathway	Benefit for my body
1-5*	Aerobic respiration	This pathway converts free fatty acids (FFA) into ATP in the presence of oxygen. There really is a fat-burning zone. *Lipolysis* is the technical term for the process of converting fat cells (triglycerides) into FFAs, which are then converted to ATP in the mitochondria of muscle cells; 1 FFA molecule can yield 129 ATP. At rest and lower-intensity activity, this is the primary energy pathway; however, it is not efficient for producing ATP for moderate- to high-intensity activity. This pathway provides ATP for low- to moderate-intensity exercise for an extended period of time. This energy pathway does not require an extended amount of time to rest between aerobic bouts of exercise.
6-8*	Aerobic glycolysis	This pathway is the process of converting glycogen to ATP with the use of oxygen; 1 molecule of glycogen can yield 38 molecules of ATP. Pyruvate, the byproduct of aerobic glycolysis, is then used to help fuel aerobic respiration. It can provide ATP for moderate-intensity exercise for 1-4 minutes. In order to allow a full recovery between work intervals, this pathway requires a rest-to-work ratio of 30 seconds to 3 minutes for every 1 minute of work. When starting to exercise at this intensity, use a longer rest interval. As your fitness level improves, gradually reduce the rest interval. For example, if you work to the point of being out of breath at the end of 1 minute, you will want to rest for 3 minutes for an optimal recovery; gradually reduce the amount of rest time from 3 minutes down to 30 seconds.
7-9*	Anaerobic glycolysis	Converts 1 molecule of glycogen into 3 molecules of ATP *without* oxygen. A byproduct of anaerobic glycolysis is an accumulation of lactate and hydrogen ions (H++), causing blood to become acidic; the burning feeling in your muscles during HIIT is an accumulation of H++. Recovery intervals are essential to allow for removal of H++ and replenishment of muscle glycogen. Too much exercise without proper recovery could lead to the use of protein for fuel instead of carbohydrate, meaning that less protein will be available to repair muscle damage. When exercising at this intensity, you should expect to be almost out of breath in approximately 30 seconds. In order to allow optimal recovery between work intervals, this energy pathway requires a rest-to-work ratio of 1 to 2 minutes for every 30 seconds of extremely hard effort. When starting to exercise at this intensity, use a longer interval for optimal recovery. As your fitness level improves, gradually reduce the length of the recovery interval. For example, if you become out of breath in 30 seconds, you will want to rest for 2 minutes; gradually reduce the rest interval down to 1 minute.
9-10*	Phosphocreatine (ATP-PC)	When a muscle needs energy immediately, it will use the ATP and phosphocreatine (PC) stored in the cells to fuel high-intensity activity without the need for oxygen. Splitting ATP into adenosine diphosphate and inorganic phosphate (ADP and Pi, respectively) produces approximately 7 calories of energy and releases H++. Due to the finite amounts of ATP and PC store in muscle cells, this system is limited to short durations of exercise lasting less than 20 seconds. During HIIT, the role of a rest or active recovery interval is to allow the muscle to remove the metabolic waste created by splitting ATP and to replace what was used during the exercise. When exercising at this intensity, you can expect to be completely out of breath in 30 seconds. This pathway requires a longer rest interval for a complete recovery. For every 30 seconds of work that leaves you breathless, rest at least 90 seconds to 2.5 minutes. When starting to exercise at this intensity, use a longer interval for optimal recovery, as your fitness level improves, gradually reduce the length of the recovery interval. For example, if you become completely out of breath in 30 seconds, rest for 2.5 minutes (150 seconds); gradually reduce the rest interval to 90 seconds.

* There is not an exact intensity when the body will transition from using one metabolic process to the next. Through consistently progressive exercise the body can become extremely efficient at tolerating higher exercise intensity while using a particular energy pathway. For example, someone can be working really hard, but due to his fitness level may be producing energy through anaerobic glycolysis as opposed to the ATP-PC pathway.

numerous options for exercising at home, at your favorite fitness facility, or in an underequipped hotel fitness center when traveling. One often-overlooked benefit of circuit training is that it uses all of the muscles in your body at the same time, while most modes of cardio training involve primarily lower-body muscles.

The most limited resource we have is time; there never seems to be enough of it to do the things that we *want* to do, let alone to do the things we *need* to do, like exercise. Having an extremely efficient way to exercise that can be done in a relatively short amount of time can help you make it a regular habit, and that's where HIIT becomes an important strategy.

HIIT is a system of organizing metabolic conditioning featuring short durations of extremely challenging activity followed by brief periods of recovery. Using a scale of 1 to 10, where 10 is the hardest exercise you can perform, HIIT work intervals should be between an 8 and 10, while the recovery intervals should be between a 4 and 6. The time period for HIIT work intervals can be as short as 10 seconds or as long as 60; the longer the work interval, the greater the level of fatigue, which requires a longer recovery period. A typical HIIT workout might feature work intervals for a period of 30 seconds followed by 30-to-60-second periods of active recovery. According to research conducted by Dr. Martin Gibala, the intensity of each bout of exercise is more important than the duration (Gibala 2017; Gibala and McGee 2008). The benefit of HIIT is that you don't need to exercise for a significant amount of time as long as the exercise you do includes periods of extremely challenging activity.

The intensity of circuit training can be progressive, making it an extremely effective format for HIIT workouts. One way of using circuit training for higher-intensity workouts is by alternating between easy, moderate, and hard exercises; a high-intensity exercise that leaves you breathless can be followed by a lower-intensity exercise that allows you to regain control of your breathing before challenging it again with the next exercise.

Doing repetitions for a set amount of time is another way to modify circuit training for HIIT. Instead of doing a certain number of reps, set a timer for 20 to 40 seconds and see how many reps you can complete in that time interval before moving on to the next exercise.

Yet another option is to determine a number of reps for each exercise, such as 10, then set a timer for a period of time—say, 15 minutes—and see how many times you can complete the circuit doing 10 reps of each exercise in the time allotted.

As you can see, circuit training provides many options for adjusting the intensity of metabolic conditioning workouts. Because circuit training transitions from one exercise to the next with minimal rest time, all exercise circuits can be considered a form of metabolic conditioning. However, not all circuit training is HIIT. It is the intensity that determines a HIIT program, not the individual exercises or the overall structure of the workout. When starting an exercise program, it may be necessary to take a little rest break of 15 to 30 seconds between each exercise in a circuit. However, as your body adapts to the intensity of the exercises, you can simply adjust one or two variables, such as increasing the number of repetitions or reducing the length of the rest interval, to make the workout more challenging. Think of it this way: If you only have a limited amount of time to invest in a workout, exercise circuits built around HIIT can provide one of the best returns on your investment. Or, if you want to exercise but aren't interested in crushing yourself, you can reduce the stress load by reducing the number of reps or taking longer rest breaks while still getting the benefits of being physically active.

Circuit training can be made more challenging and metabolically demanding by using heavy weights, moving quickly to perform a number of reps in a short period of time, or taking no rest breaks between individual exercises. Circuit training can also be made less intense by performing mobility exercises at a slower pace with longer break periods between each individual exercise.

Here are four reasons why exercise circuits based on HIIT can be an extremely efficient strategy for metabolic conditioning, allowing you to perform the most effective workout for your needs (Gibala 2017).

1. You have a busy schedule, which limits your training time. HIIT workouts can be done in 30 minutes or less, making them extremely effective for producing results in a limited amount of time.

2. You have been following the same cardio workout routine for a long time and have plateaued. Using an exercise circuit based on HIIT could give your program a significant boost by increasing the intensity so that you continue experiencing results.

3. You are exercising for weight loss. HIIT can help you burn more calories in a shorter period of time, along with providing an EPOC effect to help you continue expending energy even after the workout is over.

4. You like it. The best exercise in the world is the one you enjoy and will do on a regular basis. If HIIT works for you, go for it and have fun, but make sure you allow time for appropriate recovery because that's when the real results happen.

One significant benefit of using circuit training for HIIT instead of traditional exercises such as running or cardio machines is that it can reduce the risk of developing repetitive stress injuries, which can occur as a result of high-volume training. An indicator of the effectiveness of both circuit training and HIIT is the fact that various branches of the US military have recently rewritten guidelines for physical fitness to move away from long-distance running in favor of shorter, higher-intensity intervals of various types of exercise, including strength training with external resistance and traditional bodyweight calisthenics, performed in a circuit (US Army 2012; Heinrich et al. 2012). If the US military changes its procedures to focus on conditioning through HIIT exercise circuits, you can trust that it can be effective for your workouts as well.

HIIT can be extremely effective, but should not be a starting point for your workouts. Instead, it is a goal to work toward as your fitness level improves and you find yourself participating in exercise more frequently. Before jumping right into a metabolic conditioning workout program, it is a good idea to focus first on lower-intensity exercise like mobility training. Yes, your goals are important, but it's necessary to understand that *the* single most important thing about exercise is that consistency comes before intensity.

Before doing the challenging metabolic conditioning workouts that can deliver results, it is helpful to first learn how to move better; this can help you reach your goals with a reduced risk of injury. Your initial goal should be to complete two or three mobility workouts a week for a period of at least four to six weeks before increasing the level of difficulty and progressing to metabolic conditioning. This will do three things: (1) It will allow your body an appropriate amount of time to properly adapt to the physical stresses from exercise, (2) Focusing on mobility training before increasing intensity to metabolic conditioning will help you learn how to perform the foundational movements reflexively; the better your movement skill, the lower

What the Science Says:
The Danger of Emphasizing Duration Over Intensity

High-intensity workout programs are popular and here to stay because they're both dynamically challenging and extremely effective, helping many people achieve a variety of results, from weight loss to muscle growth. Research has found that performing only a few minutes of high-intensity work intervals can provide improvements similar to longer periods of lower-intensity cardiorespiratory exercise (Gibala and McGill 2008; Boutcher 2011).

HIIT does expend more calories per minute when compared to steady-state training. However, performing HIIT or exercising at a moderate to high intensity (where breathing is much faster than normal and saying more than a couple words at a time can be difficult) for more than 50 or 60 minutes at a time can be inefficient and, rather than burning calories from fat or carbohydrates, it could lead to the loss of muscle protein. Your muscles and liver only store a limited amount of carbohydrate as glycogen. Once it is no longer available as an energy source, the cortisol hormone initiates a process called gluconeogenesis, stimulating the liver to convert protein into glycogen to continue to fuel activity. When protein is used as a source of fuel, it is not available to repair the proteins damaged during exercise.

When doing HIIT circuits, focus on work intervals at an RPE of 7 to 10 and allow your breathing to return to almost normal during the active rest between circuits. Limit your metabolic conditioning to periods of 30 minutes or less to ensure that you are burning carbohydrates or fats and leaving protein to be used for the postexercise repair process.

the risk of injury as you increase the intensity of your workouts, and (3) It will help you make exercise a consistent habit. Once you are exercising on a regular basis, *then* you can begin to increase the intensity to help burn more calories.

Rest Intervals and Recovery

Intense exercise does produce results. Keep in mind that there is a very limited amount of fuel stored in your muscles, which is why the highest-intensity activities can only last for a short period of time before fatigue. The recovery period between exercise circuits should be long enough to allow for at least partial replenishment of that fuel. Full restoration can take up to 3 minutes, but resting for 60 to 90 seconds should provide for approximately 80 percent of ATP replacement. So, if you want to maximize the work you do within a single workout, you really do need to allow for rest intervals so your body is ready to give full effort again.

During the rest and recovery period between workouts, the body will shift to an anabolic state to repair damaged muscle proteins, as well as replace the muscle glycogen converted to ATP during the exercise session. To reduce the risk of an overuse injury and to give your body the time to produce the hormones that increase lean muscle mass, it is necessary to allow for proper recovery between workouts. Generally speaking, it is a good idea to limit the amount of HIIT you do to three sessions or less per week, with at least one full day between extremely challenging workouts. This simple step can help you move closer toward your goals.

By their very nature, HIIT workouts are designed to push you to your physical limits where you're constantly sweating, out of breath, and feeling downright uncomfortable. As fitness instructors often say, "If it doesn't challenge you, it won't change you." The reality is that our fitness improves *after* the workout, not during it. If we are constantly hammering as hard as we can with every workout, we are not allowing our bodies the necessary time to experience optimal recovery.

This doesn't mean you do nothing the day after a HIIT workout. Instead, you should plan on doing a lower-intensity mobility or core training workout. Mobility training can help with the active recovery from harder, more challenging workouts because it can help with the repair and recovery process. The lower-intensity mobility workouts (around 4-5 RPE) can help remove metabolic waste while delivering the nutrients that can help repair the muscles used in the previous day's workout. You may be a little sore from that hard workout, but that's when it's important to do some lower-intensity mobility training to help your body fully recovery. Once you push through the initial discomfort, you will feel much better by the end of that active recovery workout. The best thing is that you'll have the ability to go back and hit it hard again in your next workout, assuming you do other things for your recovery like fuel, hydrate, and rest properly.

Energy Use

When you first start to exercise, your body uses the anaerobic energy pathways and stored ATP to provide the energy for that activity. A proper warm-up is important because it can take about five to eight minutes to be able to efficiently use aerobic metabolism to produce the ATP necessary to sustain physical activity (see table 5.2).

What the Science Says: Rate of Perceived Exertion

Wearing a heart rate monitor or activity tracker is one way to monitor how hard you work during exercise, but an easier way that doesn't require an investment in technology is the use of the rate of perceived exertion (RPE). The easiest way to use RPE is with a scale of 1 to 10, where 1 is the amount of effort it takes to sit on the couch (not much) and 10 is the amount of effort it takes to run for your life (the hardest you are able to work).

RPE	Description	% of maximum effort (estimated)
1-2	The amount of effort it takes to remain in a sedentary position or perform a few easy ADLs.	10-20%
3-4	The amount of effort it takes to walk or stroll at a comfortable pace.	20-40%
4-5	The amount of effort it takes to walk at a fast pace or jog at a relatively slow pace.	30-50%
5-6	The amount of effort it takes to run at a comfortable pace for an extended period of time. Relies on aerobic metabolism to fuel activity.	40-60%
6-8	The amount of effort it takes to run at a hard pace for brief periods of time or relatively short distances. This is the intensity where the working muscles will start using anaerobic metabolism to produce ATP.	50-80%
9-10	The hardest amount of work you are able to perform—for example, running at an all-out sprint for a short distance or brief period of time. Relies on anaerobic metabolism; ATP will deplete rapidly requiring a recovery interval.	80-100%

Table 5.2   **Using Interval Training to Train Specific Energy Systems**

% of maximum power	Primary system stressed	Typical exercise time	Range of work-to-rest period ratios
90-100	Phosphagen	5-10 sec	1:12 to 1:20
75-90	Fast glycolysis	15-30 sec	1:3 to 1:5
30-75	Fast glycolysis and oxidative	1-3 min	1:3 to 1:4
20-30	Oxidative	>3 min	1:1 to 1:3

Reprinted by permission from T.J. Herda and J.T. Cramer, "Bioenergetics of Exercise and Training." In *Essentials of Strength Training and Conditioning*, 4th ed., edited by G.G. Haff and N.T. Triplett for the National Strength and Conditioning Association (Champaign, IL: Human Kinetics, 2016), 60.

Once a steady state of oxygen consumption is achieved, the aerobic energy pathways are able to provide most of the ATP needed for the workout. During periods of moderate- to high-intensity exercise when ATP is needed rapidly, the muscles involved in exercise will rely on either glycolysis or ATP-PC, where the PC is phosphocreatine that combines with ADP (adenosine diphosphate) to produce energy, known as ATP. Once those stores are diminished, fatigue will occur.

Have you ever heard of the term *skinny-fat*? That sounds like a complete oxymoron, but it does indeed describe what can happen as the result of too much HIIT, an inadequate supply of nutrition, and not enough recovery time between workouts. During moderate- to high-intensity exercise, the body will deplete the amount of glycogen available for ATP. The rest intervals in HIIT are essential because that is when muscles will replace the energy spent during the previous exercise interval. If not enough time is allowed for full replenishment of the glycogen used during a high-intensity interval, the body will begin using protein for fuel. Gluconeogenesis is the process by which the body uses amino acids to create ATP. When amino acids are used for energy, it reduces the amount available to repair damaged muscle proteins; therefore, muscle growth from HIIT is severely hampered. This is also why eating carbohydrates after a high-intensity workout is important: The carbs from your diet will be used to replace spent muscle glycogen so that you have a full tank of energy during your next hard workout. In addition, this is why it's a good idea to wait at least 48 hours between really hard, gut-busting workouts. You want to ensure a completely adequate supply of energy so that your body can use protein for repairing muscle tissue, not energy.

Metabolic Conditioning = Muscle Growth

Here is some good news, or bad news depending on your point of view: Exercise alone does not induce muscle growth. For muscle growth to occur, your body needs to experience at least one of three different conditions: metabolic or mechanical stress, more efficient glycogen storage, and stimulation of type II muscle fibers. Here, we'll look at each of these conditions and explain how they help you reach your goals.

First, if you want to increase your lean muscle mass, the exercise you do must be challenging enough to create metabolic or mechanical fatigue in order to increase the amount of lean muscle. So, if your training doesn't fatigue the muscles, you won't help those muscles grow. Let's explore how to apply the training stress in the right way to get the most out of your workout program.

Table 5.1 explains that when you exercise at the level where your body is using anaerobic glycolysis, you produce lactate and hydrogen ions (H++) as by-products of metabolic stress. The buildup of H++ is what makes you feel the burn, which is an indication that you are reaching a lactate threshold—i.e., that your blood contains more acidity and you're not going to be able to generate as much energy until your body systems get rid of those by-products of high-intensity movement. This is your sign that it's time for a lower-intensity, active-recovery interval. HIIT, in the form of circuit training, can train your body on how to tolerate working at that threshold, as well as improve your body's ability to quickly remove lactate and other metabolic waste. Metabolic stress induced by HIIT is an effective component of developing lean muscle; an exhaustive review of the research literature on training for muscle growth observed that high levels of metabolic stress can indeed lead to muscle growth (Schoenfeld 2010).

Mechanical stress, on the other hand, refers to the physical forces applied to muscle fibers. HIIT and resistance training damage the individual actin and myosin protein strands of muscle tissue, which, in turn, signal the biochemical reaction to produce new satellite cells responsible for repairing the mechanical structures via new proteins. This is one way in which exercise to the point of momentary muscle fatigue initiates muscle growth.

Like metabolic stress, mechanical stress is an important and essential stimulus for creating exercise-induced muscle growth. Similar to the age-old quandary of which came first, the chicken or the egg, we're not sure which plays a greater role in muscle growth. Both occur simultaneously, making it difficult for researchers to identify which has more influence on muscle growth. However, we do know that exercising to the point of momentary fatigue combined with short rest intervals can create both the mechanical and metabolic stimulus that could lead to muscle growth.

Determining the right type and amount of metabolic or mechanical stimulus for your needs will take some trial and error. While both result in muscle growth, the fact is that metabolic and mechanical stress can also cause muscle soreness. A moderate- to high-intensity workout should leave you slightly fatigued by the end; you don't want to be completely wasted, but you definitely want to feel like it would be tough to continue exercising at the same level of intensity. The day after a properly challenging workout should leave you feeling like you exercised the day before; you don't want to feel any extreme soreness or pain—that is an indication that you did too much work or damaged some tissue—but you definitely want to feel the muscles that you used during the workout. If you do feel any pain, it will be important to rest for a couple of days, and if it continues, it may be necessary to check with a medical professional to make sure that nothing is injured.

Besides stimulating the production of the hormones responsible for muscle repair, a second way that high-intensity, physically challenging exercise creates muscle growth is due to the amount of muscle glycogen used for ATP production. Exercise to the point of fatigue will deplete the amount of glycogen in muscle cells. As a result, the muscle cells will become more efficient at storing glycogen for future use. Glycogen storage provides necessary energy, which can help you sustain longer bouts of exercise: You improve your endurance. It's important to note that when it's stored in muscle tissue, one gram of glycogen holds approximately three to four grams of water. As your muscle cells adapt to store more glycogen, they will also store more water, leading to an increase in size (Schoenfeld 2013).

The third way that metabolic conditioning produces muscle growth is by stimulating the type II motor units and muscle fibers responsible for fast, high-velocity movements. Dynamic, power-based movements use primarily type II muscle fibers because of the requirement for immediate energy from anaerobic sources. Exercises such as jumps, medicine ball throws, and kettlebell lifts like the swing, clean, or push press maximize the power output of your muscles. The end result of a metabolic conditioning workout featuring power exercises is that you get results you can see. For example, consider sprinters who train to be as fast as possible when running 100- or 200-meter races. Sprinting requires fast, power-based muscle actions, leading to activating more type II fibers, ultimately resulting in sprinters having lean, muscular physiques.

To optimize your aerobic efficiency during exercise, you should try to work at an intensity where your breathing is quick but under control, and you can talk without too much difficulty. On a scale of 1 to 10, where 10 is the hardest, this would be about 5 or 6. Staying at this intensity means that you will optimize your aerobic efficiency instead of simply trying to work as hard as possible.

What the Science Says: Talk Test

You can easily determine the appropriate intensity for your metabolic conditioning workouts by using the talk test. When you can talk comfortably during exercise, you are working at an intensity where your aerobic energy system is using oxygen to help metabolize fat into ATP to fuel muscle activity. As the intensity of exercise increases, your energy demands become more immediate and your body will start using glycogen stored in the muscle cells to supply energy. As your work rate increases, your body needs more oxygen and, because it's burning more carbohydrate, it is expiring (breathing out) more carbon dioxide, causing your breathing rate to increase, which limits your ability to talk. To ensure that you are doing enough exercise to burn a significant number of calories when you are doing your metabolic conditioning circuits, you want to make sure you are moving at an intensity that makes talking, or saying more than a few words at a time, difficult. At the end of the circuit you should take a long enough rest that allows you to regain control of your breathing (and your ability to speak). As you progressively increase the intensity to do more interval training, the exercises (work intervals) should be hard enough to leave you almost breathless, or, at the very least, unable to say more than a couple words. During the recovery period, you want to focus on getting your breathing back under control. Once you feel that you can talk comfortably again, guess what. It's time to get back to work!

What the Science Says:
Using Fitness Trackers to Measure Intensity

In the story of Goldilocks and the three bears, Goldilocks found that Papa Bear's porridge was too hot, Mama Bear's was too cold, but that Baby Bear's was just right. This is how many people approach cardiovascular exercise: Some people are Papa Bear and exercise at too high of an intensity. Others are Mama Bear and don't work hard enough. The smart ones, like Baby Bear, are training at the appropriate intensity for their needs.

Knowing how to measure and use your heart rate could help you get the best results from your exercise program. Here are a few considerations for how to use heart rate to identify the most appropriate exercise intensity for your needs.

First, invest in a heart rate monitor. If you are serious about your fitness, wearing a monitor can help ensure that you're training at the right intensity to reach your goals. The most affordable monitors will only measure your heart rate during exercise, while the most expensive models can include a GPS system to track your distance covered, measure calories burned during a workout (it's an estimate determined by an algorithm based on age, weight, gender, and heart rate), as well as connect with mobile apps to store all of your training information in a central location.

There are different types of monitors. Some use a strap around your chest to read the frequency of your heart rate and then send that information to a watch, allowing you to see the heart beat in real time. A second kind can be worn on the wrist without any need for a strap. There is a slightly larger margin of error for a monitor worn on your wrist, but wearing a strap around the chest can be uncomfortable.

The benefit of using a fitness tracker is that you can monitor your heart rate so you know exactly how hard you are working during a hard exercise interval and whether you have recovered during the rest period. Watching your heart rate rise and fall helps you understand how hard you can exercise during a work interval and how quickly you recover during the rest period. The fitter you are, the faster you can recover between individual work intervals; a tracker can help you monitor the process of shortening your recovery times.

Metabolic Conditioning Workouts

The primary purpose of metabolic conditioning is to improve your body's ability to produce and use energy to fuel muscle activity during exercise. Another purpose is to burn calories to either remove excess energy from the body (fat is stored energy) or to maintain a healthy body weight. These workouts are designed to be performed as circuits where you move from one exercise to the next with minimal time in between; the rest period occurs once all exercises are completed. A countdown timer is necessary to help you monitor the length of each exercise.

The initial goal of these circuit workouts is to simply move at a consistent pace for the entire duration of the interval, which should begin with 25 seconds. As your fitness level improves, add more time to the interval; specifically, add 5 seconds every 2 to 3 weeks until you are doing intervals for 45 seconds at a time. In addition, exercise is no fun unless you're able to quantify your progress. Therefore, start counting how many reps you do during each set, especially the first time through the circuit. Your goal for the next times through the circuit is to meet or beat your initial number. This can be helpful for challenging yourself from workout to workout. For example, the first time through the kettlebell metabolic conditioning circuit, you may only perform 12 reps in 25 seconds, but before long you will be able to do 15 to 20 reps, a significant improvement. Start by completing two circuits. As you feel yourself getting stronger, feel free to add additional circuits. The end goal for each of these workouts is to reach a point where you are doing exercises for 45-second intervals for a total of 5 circuits.

Two ways to modify circuit training are to increase intensity by doing reps for time and to complete as many circuits as possible in a given period of time. Other ways to make metabolic conditioning programs more challenging will be addressed in chapter 6. For easier reference, flip to the green-colored tabs on the sides of the pages to help you quickly identify the metabolic conditioning exercises in this book.

BODYWEIGHT EXERCISES FOR METABOLIC CONDITIONING

The primary benefits of bodyweight exercises are that no time is lost switching weights or moving from machine to machine. Heck, you don't even need to be in a gym, making this workout an excellent option if you travel frequently. Simply find 8 to 10 square feet of floor space and you have all you need to perform a metabolic conditioning circuit of bodyweight exercises. Use a countdown timer set to 25 seconds. Your goal is to do as many repetitions as possible in 25 seconds. Transition from one exercise to the next with minimal rest in between. Once you have completed all exercises, rest for 60 to 90 seconds, then repeat the circuit. Start with 1 to 2 circuits and gradually progress (every 2 weeks or so) to 5 circuits. Once you are doing 4 or 5 circuits, increase the length of time from 25 to 30 seconds. Add 5 seconds to each exercise every 2 weeks up until you're doing sets of 45 seconds. As you feel yourself getting stronger, keep track of the number of reps you do during your first time through the circuit, and then try to meet or beat that number each additional time you do the exercise. Your goal is to complete as many repetitions as possible (AMRAP) during the work interval.

Exercise	Time*	Circuits+
Alternating lateral lunges with reach	25 sec	2-5
Plank to knee tap	25 sec	
Speed squats	25 sec	
Step-through	25 sec	
Rollerblader (ice skater)	25 sec	
Lateral crawling	25 sec	
Slow-motion burpee	25 sec	
Rest and recovery	45-90 sec between circuits after all exercises	

*Add 5 seconds to the work interval every 2-3 weeks until you are doing 45 seconds for each exercise.

+Once you are able to do 2 circuits of 45 seconds, start adding additional circuits until you are doing 5 circuits of 45-second intervals.

Alternating Lateral Lunges With Reach

Benefits

Lower-body exercises such as lunges and squats engage a number of large muscles, making them an excellent option for metabolic conditioning. These lateral lunges with reach will help improve hip mobility and strength, while the alternating, right-to-left movement will increase the heart rate.

Instructions

1. Start in a standing position with your feet hip-width apart. Step directly to your left. Keep your left foot parallel to your right as it hits the ground, and push your left hip back as you reach for the left foot with the right hand. (This motion helps engage the glutes.)
2. To return to standing, pull back with your right arm and push your left foot into the floor while pressing your right foot into the ground to pull yourself up with your right inner thigh muscles.
3. Alternate legs, reaching across the body to touch the foot each time. Your goal is to alternate to each side for the duration of the work interval.

Correct Your Form

- Reaching for your foot with the opposite hand increases the load on the hip, helping you activate more of your gluteal muscles.
- Reach to your knee or in front of your knee if you can't reach all the way to your foot.
- When placing your foot on the floor (the left foot in the instructions), make sure both feet are parallel and pointing in the same direction.

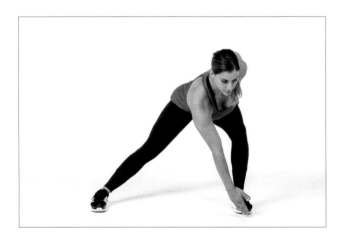

Plank to Knee Tap

Benefits

High planks help improve arm, shoulder, and upper-back strength. Adding movement like a hip hinge to knee tap requires muscles to do more work during the exercise, which helps increase energy expenditure. This variation of a plank is also great for core strength, and pressing into the ground with one arm while reaching for the opposite leg with the other arm can help improve shoulder strength.

Instructions

1. Start in a high plank position (the up position of a push-up) with your hands directly under your shoulders and your elbows rotated to point back toward your feet. Push your hands into the ground and upper back upwards into the shoulder blades to increase stability.
2. Lift both hips into the air (like the yoga pose downward facing dog). Push your left hand into the ground as you reach for your left knee with your right hand. Pull your hand back and place it back on the floor, then alternate so your left hand reaches for your right knee.
3. Your goal is to alternate to each knee for the duration of the work interval.

Correct Your Form

- If you find it hard to keep moving during the entire duration of the work interval, just focus on holding the high plank.
- To increase stability with the one hand on the ground (the left hand in the instructions), think about pushing the floor away from you while pressing the tops of your toes into the ground.

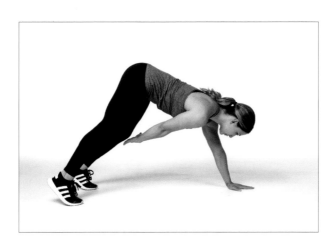

Speed Squats

Benefits

Moving at a faster pace requires the muscles to work harder while also improving the resiliency and strength of the fascia and elastic connective tissues that surround each joint.

Instructions

1. Stand with your feet approximately shoulder-width apart and your arms hanging down along the side of your body. Keep your spine long and straight and push your hips back to begin the lowering phase of a squat. As your body sinks lower, raise your hands to reach in front of you at approximately waist height.
2. Continue to push your hips back while lifting your arms and keep your chest raised as you descend to a comfortable depth with your hips. To return to standing, push both feet into the floor and your hips forward as you pull your arms back to the sides of your body.

Correct Your Form

- If you feel your knees becoming sore, emphasize the motion from your hips by pushing your tailbone behind you as you lower into the squat.
- Keep your spine long during both phases of the movement to ensure that the movement is coming from the hips, not the spine.

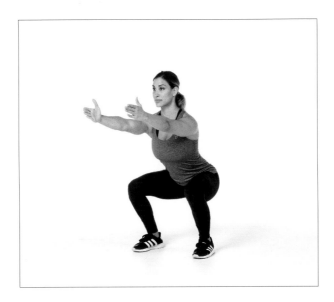

Step-Through

Benefits

Holding your bodyweight with only one arm and foot while completing the movement requires a significant amount of energy from the working muscles. This move may look easy, but it will get your heart rate up while strengthening your arm, shoulder, and core muscles.

Instructions

1. Start in a quadruped position with your hands directly under your shoulders and the tops of your toes on the ground, keeping your knees off the ground.

2. Pick up your left arm and pull it back as you rotate on your right shoulder and kick your right leg across your body. Pause for a moment, then rotate back to place your left hand and right foot on the floor before rotating to the other side by pulling your right hand back and kicking your left leg across your body so that your left hand and right foot are the only points of contact on the ground.

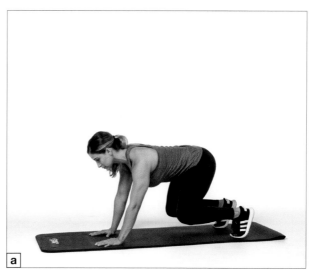

Correct Your Form

- If you feel your wrists getting sore while rotating, focus on just holding the position on your hands and toes for the duration of the work interval.

- Pressing your hand into the ground and squeezing the arm in the air (the left arm in the instructions) will help you maintain stability during the exercise.

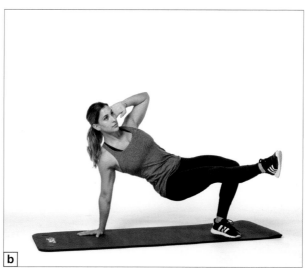

Rollerblader (Ice Skater)

Benefits

This exercise, also known as *ice skaters*, depending on where you're from, consists of lateral, side-to-side movement, which is both relatively easy and fun to do. Because it uses the larger muscles of the upper thighs, it is extremely efficient at elevating your heart rate and burning calories.

Instructions

1. Stand with both feet under your hips. Pick your left foot up off of the floor as you explosively press your right foot into the ground to initiate the jump to your left.

2. The ball of your left foot should be the first point of contact to hit the ground. Land on the ball of your foot and allow your heel to roll all the way down to touch the floor. As you do, push your left hip back so that the larger hip and thigh muscles are doing most of the work to decelerate and stabilize your leg.

3. Stay on your left leg and bring your right leg close to your left before pushing off with the left foot to leap back to your right foot. Start with small jumps while moving in a slow, steady tempo; as you become stronger, increase the speed and distance.

Correct Your Form

To protect your knees make sure that you push your hip back as you land on the floor. If necessary, use the opposite hand to reach across your body at waist height. This will help activate the larger muscles of the glutes to enhance stability and control.

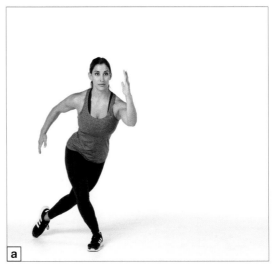

a

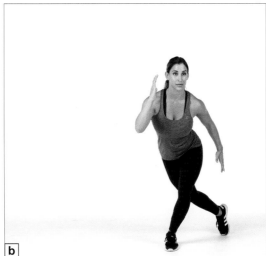

b

Lateral Crawling

Benefits

Supporting your body weight with your shoulder, leg, and core muscles requires a lot of energy; maintaining that position while moving side to side challenges your muscles to work harder, which increases overall oxygen consumption and caloric expenditure.

Instructions

1. Start in a high plank position with your hands directly under your shoulders and your arms rotated so that your elbows are pointed toward your feet.
2. To increase stability, keep your feet slightly wider than shoulder-width. Press your back upwards into your shoulder blades with your toes digging into the ground as you squeeze your thigh and glute muscles while pushing your hands into the floor.
3. Pick up your left hand and place it further to your left. Once your hand is back on the ground, pick up your left foot and move it further to the left before you bring your right leg closer to your left and your right hand back, directly under the right shoulder.
4. Move as far as you can to the left, then move back to your right. Keep moving for the duration of the work interval.
5. Start with small movements at a slow, steady tempo; as you become stronger, increase the speed and distance.

Correct Your Form

- If you feel your hips sagging, squeeze your glute and thigh muscles as you lift your tailbone up toward the ceiling.
- If you don't have much space in your exercise area, move side to side: left hand and left foot to the left side, then right hand and right foot back to the initial starting position.

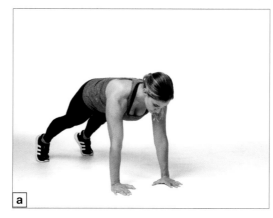

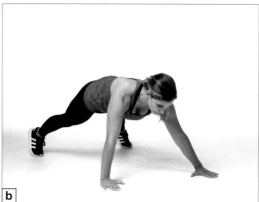

Slow-Motion Burpee

Benefits

The burpee is named after Royal Burpee, an exercise physiologist who helped the US military develop conditioning programs in the 1930s. A burpee requires a number of muscles to work together to create the movement, which burns a significant amount of calories; this explains why these are a popular exercise in many high-intensity conditioning workouts. Even though this version slows down your speed, because you use so many muscles, it is still effective for burning a lot of calories, especially if you add a small jump once you return to standing.

Instructions

1. Stand with your feet approximately shoulder-width apart, and hang your arms down along the front of your body. Keep your spine long as you push your hips back to lower yourself into a squat. As your body sinks lower, place both hands on the ground in front of you. Once you lower your hips as low as possible, start walking your hands forward to move into a full plank position. Pause at the end before walking your hands back toward your feet.

2. As your hands move back toward your body, bend your knees and drop your hips so you end of at the bottom position of a squat.

3. Pick your hands up off the ground as you raise your chest and push both feet into the floor to return to the initial standing position. (*Optional*: As you return back to the initial standing position, perform a jump at the top of the movement before descending back into a deep squat).

4. Your goal is to complete AMRAP during the work interval. As you feel yourself getting stronger, keep track of the number of reps you do during your first time through the circuit, and then try to meet or beat that number each additional time you do the exercise.

Correct Your Form

If lowering yourself into a squat is a challenge, do an inchworm by folding over at the hips to place your hands on the floor, keeping your knees slightly bent, before walking your hands out to move into a high plank position.

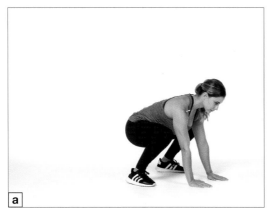

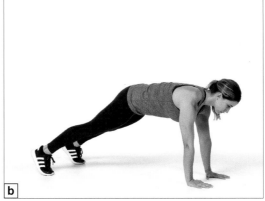

STABILITY BALL EXERCISES FOR METABOLIC CONDITIONING

Stability ball exercises create a unique physiological challenge that engages a significant number of muscles. Using more muscles during a workout increases the overall oxygen consumption and energy expenditure, which in plain English means burning more calories. To increase the number of calories burned, keep the time between each exercise as short as possible, but allow enough time at the end of the circuit to bring your breathing back under control.

When selecting a stability ball, use a 55-centimeter ball if you're 5'7" or shorter. Select a 65-centimeter ball if you're between 5'7" and 6'4". Select a 75-centimeter ball if you're taller than 6'4". The ball should be inflated until it's firm and you can sit on it so your knees and hips can comfortably hold a 90-degree bend. Your goal is to complete AMRAP during the work interval. As you feel yourself getting stronger, keep track of the number of reps you do during your first time through the circuit, and then try to meet or beat that number each additional time you do the exercise.

Exercise	Time*	Circuits+
Knee tuck	25 sec	2-5
Hip bridge to hamstring curl	25 sec	
Prone hip roll	25 sec	
Roll-out	25 sec	
Diagonal lift	25 sec	
Reverse back extension	25 sec	
Russian twist	25 sec	
Ball pass crunch	25 sec	
Rest and recovery	45-90 sec between circuits after all exercises	

*Add 5 seconds to the work interval every 2 to 3 weeks until you are doing 45 seconds for each exercise.

+Once you are able to do 2 circuits of 45 seconds, start adding additional circuits until you are doing 5 circuits of 45-second intervals.

Knee Tuck

Benefits

Knee tucks use the deep muscles of the core responsible for stabilizing the spine, upper-arm and shoulder muscles to support your body weight, and muscles that move your hips and core, making this an excellent option for both strength training and calorie burning.

Instructions

1. Face the stability ball so that your chest is on the top of the ball and your knees are on the ground.
2. Walk your hands forward until the tops of your thighs are on the ball.
3. Keep your hands directly under the shoulders and pressed into the floor throughout the exercise for the stability. Rotate your elbows back toward your feet.
4. To start the movement, lift your hips into the air as you bring your knees up toward your waist. Think about pulling in your belly button and rolling your pelvis up toward your rib cage.
5. Pause at the end of the movement before straightening your legs to return to the starting position.

Correct Your Form

- In the starting position, the closer the ball is to your hands, the more control you will have. The further the ball is from your hands, the more challenging the exercise will be.
- Start with the ball under your knees. If that's too difficult, start with the ball under your thighs.
- To enhance stability of your upper body, have your hands at least shoulder-width apart.

TIP Progress to doing a push-up to knee-tuck after 3 to 4 weeks.

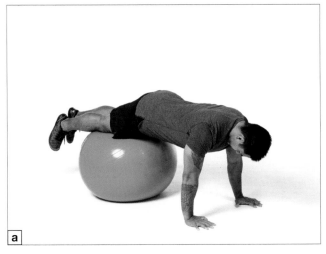
a

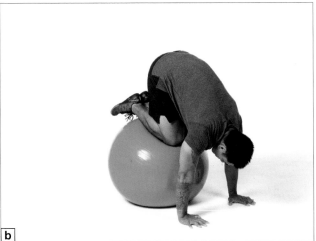
b

Hip Bridge to Hamstring Curl

Benefits

This move uses the entire posterior chain of your lower body, especially the large hip extensor muscles, including the gluteus maximus, adductor magnus, and hamstring muscles, making the exercise effective for both strength training and burning calories.

Instructions

1. Start by lying flat on your back with your arms by your side and the backs of your lower legs on top of the ball. Pull your toes up toward your shins, squeeze your glutes, and lift your hips in the air. Press both arms into the ground to create stability.
2. Once your body is in a straight line, pull your heels up to your tailbone, bringing the ball closer to your body. Slowly extend your legs back to a straight position before slowly lowering your hips to the ground.

Correct Your Form

- If you feel your calves tightening and cramping up, make sure you are pulling your toes up to your shins. This increases the length of your calf muscles, reducing the risk that they become tight during the exercise.
- If you feel a strain in your lower back, move the starting position of the ball closer to your body so the backs of your calves are resting on the top, not the heels.
- To increase stability with your hips off the ground, place your arms wider and keep them pressed into the ground.

> **TIP** As you learn the exercise, raising the hips up as you bring your heels toward your tailbone should be a single, fluid motion.

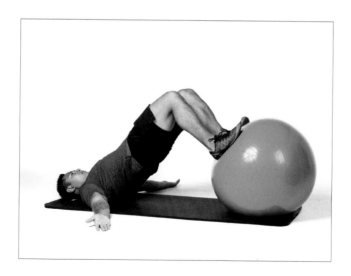

Prone Hip Roll

Benefits

This exercise is tricky to learn, but once you can easily perform it, you will notice that it helps strengthen your hip and shoulder muscles while your deep core muscles work hard to keep the spine stable.

Instructions

1. Face the stability ball so that your chest is on the top of the ball and your knees are on the ground.
2. Walk your hands forward until the tops of your lower thighs (just above your knees) are on the ball. Keep your hands directly under the shoulders and pressed into the floor throughout the exercise for the stability. Rotate your elbows back toward your feet.
3. When your thighs are on top of the ball, squeeze your legs together as though you are holding a coin in between them. To start the movement, press your hands into the ground while lifting your right hip so that the side of your left hip rolls on to the top of the ball. Pause, then roll to the other side. Pick up your left hip as the side of your right hip rolls on to the top of the ball. Alternate sides.
4. Start with 3 to 4 reps on either side, for a total of 6 to 8. As you get stronger, add 2 reps per week until you are able to do 8 to 10 reps on each side, for a total of 16 to 18.

Correct Your Form

- If you have a hard time starting the rolling movement, move the ball closer to your waist to shorten the lever arm.
- To improve the efficiency of movement, think about lifting the right hip up as you roll on to the side of your left hip. Moving from the hips is the key to the exercise.

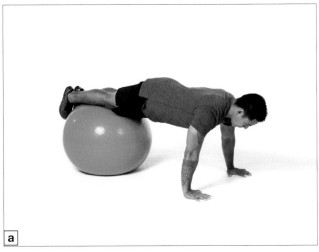

a

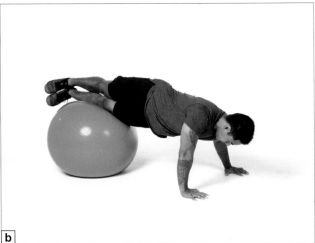

b

Roll-Out

Benefits

This move lengthens your abdominal muscles and fascia, which can be extremely effective for strengthening those tissues. Because you are using so many muscles, you will burn a lot of calories while strengthening your core.

Instructions

1. Start facing the stability ball so that your chest is close to the top of the ball. Your elbows should be directly under your shoulders. Place your knees on the ground. (It may be necessary to lay a pad or stretch mat under your knees to increase comfort.)
2. Keep your hips pressed forward so that your body remains in a straight line from your knees up to your shoulders.
3. With your elbows on the ball, fall forward as you push the ball away with your arms, and go as low as comfortably possible. To return to the starting position, shift your hips back while pulling your elbows back toward your body.

Correct Your form

If this feels uncomfortable on your back, it might be necessary to start close to the ball. Focus on keeping your spine long and extended during the exercise. Don't worry about how far forward you go; instead, go to a comfortable ROM. As you become stronger, you can start with the ball further away from you to increase the level of difficulty and the amount of force placed on the abdominals.

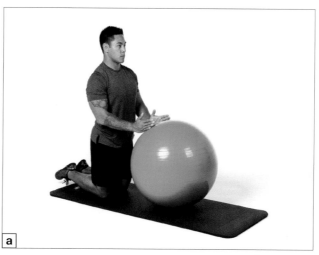

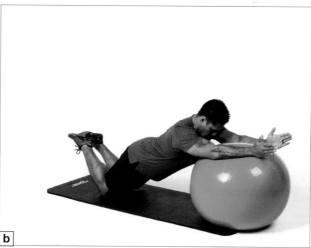

Diagonal Lift

Benefits

When humans walk, the core muscles are lengthened as the shoulders rotate over the hips. This rotational movement with a small squat is effective for strengthening the hip, core, and shoulder muscles all at the same time. Because a stability ball is relatively light, this movement can be done at a fast tempo to increase the heart rate and overall energy expenditure.

Instructions

1. Stand with your feet shoulder-width apart and your right foot forward so that the heel of your right foot is even with the toes of your left foot.
2. Hold the stability ball between your hands by your right hip. Sink back into your hips to squat down. As you return to standing, push your left foot into the floor as you rotate your right hip and foot to point toward the midline of your body. The stability ball should travel in a diagonal line from your right hip to above your left shoulder and end up with your right shoulder facing the wall to your left.
3. As you lower the ball, sink back into the squat and allow your right foot to rotate back to point straight ahead.

Correct Your Form

- When starting the diagonal lift, you should be lowered into a partial squat with a straight spine (lowered into the right hip as demonstrated by the photo).
- When returning to standing, push with both legs into the ground while letting the outside leg (the right leg in the instructions) rotate to face the midline of your body.
- The rotational movement should come from your hips and feet so the spine can remain long and straight during the exercise.

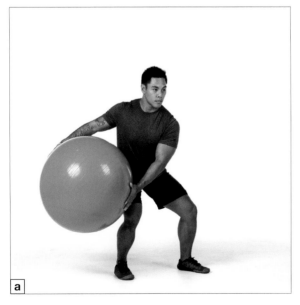
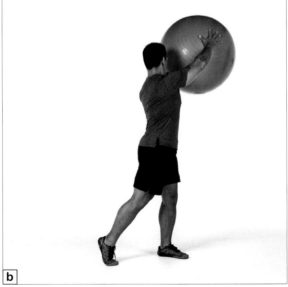

Reverse Back Extension

Benefits

This unique move strengthens the extensor muscles of your posterior chain by lifting the lower half of your body up against the downward pull of gravity. This can help strengthen the lower back and hip muscles without putting too much force on the spine.

Instructions

1. Face the stability ball so that your chest is on the top of the ball and your knees are on the ground.
2. Walk your hands forward until the front of your hips are on top of the ball. Keep your hands placed on the ground in front of you for stability, and keep your legs pressed together throughout the exercise for more control.
3. Keeping your hips on the top of the ball, squeeze the muscles of your glutes and along the backs of your legs to lift them into the air. Bring your legs up until your entire body is a straight line, then slowly lower them.
4. When learning this exercise, focus on control of the movement by using your glute and hamstring muscles.

Correct Your Form

It's important that you feel the work from this exercise in your glutes and backs of the legs. If you feel it in your lower back, move forward on the ball to shorten the lever arm of your lower body.

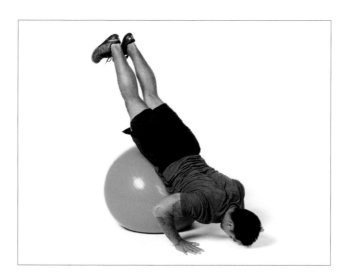

Russian Twist

Benefits

Because the Russian twist rotates your shoulders while your hips remain stable, it strengthens many of the core muscles between your trunk and hips, helping improve strength and coordination between your upper and lower body. Once you develop a foundational level of strength when performing this movement, you can increase the speed and number of reps to increase the overall energy expenditure.

Instructions

1. Start in a seated position on top of the ball. Slowly walk forward until the widest part of your back—between your shoulders—is directly on top of the ball.

2. Clasp the fingers of both hands directly over the top of your chest and press your hands together. Move your shoulders by dropping your hands to the left and lifting the right shoulder so that you roll on to your left shoulder. As you do this with your upper body, push your left foot into the ground and right hip into the air to create stability. Briefly pause on your left shoulder before rolling your back over the top of the ball to move over to your right shoulder. As you move to your right shoulder, pick up your left shoulder and allow the top of your right arm to roll on to the ball. Push your right foot into the ground and left hip into the air to enhance stability.

3. Start with 3 to 4 reps on either side, for a total of 6 to 8. Once you can do those with control, start adding 2 reps every week until you can do 8 to 10 reps on either side, for a total of 16 to 20.

Correct Your Form

- This is a challenging exercise that requires a lot of control from your hips and lower body, especially when moving at a faster pace. Pressing your feet into the ground and squeezing your glute muscles throughout the entire movement will help create stability and allow you to rotate your trunk and upper body at a faster pace.

- Keeping your arms straight with both hands pressed together will create more stability through your upper body, allowing it to roll over the top of the ball.

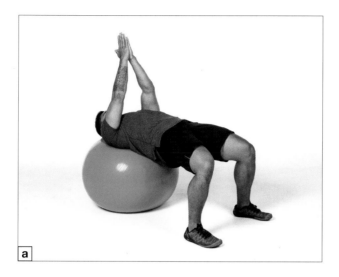

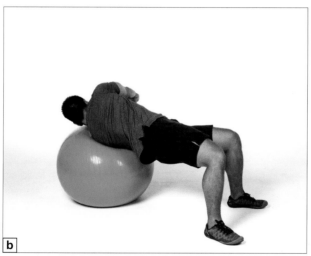

Ball Pass Crunch

Benefits

This exercise combines movement from both your upper and lower body to increase the number of muscles activated and the overall energy expenditure. Passing the stability ball between your feet and hands can help improve coordination and dexterity between the upper- and lower-body appendages.

Instructions

1. Lie flat on your back with your legs extended straight and your arms overhead holding the stability ball between both hands. Bring your arms toward your chest. As the ball is passing over your head, draw your belly button toward your spine as you roll up on your spine to perform a crunch. At the same time, lift your legs up toward your hands to grab the ball with your feet. Keep the ball between your feet as you lower them toward the floor.
2. Keeping the stability ball between your feet, lift your legs and bring them toward your body as you curl up with your abdominals and reach with your arms to grab the stability ball with your hands to move it into an overhead position.
3. When starting this exercise, move at a steady pace, and focus on controlling the movement from your abdominals.

Correct Your Form

- To help stabilize your neck during the crunch portion of the exercise, press your tongue into the roof of your mouth to activate the muscles that stabilize the vertebra of the cervical spine.
- As you perform the crunch, roll up on your spine by contracting the abdominal muscles. Think about shifting the bottom of your rib cage toward the top of your pelvis.
- If necessary, instead of grabbing the stability ball with your feet from your hands, think about squeezing the ball in between your knees. This shortens the lever arm and reduces the intensity of the exercise.

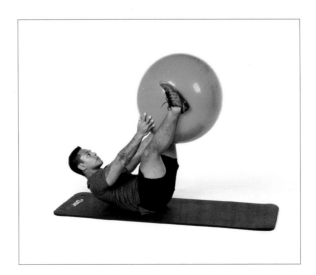

MEDICINE BALL EXERCISES FOR METABOLIC CONDITIONING

A major benefit of using a medicine ball includes strengthening both muscle and elastic connective tissues by moving a weight *through* gravity as opposed to directly against gravity. Additionally, most fitness facilities have medicine balls, so if the gym is really busy, you can use just one piece of equipment to experience a great workout. When selecting a medicine ball, choose one that is approximately 5 to 7 percent of your bodyweight. As you get stronger, you can gradually progress to ones that weigh 10 percent of your bodyweight. Your goal is to complete AMRAP during the work interval. As you feel yourself getting stronger, keep track of the number of reps you do during your first time through the circuit, and then try to meet or beat that number each additional time you do the exercise.

Exercise	Time*	Circuits+
Straight-arm slam	25 sec	2-5
Standing rotation	25 sec	
Squat to forward press	25 sec	
Push press to bounce catch	25 sec	
Reverse crossover lunge with reach	25 sec	
Full-body crunch	25 sec	
Lateral skater with forward reach	25 sec	
Reverse lunge with overhead lift	25 sec	
Rest and recovery	45-90 sec between circuits after all exercises	

*Add 5 seconds to the work interval every 2 to 3 weeks until you are doing 45 seconds for each exercise.

+Once you are able to do 2 circuits of 45 seconds, start adding additional circuits until you are doing 5 circuits of 45-second intervals.

Straight-Arm Slam

Benefits

High-speed movements use the type II muscle fibers responsible for definition. Slamming a medicine ball into the ground is a safe and effective power exercise that recruits most of the muscles in your upper back and arms. The rapid action of the muscles increases the overall work rate and energy expenditure of the exercise.

Note: If you exercise in a location where you are not able to slam the ball on the ground, perform the same movement pattern but stop at the bottom of the pattern before releasing the ball (this is the exercise in the pictures). Pulling the ball downwards rapidly from an overhead position will create an effective overload in the hip and back muscles of the posterior chain.

Instructions

Slams

1. Stand with your feet hip-width apart and knees slightly bent. Hold the medicine ball between both hands in front of your waist. Quickly raise both arms overhead, then keep both elbows extended (so the arms are long) as you rapidly bring the ball down in front of you to slam it on the floor between your feet.

2. As you slam the ball down, sink into your hips to generate more force. Rapidly push your feet into the ground to return to standing and catch the ball in your hands on the way back up, and quickly allow it to go back to the overhead position. If you do NOT release the ball, quickly return to the standing position and return your hands holding the medicine ball to an overhead position as fast as possible. You should feel this exercise in the muscles of your upper back.

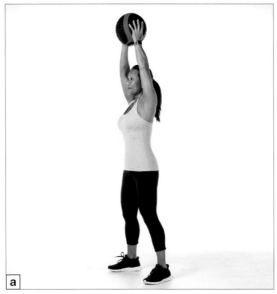
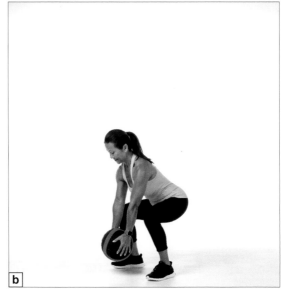

a   b

Straight-Arm Slam *(continued)*

If you can't slam a ball, do the following exercise.

Explosive Chop Without Release

1. Stand with your feet hip-width apart and hold a medicine ball over your head. Keep your spine long as you quickly sink back into your hips while performing a squat.
2. Bring the medicine ball down in front of your body and stop the ball at the bottom of the movement before releasing it; this will increase the energy and strength transferred into the hip muscles.
3. Quickly return to standing and repeat.

Correct Your Form

Slams

- Keep your arms straight as you lift the ball overhead and slam it down. This will keep all of the work in the back muscles, as opposed to the triceps muscles of your upper arms.
- Sinking into your hips as you slam the ball allows you to apply more energy to the move.

Standing Rotation

Benefits

During upright movements, rotation should come from the feet, hips, and shoulders, not the spine. This exercise strengthens the muscles of the hips, core, and upper shoulders by using all of them together during this movement. Because so many muscles are involved, moving at a fast pace can increase your heart rate and the amount of calories you burn.

Instructions

1. Stand with your feet hip-width apart and your knees slightly bent. Hold the medicine ball between both hands directly in front of your chest.
2. Keep your spine long, push your left foot into the floor, and rotate your left foot toward the midline of your body to rotate your shoulders toward the right. At the end ROM, quickly push your right foot into the floor and rotate it to your left as you turn your shoulders and hips to your left. The goal for this exercise is to move quickly from side to side by turning the feet and the hips.

Correct Your Form

- Rotation comes from your feet and hips, so to perform this movement correctly (and to protect your knees and spine), focus on turning your feet and hips quickly during this exercise. Your feet should rotate on the ground as though you're putting out a cigarette (that someone else left burning).
- Your spine should remain long and straight as you move your feet, hips, and shoulders.

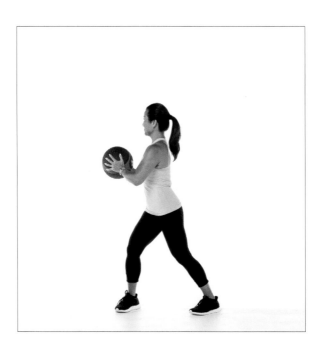

Squat to Forward Press

Benefits

Holding a medicine ball as you extend both arms in front of your body helps create a counter-weight for your hips so that as you lower toward the ground, you can push your hips back further and sink deeper into the squat to activate more muscles.

Instructions

1. Stand with your feet hip-width apart while holding a medicine ball in front of your chest with both hands. Keep your spine long as you push your hips back to lower yourself into a squat. The first movement should be your hips moving back, behind you.
2. As you lower into the squat, extend both arms in front of your body. At the bottom of the movement, pause briefly, then push both feet into the floor to return to the standing position. As you're standing, pull the medicine ball back in to your chest.
3. Your movement during this fast-paced exercise should be fluid as you move up and down while pushing your arms forward and pulling them back.

Correct Your Form

Like *any* squat variation, it is important that most of the movement come from your hips as opposed to your knees moving forward. The benefit of pushing the medicine ball in front of you is that it creates a counterbalance that allows you to sink deeper into your hips at the bottom of the squat.

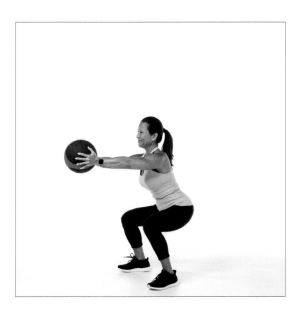

Push Press to Bounce Catch

Benefits

Power exercises can help increase the total caloric expenditure while using the larger type II muscle fibers responsible for generating a high magnitude of force in a short period of time. Because type II fibers play a role in muscle definition, using power exercises may help improve muscle definition without adding additional muscle size. Dropping your hips quickly as you're catching the ball helps improve your hip mobility while strengthening your hip extensors, specifically, the gluteals and hamstrings.

Note: This exercise can only be performed outdoors or in a location with high ceilings. If working indoors, focus on the speed of the movement from squat to overhead press without releasing the medicine ball at the top of the movement. If you exercise in a location where you are not able to slam the ball on the ground or in an indoor location with low ceilings, perform a push press to catch.

Instructions

Push Press to Bounce Catch

1. Stand with your feet hip-width apart while holding a medicine ball in front of your chest with both hands. Keep your spine long as you push your hips back to lower yourself into a quarter-squat, moving down only enough to feel a stretch in your glute muscles. Quickly push your feet into the ground and snap your hips forward as you rapidly press both arms directly overhead.
2. As your arms reach full extension, release the medicine ball so that it travels straight up. You should push it in a trajectory slightly in front of your body so that it hits the ground about 12 to 18 inches (30-46 cm) in front of you.
3. Allow the ball to bounce. As it hits the highest point of the bounce, drop your hips into a squat to catch it as it comes down.

Squat to Overhead Press

If you're inside and don't have the room overhead required to throw the medicine ball upwards, perform the same pattern from the squat to overhead press but do NOT release the ball at the top of the move. Instead, press the ball directly overhead for a shoulder press. To increase the metabolic effect, move up and down as fast as possible while extending your arms directly overhead.

For either version, focus on moving quickly so your hip and thigh muscles act like rubber bands, allowing you to snap down and up quickly.

Correct Your Form

- The power for this exercise comes from your legs and hips. The energy travels from the floor through your body and is released into the ball through your arms.
- When catching the ball from the bounce, time your squat so that you get under the ball as it starts traveling down from the initial bounce. When lowering into the squat, you want to feel the weight of the medicine ball help you lower into the squat.

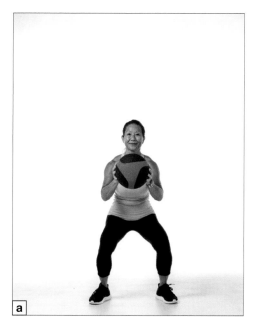

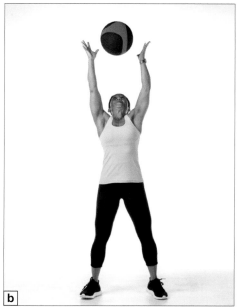

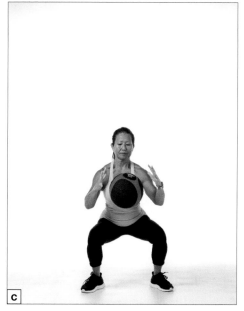

Reverse Crossover Lunge With Reach

Benefits

Muscle, fascia, and elastic connective tissue can become stronger as a result of lengthening under resistance. This action lengthens the muscles of the outer thigh to improve their strength and resiliency, while reaching for the ground with the medicine ball increases the force into the tissues, making them stronger. Performing this exercise at a rapid pace can increase strength while elevating heart rate, providing multiple benefits with just one move.

Instructions

1. Stand with your feet hip-width apart while holding a medicine ball in front of your waist with both hands.
2. Keep your spine long as you move your left leg behind your right, guiding your left foot toward the four or five o'clock position). As the ball of your left foot hits the ground, hinge forward at your hips and with the medicine ball, reach only as far as your hips will allow.
3. To return to standing, press your right foot into the ground as you pick up your left leg and place it back in the start position. Alternate legs.

Correct Your Form

The idea of this exercise is to use the position and leverage from one leg (the right leg in the instructions) to help increase flexion in the stationary hip (the left leg in the instructions). When sinking into the lunge, think about pushing your hips back so that your weight goes back into your glutes as opposed to forward in your knee.

> **TIP** During the first few workouts focus on learning this exercise so you feel it in your hips.

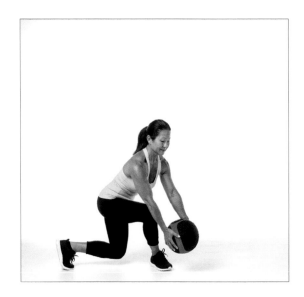

Full-Body Crunch

Benefits

Using your entire body for crunches increases the lever arm, which, in turn, increases the number of muscles engaged for the exercise. This movement uses the abdominals to move both the upper- and lower-body segments to increase total energy expenditure.

Instructions

1. Lie on the ground on your back with your legs out straight, and extend your arms overhead while holding the medicine ball between your hands so that your thumbs are close to the ground with your palms facing each other.
2. As your arms reach the top of your chest, draw your belly button in toward your spine and roll your back off the ground to perform a crunch as you pull your knees toward your chest. As you lift your knees toward your chest, lightly touch the medicine ball to the tops of your knees before returning your arms and legs back to the original starting position.

Correct Your Form

- To reduce soreness in your neck and to maintain good form through the front of your core, press your tongue into the roof of your mouth. This will engage the muscles that help stabilize the cervical spine.
- If you feel any discomfort in the low back, start with your knees bent and your feet flat on the floor, which places your lower back in a more neutral position and shortens the lever arm. As you get stronger you can extend your legs longer at the start.

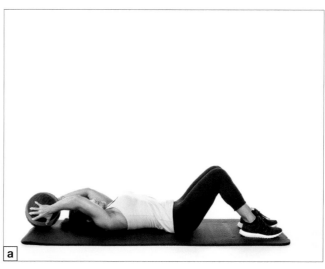

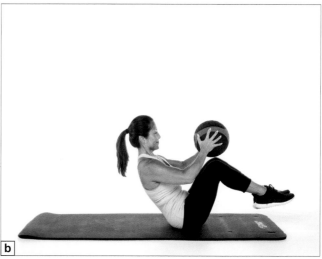

Lateral Skater With Forward Reach

Benefits

When done properly, the lateral skater can help strengthen the hips while increasing the heart rate. The forward movement of the medicine ball while you balance on one leg can also improve hip strength to help increase stability because the hip and core muscles will have to work harder to create stability as the ball moves away from your body. Performing power exercises standing on one leg at a time are useful for working with runners because they can help improve velocity of force production and the ability to rapidly stabilize the body as the foot hits the ground.

Instructions

1. Stand with your feet hip-width apart while holding a medicine ball in front of your waist with both hands. Keep your spine long as you sink into your hips in a partial squat. Lift your left foot off the floor as you push off with your right to quickly move to your left.
2. Let your left foot hit the ground with the ball of the foot first before rolling down to the heel. (When landing from any jump, the sequence should be ball of foot, heel of foot, then hip moving back.) As you are sinking into your left hip, press the medicine ball forward directly in front of your chest.
3. Quickly pull the medicine ball back as you push off with your left foot to return to the right. You are trying to push the medicine ball in front of you as you land on each foot; this motion will increase the amount of force in your glutes.

Correct Your Form

- When learning this exercise, start with small movements at a steady pace. As you improve, feel free to increase the ROM or move at a faster pace.
- The ideal way to do this move is to fluidly push the medicine ball in front of you each time you land on one leg. This will increase the activation of the glutes to enhance overall hip strength.

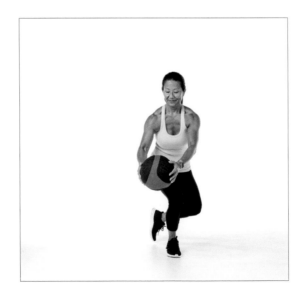

Reverse Lunge With Overhead Lift

Benefits

The muscles of the core region are designed to work most effectively when strengthened in an upright, standing position. The movement of the arms overhead with the leg stepping back increases the use of your core muscles from both the bottom and top, making it an effective exercise for both burning calories and increasing strength.

Instructions

1. Stand with your feet hip-width apart while holding a medicine ball in front of your waist with both hands. Keep your spine long as you step back with the left foot. Place the ball of your left foot directly behind you and lower your left knee toward the ground while bending your right hip and knee.
2. As you're lowering your body, use both arms to swing the medicine ball directly overhead. You should feel all of the muscles along the front of your body being lengthened. Pause at the bottom with your arms overhead before swinging both arms back down to return the medicine ball to the starting position in front of your waist.
3. As you're lowering the medicine ball, press your right foot into the ground and push off with the left foot to return to the standing position.

Correct Your Form

- Keep your chest raised and spine long during the movement. Maintaining good posture can increase the strength of the abdominals as you're raising the medicine ball overhead.
- When returning from the bottom of the lunge to the standing position, think about pulling the knee of the forward leg backward (the right leg the instructions) to help strengthen the muscles along the back of the leg.

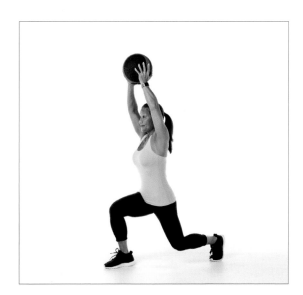

SANDBAG EXERCISES FOR METABOLIC CONDITIONING

Like a medicine ball, a sandbag helps improve the strength of both muscle and elastic connective tissues because you can move a sandbag in multiple directions as opposed to moving in only a single, linear path of motion. Additional benefits of sandbags include a pliable surface that helps develop grip strength and, unlike medicine balls, it won't roll away from you when you set it down. Select a weight that is approximately 5 to 7 percent of your body weight when starting this circuit. As you get stronger, you can gradually progress to ones that weigh 10 to 15 percent of your body weight. Your goal is to complete AMRAP during the work interval. As you feel yourself getting stronger, keep track of the number of reps you do during your first time through the circuit, and then try to meet or beat that number each additional time you do the exercise.

Exercise	Time*	Circuits+
Crunch with resistance	25 sec	2-5
Push press throw to catch	25 sec	
Forward to reverse lunge with overhead lift	25 sec	
Swing (alternating hands)	25 sec	
Reverse overhead slams	25 sec	
Reverse crossover lunge with reach	25 sec	
Half Turkish get-up	25 sec	
Rest and recovery	45-90 seconds between circuits after all exercises	

*Add 5 seconds to the work interval every 2 to 3 weeks until you are doing 45 seconds for each exercise.

+Once you are able to do 2 circuits of 45 seconds, start adding additional circuits until you are doing 5 circuits of 45-second intervals.

Crunch With Resistance

Benefits

The reverse crunch movement emphasizes bringing your hips up toward your rib cage, which strengthens the abdominals from the bottom (where they attach to the pelvis) to the top (to the attachment point at the bottom of the ribs). This movement can strengthen the abdominals while reducing the stress on the lower back that can occur during standard crunches.

Instructions

1. Lie on your back with your knees bent and feet flat on the floor. Hold a sandbag between both hands, and start with your arms overhead so that they are resting on the floor.
2. Keep your arms straight and pull them from an overhead position to a point where the sandbag is directly over your chest.
3. With the sandbag directly over your chest, pull your belly button in toward your spine and shift your rib cage down toward your pelvis to perform a crunch by rolling up slowly.

Correct Your Form

- Make sure to allow your body to return to a fully extended, lying position after the completion of each rep. This will use the muscles in a complete ROM, helping them become stronger.
- When doing this exercise think about bringing the top of your pelvis closer to the bottom of your rib cage. Thinking about this movement can help improve your skill as you are doing the exercise.

> **TIP** Slowly lower your back down to the floor, and slowly lower both arms to extend them overhead. To increase the level of difficulty, as you become stronger, hold both legs off the floor.

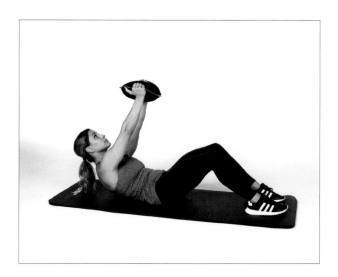

Push Press Throw to Catch

Benefits

This exercise uses rapid movements, which help increase the total caloric expenditure, and these movements are generated from the larger type II muscles fibers, which play a role in muscle definition. Extending your hips quickly as you're throwing the sandbag helps improve the explosive strength and power of your hip extensors, specifically, the gluteals and hamstrings.

Note: This exercise can only be performed outdoors or in a location with high ceilings. If working in an indoor location with low ceilings, focus on the speed of the movement from squat to overhead press without releasing the medicine ball at the top of the movement.

Instructions

1. Stand with your feet hip-width apart and hold a sandbag in front of your chest with both hands. Keep your spine long as you push your hips back to quickly lower yourself into a quarter-squat, moving down only enough to feel a stretch in your glute muscles.
2. Quickly push your feet into the ground and snap your hips forward as you rapidly press both arms directly overhead.
3. As your arms reach full extension, release the sandbag so that it travels straight up. You should push it in a trajectory slightly in front of your body so that it hits the ground about 12 to 18 inches (30-46 cm) in front of you.
4. Allow the sandbag to hit the ground. When it is on the ground, quickly drop into a squat to pick it up and repeat the movement.

If you're inside and don't have much room overhead, don't release the sandbag at the top of the move; instead move up and down as quickly as possible while extending your arms directly overhead in a shoulder press movement.

For either version, focus on moving quickly. Your hip and thigh muscles should feel as though they are made of rubber bands, allowing you to snap down and up quickly.

Correct Your Form

- When lowering into the squat, the first movement should be your hips moving back. To return to standing, quickly press your feet into the ground like you're trying to push the floor away from you.
- When extending both arms overhead, your palms should face each other, with your elbow pointed directly forward, in front of your body.

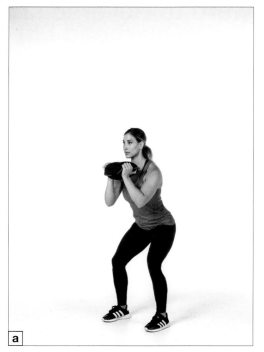

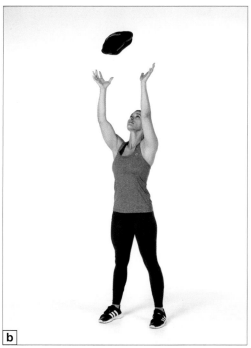

Forward to Reverse Lunge With Overhead Lift

Benefits

Because you're quickly stepping forward and backward with the same leg, this exercise is challenging but very effective. Fast movements with the larger muscles of your legs can help elevate your heart rate while increasing strength.

Instructions

1. Stand with your feet hip-width apart and hold a sandbag in front of your waist with both hands. Keep your spine long as you step back with the right foot. Place the ball of your right foot directly behind you and lower your right knee toward the ground while bending your left hip and knee.

2. As you're lowering your body, use both arms to swing the sandbag directly overhead; you should feel all the muscles along the front of your body being lengthened. Pause at the bottom with your arms overhead before swinging both arms back down to return the sandbag to the starting position in front of your waist.

3. As you're lowering the sandbag, press your left foot into the ground and push off with the right foot to return to the standing position.

4. Immediately step forward with the right foot, place your right foot on the ground, and sink into your right hip by keeping your spine long and leaning forward slightly. Lower your left knee toward the ground and keep both arms straight as you raise the sandbag directly overhead. When stepping back with the right leg, the right abdominals are strengthened (when both arms go overhead); and when stepping forward with the right leg, the abdominal muscles in the left side are strengthened as the arms go overhead, making this an excellent move for both the abs and glutes.

5. Perform the first set with one leg, and complete AMRAP during the work interval. Take only a brief rest—no more than 5 to 10 seconds—before doing the second set using the left leg (keeping the right foot planted in place).

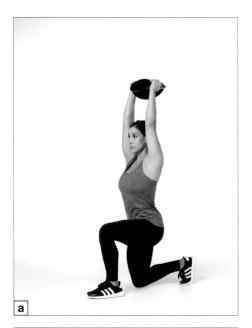

a

Correct Your Form

• When doing forward lunges, the movement should come from the hip flexing, not the knee moving forward. As your foot hits the ground (the right foot in the above instructions), push your right hip back so the gluteus maximus does most of the work.

• When doing the forward lunge, reach the sandbag in front of you at about knee to waist height. This will increase the flexion of the hip, which strengthens the hip extensor muscles by lengthening them under resistance.

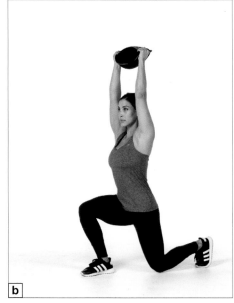

b

Swing (Alternating Hands)

Benefits

Swings are a rhythmic movement that are efficient for strengthening your hips while elevating your heart rate.

Instructions

1. Stand with your feet hip- to shoulder-width apart and hold a sandbag in your right hand. *Note*: If you have a larger sandbag, you may have to hold it in both hands simultaneously.

2. Quickly lower the sandbag and swing it through your legs toward the back side of your body. When the sandbag is traveling in between your legs, hinge forward at the waist and push your hips back.

3. To move the sandbag forward into the up phase, press both feet into the floor while snapping your hips forward. It is this forward movement of the hips, as opposed to your arm, that generates the force to move the sandbag.

4. As the sandbag reaches the top of the swing, let go and switch hands, catching it in your left hand so that you are alternating hands for every swing. When first learning this move, focus on making a clean switch between hands. As you improve your skill, increase your speed of movement.

5. Once you have the coordination and rhythm to control a steady tempo of swings while switching hands, your goal is to complete AMRAP during the work interval.

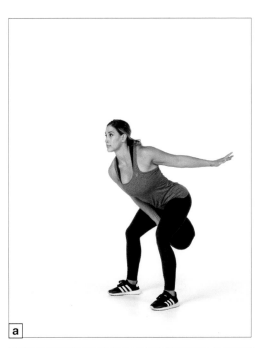

a

Correct Your Form

- A swing is a forward and backward motion of the hips hinging and extending, not a squatting motion.

- During the swings, your lower legs should remain relatively vertical with only a slight amount of movement.

- If switching hands is too challenging, focus on holding the sandbag between both hands simultaneously.

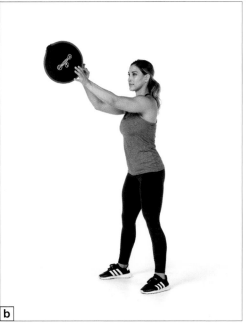

b

Reverse Overhead Slams

Benefits

This explosive move uses the larger muscles responsible for extending the knees and hips. The rapid force production from this exercise helps strengthen the muscles of your lower body while increasing the heart rate, making it an effective option for metabolic conditioning.

Instructions

1. Stand with your feet hip-width apart and hold a sandbag in front of your waist with both hands. Keep your spine long as you quickly push your hips back to lower yourself into a squat, bringing the sandbag down between your legs.

2. From the bottom of the squat, quickly push your feet into the ground as you drive your hips forward and swing your arms overhead. This should result in a full extension of your body as you roll up on the tips of your toes.

3. Your arms should travel behind your head as you release the sandbag to slam it down toward the ground behind you. (Think about performing a reverse slam dunk in basketball.)

4. Once you've released the sandbag, quickly turn around, squat down to pick it up, and continue repeating the exercise for the duration of the work interval.

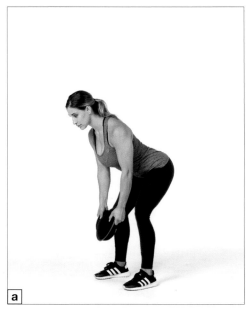

a

Correct Your Form

When swinging the sandbag overhead, focus on driving your hips forward and fully extending the spine as you move to release the sandbag behind your head.

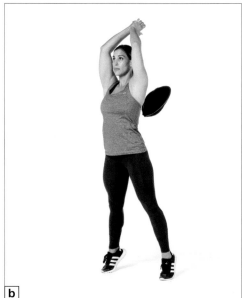

b

Reverse Crossover Lunge With Reach

Benefits

The alternating lunging action of the legs can help to increase both strength and overall energy expenditure. Moving the hips in all directions could help strengthen all of the muscles for controlling motion at the hip.

Instructions

1. Stand with your feet hip-width apart and hold a sandbag in front of your chest with the right hand. Keep your spine long as you move your right leg behind your left, guiding your right foot toward the seven or eight o'clock position. As the ball of your right foot hits the ground, hinge forward at your left hip and lower the sandbag toward your left foot allowing it to sink as far as possible; this will create a counterbalance, allowing you to sink a little deeper into your left hip.

2. To return to standing, press your left foot into the ground as you pick up your right leg and place it back in the start position, then alternate legs.

Correct Your Form

- To ensure that your hip muscles are doing most of the work, place your right foot back behind you as you move it to the left side of your body. This will ensure that the muscles of the left hip are doing most of the work as you lower yourself during the exercise.

- To increase the level of difficulty, aim a little lower—at about knee height—as you push the sandbag forward. This will increase the amount of flexion in the left hip, placing more force into the hip extensor muscles.

- As you return to standing, press your stance foot into the ground and move that hip forward (the left foot and hip in the instructions above).

TIP During the first few workouts focus on learning this exercise so you feel it in your hips.

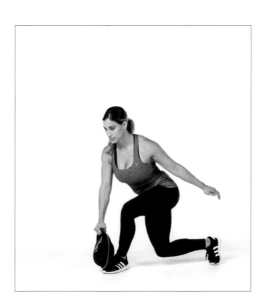

Half Turkish Get-Up

Benefits

This exercise uses a number of core, hip, and shoulder muscles together to help initiate the body moving directly off the ground. The more muscles involved in an exercise, the more calories you will burn! Besides burning calories, the half Turkish get-up can strengthen both the gluteal muscles responsible for extending the hips, the deep core muscles that stabilize the spine, and the muscles that control motion at the shoulder and upper back.

Instructions

1. Lie flat on the floor with your left leg straight and your right knee bent so that your right foot is flat on the floor. The left leg should be lying a little to the left, and the right foot should be planted a little to your right.
2. Place the sandbag in the palm of your right hand as you extend the arm straight up. You want to keep the right arm extended all the way through the exercise. Place your left arm directly out to your left side.
3. To start the exercise, roll on to your left elbow as you lift your right shoulder off the ground and curl your trunk. As you lift your upper body off the ground, push your left hand into the floor so your left arm is fully extended.
4. You should be in a seated position with your right arm overhead and your left hand and right foot on the floor. Push your right foot into the floor as you straighten your left hand to lift both hips off the floor.
5. Hold this bridge position between your left hand, left leg, and right foot for a brief pause before slowly lowering your hips to the ground and rolling all the way back to the original, lying position.
6. When learning this exercise, focus on a fluid motion between the sit-up and hip bridge. Once you have the movement down, do as many reps as possible with the right arm overhead before doing as many reps as possible with the left hand overhead.

Correct Your Form

- When pushing up off the floor, use your arm and hip together (the left arm and right hip in the instructions above).
- To ensure proper position of your spine and trunk, keep your eyes looking up toward the sandbag balanced in your hand.

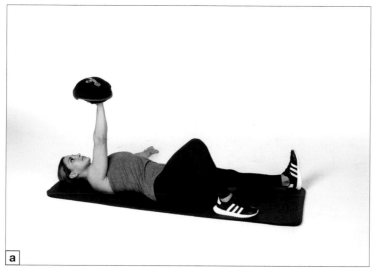

a

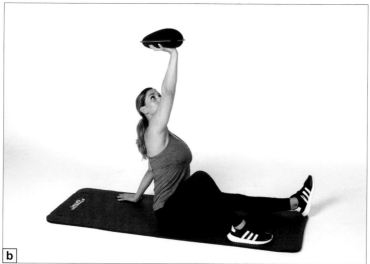

b

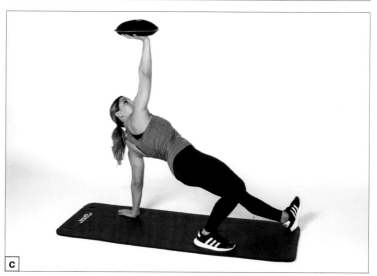

c

TWO-ARM RESISTANCE TUBING EXERCISES FOR METABOLIC CONDITIONING

The cable machines in a gym provide a number of unique exercise options that can help improve overall total body strength. Cable machines take up a lot of space and are expensive, so they are not a practical solution for home workouts. Using two-arm resistance tubing is an extremely affordable option that allows you to recreate the benefits of cable machines in the comfort of your own home. One of the best parts is that they are extremely portable, making them an excellent option for road warriors who do a lot of travel for work. Among the many benefits of doing standing band exercises are using both upper- and lower-body muscles at the same time, which helps increase overall strength with a specific emphasis on the muscles responsible for stabilizing the spine and moving the hips. Like other equipment, resistance tubing allows you to move in multiple directions as opposed to just a single, linear path of motion. The longer the tubing stretches, the greater the resistance. If a band feels too easy, it will be necessary to invest in a new one. The design of the tubing allows you to anchor it in a doorframe, giving you a number of training options.Your goal is to complete AMRAP during the work interval. As you feel yourself getting stronger, keep track of the number of reps you do during your first time through the circuit, and then try to meet or beat that number each additional time you do the exercise.

Exercise	Time*	Circuits+
Squat-to-row	25 sec	2-5
Straight-arm pull-down	25 sec	
Transverse lunge with pull	25 sec	
Alternating punches	25 sec	
Lateral lunge with straight-arm pull-down	25 sec	
Lateral lunge to band chop	25 sec	
Fast band pull	25 sec	
Rest and recovery	45-90 sec between circuits after all exercises	

*Add 5 seconds to the work interval every 2 to 3 weeks until you are doing 45 seconds for each exercise.

+Once you are able to do 2 circuits of 45 seconds, start adding additional circuits until you are doing 5 circuits of 45-second intervals.

Squat-to-Row

Benefits

A common complaint of the squat exercise is that it can cause knee discomfort, which can occur if the knees move forward before the hips move backward during the lowering phase of the exercise. Holding on to the handles of the band makes it easier to push your hips back as your lower yourself into the squat. The squat uses many of the large muscles in the lower body along with the larger muscles of the upper back, helping to make this a very energy-expensive exercise (i.e., it burns a lot of calories).

Instructions

1. Place the anchor point of the band in the doorframe or attach it to a stable machine at or a little above shoulder height. Face the anchor point of the band and stand far enough away so there is slight tension with no slack in the band when you start the exercise.

2. Your feet should be hip-width apart, and your arms should extend in front of you holding one handle in each hand. Keep your arms out in front of you and your spine long and straight as you push your hips back behind you to lower into the squat. At the bottom of the squat, push your feet into the ground and press your hips forward to return to the initial standing position.

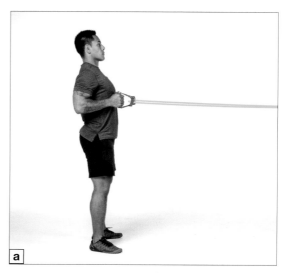

3. Once you reach the standing position, pull both hands toward your chest, keeping your elbows by your side, to perform the rowing motion.

4. This should be a fluid motion. As you finish standing in the squat, pull your arms toward your body for the row, and extend your arms in front of you before lowering yourself into the next squat.

a

Correct Your Form

- Keeping tension on the band as you start the exercise will allow you to push your hips back further to increase the amount of work your hip and back muscles do during the exercise.

- If dropping into a deep squat causes discomfort, lower yourself to a comfortable ROM and focus on the rowing motion of the arms during the exercise.

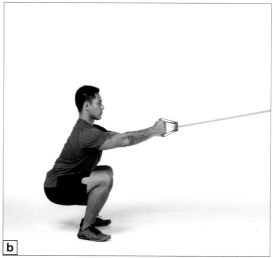

b

Straight-Arm Pull-Down

Benefits

This exercise uses the large muscles of the upper back and arms and can be done very quickly to increase your heart rate and overall energy expenditure.

Instructions

1. Place the anchor point of the band at or above your shoulder height.
2. Stand facing the anchor point at a distance far enough away so there is a slight tension on both arms of the resistance band. Sink into your hips, press your feet into the ground to create stability, and keep both arms straight with your palms facing the ground. Press both arms down toward your hips at the same time as fast as you can.
3. Your hands should travel from approximately shoulder height to your hips; they can go a little past both hips, but not too far.

Correct Your Form

- Keep your chest lifted high and your spine long so that your upper-back and arm muscles do the majority of the work.
- Sink into a quarter-squat to engage your hips, and press your feet into the ground to create stability for your lower body while your arms move rapidly during this exercise.

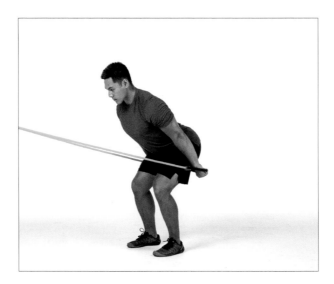

Transverse Lunge With Pull

Benefits

By creating a lot of rotation through the joint where the thigh bone connects with the pelvis, this unique move uses the hips in a way they don't move during many other exercises. Additionally, the pulling motion engages the large muscles of the upper back to make this exercise very energy-expensive.

Instructions

1. Place the anchor point of the band at or above your shoulder height.
2. Stand facing the anchor point at a distance far enough away so there is a slight tension on both arms of the resistance band. Hold both arms in front of your body at shoulder-height with your palms facing each other and feet hip-width apart.
3. With your left foot, step back and to the left so that it is pointing in the eight o'clock position. As you step back with the left leg, keep your right foot pressed into the floor, and contract your right thigh muscles to stabilize and protect the right knee. Once your left foot is on the ground, shift your weight into your left hip as you pull your left hand back toward your left shoulder.
4. Push off the ground with your left leg and return to standing. Then alternate sides: Step back with your right foot while pulling back with your right hand.

Correct Your Form

- It is important to keep the planted leg pressed into the ground while pointed toward the anchor point when stepping back with the moving leg. This will keep the knee stable, allowing the hips to do most of the rotation necessary for the movement.
- Throughout this entire exercise, it is important to keep your chest lifted and spine straight so that the rotation for the movement comes from your hips and thoracic (upper) spine.
- When pulling on the bands, hold on to the handles, but focus on pulling from your elbows. Your back muscles attach to the upper arms, so this can help increase the activation.

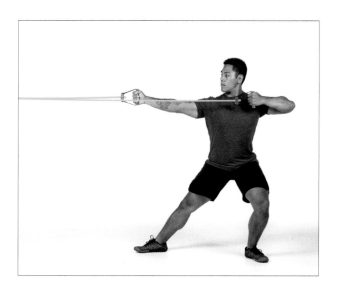

Alternating Punches

Benefits

Push movements from a standing position require the core and lower-body muscles to engage to create stability for the chest and shoulder muscles of the upper body to do the work. Punches are pushing movements; using the band for resistance can help engage the muscles of the lower body, core, and upper body, helping to increase overall energy expenditure.

Instructions

1. Place the anchor point of the band at approximately chest to shoulder height. Stand facing away from the anchor point at a distance that places slight tension on each arm of the band. Keep your feet hip-width apart, and hold the handles of the bands in your hands directly in front of your shoulders so that the band is running along on the tops of your forearms.

2. Press both feet into the ground, squeeze your glute muscles, and keep your spine long. Punch your hands forward, alternating left and right, and rotate your shoulders while punching; the left side of your body should come forward as you punch your left arm, and the right side of your body should come forward with the right punch. Pressing into the floor and squeezing your glutes will activate the core muscles to keep your spine stable.

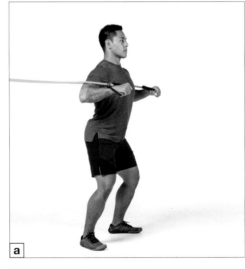

Correct Your Form

- Your spine should be long and straight to allow for proper rotation as you press forward with each hand into the punches.

- Start with your feet parallel. *Note:* The normal boxing stance has one foot slightly forward while both feet remain in a parallel position. Keeping both feet parallel allows your shoulders to rotate more easily as you throw the punches.

- To increase the level of difficulty, bring your feet closer together for a narrower base of support.

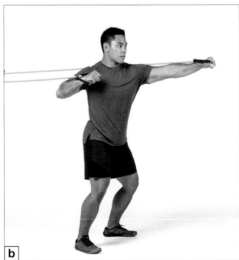

Lateral Lunge
With Straight-Arm Pull-Down

Benefits

This move combines the pulling motion from the large muscles of the upper back with the lunging action of the leg and hip muscles. Alternating legs from side to side increases overall energy expenditure.

Instructions

1. Place the anchor point of the band at or above your shoulder height.

2. Stand facing the anchor point at a distance far enough away so there is slight tension on both arms of the resistance band. Extend both arms straight out at approximately chest height with your palms facing the ground. Push your right foot down into the ground as you pick up your left foot and step directly to your left.

3. When your left foot hits the ground, keep your spine straight and push your left hip directly behind you. Once your left foot is anchored to the ground and the left hip is in a flexed position, pull both arms down toward the floor, with your right hand on the inside of your right thigh and your left hand on the outside of your left shin.

4. As your arms lift up to return to the starting position, push off with your left foot and pull your body up by pressing your right foot into the ground and by using the muscles of your right inner thigh.

5. You should return to standing position with both feet together and arms at chest height before alternating legs to do the next lunge into your right leg.

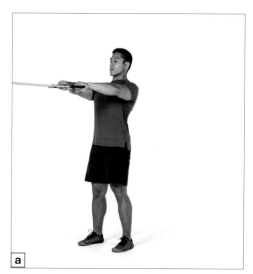

a

Correct Your Form

• When your foot hits the floor as you step into the lateral lunge, push your hip back so the primary movement is from your hip, not your spine.

• To ensure that you properly engage the larger muscles of your upper back, keep both of your arms straight when pulling the band down at the bottom of the lunge.

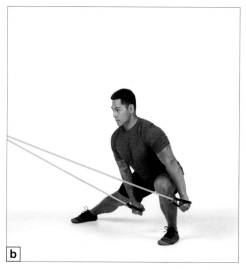

b

Lateral Lunge to Band Chop

Benefits

Many exercises focus on moving forward and backward or up and down. This exercise combines two movements—lateral lunging and trunk rotation—that are often overlooked, as both individual and integrated exercises. Rotating the trunk over the hips moves the body the way it is designed to move, and because it uses so many large muscles, it is very effective for burning calories.

Instructions

1. Place the anchor point of the band at or slightly above shoulder height. Grab only one of the two handles between both hands and interlace your fingers, holding it in front of your chest at shoulder height. Stand with your right side facing the anchor point at a distance where there is a slight tension on the band with minimal to no slack.
2. Pick up your left foot as you press your right foot into the ground to start the lateral lunge. Make a wide step to your left before you plant your left foot on the ground parallel to your right foot.
3. As you lean your weight to your left, push your left hip back, and initiate the rotation by rotating both hands to your left while keeping your spine extended and straight.
4. As you rotate the band in front of your body, shift your weight from your right to your left side, and finish the rotation by pointing your chest and shoulders directly to your left.
5. Allow your hands to rotate back to the front of your body, then push off the ground with your left foot and bring both feet together in a standing position so your hands are directly in front of your chest.

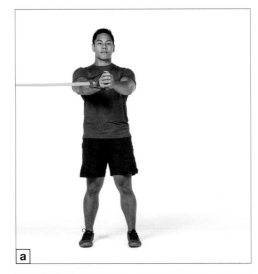

a

Correct Your Form

- Having tension in the band when starting will ensure the muscles are properly engaged all the way through the movement.
- When planting your foot into the lunge (the left foot in the instructions above), press the foot into the ground and pull your weight from your right to left leg to control the weight shift. You should feel the work in your inner thigh and gluteal muscles.

Note: Due to the tension in the band, it may not be possible to rotate all the way over the plant leg (the left leg in the above instructions). This is OK; it is more important to have tension in the band at the start of the exercise because this will increase the overall muscle activation and energy expenditure.

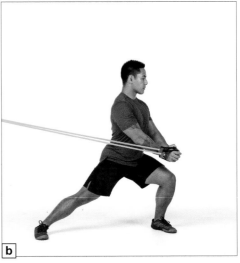

b

Fast Band Pull

Benefits

One benefit of using elastic resistance is that the faster you pull it, the more work you do and the more calories you burn. Because it challenges you to use your arms to pull on the bands as fast as possible, this exercise is similar to using a rowing machine (and is NOT recommended for a cable machine in a health club).

Instructions

1. Place the anchor point of the band at or above your shoulder height.
2. Stand facing the anchor point at a distance far enough away so there is a slight tension in both arms of the resistance band. Extend both arms straight out at approximately chest height with both palms facing each other.
3. Press both feet into the ground and sink into your hips while keeping your chest lifted and spine long as you rapidly pull both arms back as fast as possible. Pull only until your elbows have gone just past your rib cage before returning your arms to the starting position.
4. The goal is to move as fast as you can to perform as many repetitions as possible in the time interval.

Correct Your Form

To increase activation of your hip and core muscles, keep your right knee slightly bent and push your right hip back so you remain in a quarter-squat position for the duration of the exercise.

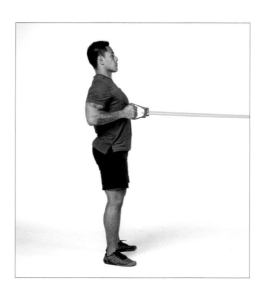

DUMBBELL EXERCISES FOR METABOLIC CONDITIONING

Dumbbells are one of the smartest ways to do a total-body workout if they are used correctly. One of their best traits is that they are compact and easy to store, making them an excellent conditioning tool if you have only a limited amount of space and time for exercise. For best results, invest in two sets of dumbbells: one relatively light, and the other heavy enough to cause fatigue at the end of the allotted time frame for each circuit.

Exercise	Time*	Circuits+
Alternating-arm bent-over row	25 sec	2-5
Lateral lunge to overhead press	25 sec	
Rotating uppercut	25 sec	
Cross-body rotating shoulder press	25 sec	
Triceps extension	25 sec	
Single-leg alternating biceps curl	25 sec	
Transverse plane lunge with reach to ground	25 sec	
Rest and recovery	45-90 sec between circuits after all exercises	

*Add 5 seconds to the work interval every 2 to 3 weeks until you are doing 45 seconds for each exercise.

+Once you are able to do 2 circuits of 45 seconds, start adding additional circuits until you are doing 5 circuits of 45-second intervals.

Alternating-Arm Bent-Over Row

Benefits

The large oblique muscles, both internal and external, help to rotate the trunk and spine during upright movements, while the large latissimus dorsi muscles of the upper back help pull the arms back during rows. Using these muscles together during an exercise increases overall energy expenditure.

Instructions

1. Stand with your feet approximately hip- to shoulder-width apart and knees slightly bent. Hold one dumbbell in each hand so that your arms are hanging along the side of your body with your palms facing in.
2. Hinge at your hips by pushing your tailbone back and keeping a straight spine with a slight bend in your knees. Lower both hands toward the floor until your elbows are fully extended.
3. Keep your spine long with your chest lifted up, palms facing each other, and feet planted firmly into the floor as you pull the dumbbells back toward your belly button. Alternate between the right and left arm. As you pull the right arm back, allow your trunk to rotate slightly to your right. Let your trunk return to neutral as you return your right arm to the starting position. As you pull your left arm back, allow your trunk to rotate to your left.

Correct Your Form

- The thoracic spine (the upper part of your back) allows for rotation. To ensure proper rotational movements, keep your chest lifted and spine long as you do this exercise.
- As you pull with each arm, turn your shoulders and chest toward the side of the arm you are pulling with so that you are flowing from left to right during this exercise.
- Hold on to the dumbbells with your hands, but when pulling the weights back during the rows, think about pulling from your elbows. The latissimus dorsi muscles attach to your upper arms; focusing on them during this exercise can help increase their activation.

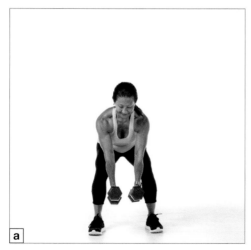
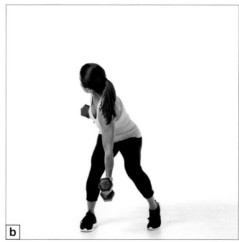

Lateral Lunge to Overhead Press

Benefits

Lateral lunges use the larger muscles of the hips and thighs to increase the overall energy expenditure of the workout. The overhead press component uses the upper body to increase muscle activity and overall caloric expenditure.

Instructions

1. Stand with your feet hip-width apart and hold one dumbbell in each hand. Step directly to your right. Keep your right foot parallel to your left as it hits the ground, and push your right hip back as you reach for the right foot with both hands.

2. To return to standing, pull your arms up and push off the floor with your right foot while pressing your left foot into the ground to pull yourself up with your left inner thigh muscles.

3. When you return to the full standing position, bend both elbows to perform a biceps curl with each arm before pressing them directly overhead to a shoulder press. Lower the weights back to your waist before performing the next repetition. Alternate legs and perform a shoulder press every time you return to the upright, standing position.

Correct Your Form

- When reaching for your foot at the bottom of the lunge, make sure the first movement comes from pushing your hip back. Once your hip is flexed you can bend your spine to reach for the foot. Bending your spine first without properly using the hip could cause minor discomfort in your lower back.

- The goal is to flow from right to left while performing an overhead press every time you are in a full, standing position.

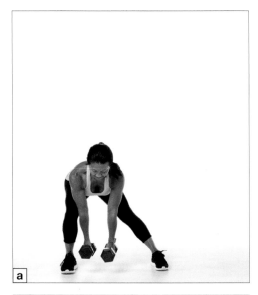

a

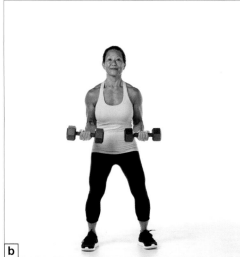

b

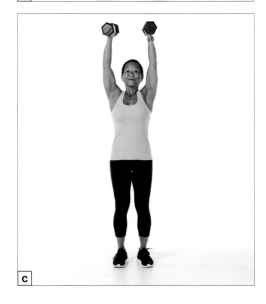

c

Rotating Uppercut

Benefits

The rotational movements of the hips and trunk combined with the motion of the arms during the uppercuts use a number of the larger muscle groups in the core and upper body, increasing overall caloric burn of this circuit.

Instructions

1. Stand with your feet shoulder-width apart, and hold one dumbbell in each hand with your palms facing up. Keep your elbows tucked in by each side while sinking your hips back into a quarter-squat.
2. Press your right foot into the ground to turn your right leg toward the midline of your body to rotate to your left. Keep your left foot pressed firmly into the ground so that you rotate around your left hip. Keep your right elbow bent as you perform an uppercut with your right arm by swinging your right elbow up to shoulder height.
3. Lower your right arm and rotate back to center, then push your left foot into the ground to rotate around your right hip while swinging your left arm up in an uppercut.

Correct Your Form

- During the uppercut portion of this exercise, the elbow should travel from your hip to shoulder height while remaining bent at a 90-degree angle. This ensures the movement comes from your shoulder.
- To rotate your hips, focus on pushing and twisting your feet into the ground, as though you are putting out a cigarette someone left burning.
- Keep your chest lifted and your spine straight so that the rotational movements come from your hips, not your back.

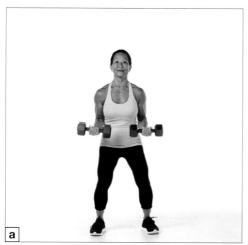
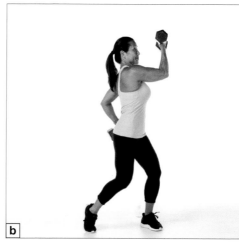

Cross-Body Rotating Shoulder Press

Benefits

Your internal and external obliques are located on the back and front, respectively, of your trunk. Performing trunk rotations as you twist before performing a shoulder press will use both obliques at the same time while strengthening the shoulders, making this an effective exercise for both burning calories and strengthening your core muscles.

Instructions

1. Stand with your feet hip-width apart, and hold one dumbbell in each hand so that your elbows are tucked in by your rib cage. The weights should be in front of your shoulders, and your palms should face each other.
2. Maintain a long spine as you rotate to your left. When finishing the rotation of your trunk, you should be facing toward the nine o'clock position. Press your right hand into the air across your body before quickly pulling your elbow back to your rib cage to lower the weight. Keep your spine tall and rotate to your right.
3. As you face the three o'clock position, press your left hand across your body before pulling the weight down by pulling your left elbow to your rib cage. When doing this exercise, alternate sides.

Correct Your Form

- Any time you rotate your trunk, make sure your spine is long and extended so the rotation comes from the intervertebral segments of the thoracic spine as opposed to the lumbar segments of the lower back.
- Rotating your feet and legs as you rotate your trunk will help ensure that the right muscles are controlling the trunk rotation.

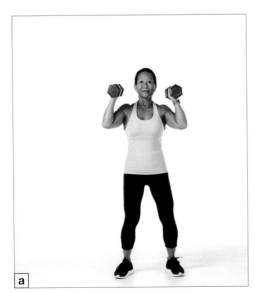
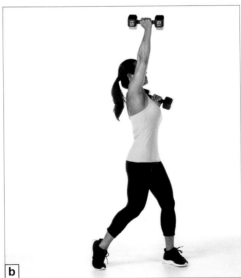

Triceps Extension

Benefits

The triceps muscles help extend the shoulder and control movement of the arm. Doing specific exercises for this muscle can increase upper-body strength while burning calories.

Instructions

1. Stand with your feet hip-width apart, and hold one dumbbell in each hand. Keep your spine long and extended as you push your hips back into a quarter-squat and hold.
2. To increase stability, press both feet firmly into the floor and keep both elbows by your side. Push both hands straight back at the same time until the arms are fully extended, then use the biceps muscles to return your hands to their initial starting spot.

Correct Your Form

- When in the hips-flexed, hinge position, make sure your spine is long and extended. To enhance stability, squeeze your glute muscles as you push your feet into the floor.
- As you extend both arms, think about squeezing the back of your upper arms to help increase overall muscle activation.

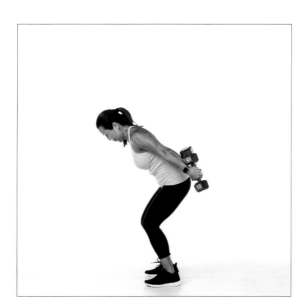

Single-Leg Alternating Biceps Curl

Benefits

Rotating the wrist to face the ceiling uses the smaller muscles under the biceps. As these muscles become stronger, they can help improve the appearance of definition and size. In some cases, doing an exercise while balanced on a single leg can increase overall work rate because the core and hip muscles have to work very hard to maintain stability.

Instructions

1. Stand with your feet hip-width apart. With both arms hanging by your side hold on to dumbbells with the palms of your hands facing the midline of your body.
2. Push your left foot into the ground and pick up your right foot so that you are balancing on your left leg. Keep your right leg slightly off the ground, but if necessary, let the toes of your right foot rest on the floor to help you maintain stability and control.
3. Bend your left elbow to bring the weight toward you shoulder. As the left dumbbell passes the height of your belly button, begin rotating your wrist so that you finish with your left palm facing the ceiling.
4. Lower your left hand down and allow your hand to rotate back to a position where it is facing the midline of your body. Alternate arms from left to right.

Correct Your Form

- To maintain control while balancing on one leg, contract the thigh and glute muscles on the stance leg, the right leg in the instructions.
- As you do these curls, work on flowing with the movement so that as one arm is extending to return to the starting position, the other arm is bending to perform the exercise.

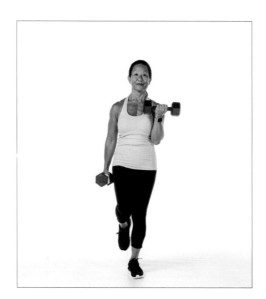

Transverse Plane Lunge
With Reach to Ground

Benefits

This movement helps engage the larger muscles of the hips and legs, making it a very effective option for burning a number of calories. The movement of the hips helps strengthen all of the muscles responsible for controlling rotation between the thigh and pelvis.

Instructions

1. Stand with your feet hip-width apart. With your arms hanging by your side, hold one dumbbell in each hand so that your palms are facing the midline of your body.

2. Press your left foot into the ground so that your toes are pointed straight ahead toward the twelve o'clock position. Squeeze your left thigh; the contraction of the muscles helps protect the knee as the hip rotates.

3. Pick up your right foot and rotate your pelvis to the right so the right hip faces the three or four o'clock position.

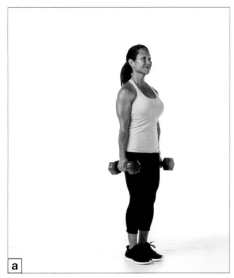

4. Place your right foot on the ground and shift your weight into the right hip as you push your right hip directly behind you. Hinge at the hip as you reach down with both hands to increase the amount of hip flexion. Reach down for your right foot and keep both hands on the inside edge of the foot (this will cause greater activation of the outer right thigh). As long as your hip moves into flexion first, you can allow your spine to bend as your reach with both hands.

5. To return to standing, pull both hands back up and extend your spine as you push off with your right leg to return to standing. As you push off with your right leg, press your left foot into the floor and think about bringing your foot up so you can return it to the initial position with both feet facing straight ahead. Alternate legs.

a

Correct Your Form

- Make sure your hip is properly flexed and hinged forward before bending the spine to reach for the floor. It doesn't matter if you actually reach the floor; the important thing is to ensure the flexion comes from the hip first and the spine second.

- When returning to the starting position, pressing the foot into the ground while squeezing the inner thigh muscles engages a number of muscles at the same time, which increases overall caloric expenditure.

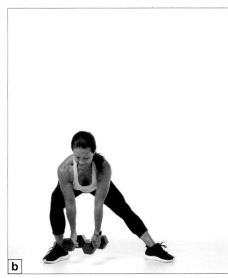

b

KETTLEBELL EXERCISES FOR METABOLIC CONDITIONING

Even though they have experienced a surge in popularity in recent years, kettlebells have been used for many years in strength training and metabolic conditioning because the movements are easy to learn. One of their best traits is that they are compact and easy to store, making them an excellent exercise option if you have only a limited amount of space and time for exercise. For best results, invest in two kettlebells: one relatively light, the other heavy enough to cause fatigue by the end of the allotted time frame for each circuit. For most people, the heavy kettlebells are 10 to 12 kilograms (22 to 26 lbs).

Exercise	Time*	Circuits+
Goblet squat	25 sec	2-5
One-arm high pull	25 sec each side	
Reverse crossover lunge with reach to ground	25 sec	
Two-hand swing	25 sec	
One-arm clean	25 sec each side	
One-arm push press	25 sec each side	
Transverse plane lunge with reach to ground	25 sec	
Rest and recovery	45-90 sec between circuits after all exercises	

*Add 5 seconds to the work interval every 2 to 3 weeks until you are doing 45 seconds for each exercise.

+Once you are able to do 2 circuits of 45 seconds, start adding additional circuits until you are doing 5 circuits of 45-second intervals.

Goblet Squat

Benefits

Holding a weight in front of your body when doing squats requires the muscles of the deep core to be engaged to control position and maintain stability of the spine. Squats also use the larger muscles of the legs to initiate and control movement. Involving so many muscles in an exercise increases the overall energy expenditure.

Instructions

1. Stand with your feet shoulder-width apart and hold a kettlebell in both palms with the handle between your forearms and the bottom facing the ceiling.
2. Keep your elbows tucked next to your rib cage and your spine long as you push your hips back to begin the lowering phase of a squat.
3. Continue to push your hips back while you allow your knees to come forward as you descend to a comfortable depth. To return to standing, push both feet into the floor and pull your knees back.

Correct Your Form

- Pushing the hips back to initiate the start of the squat movement can help ensure that the right muscles are working to control movement of the hips. Moving the knees forward before the hips could be a potential mechanism of injury.
- Press both feet into the floor as though you are trying to push it away from you when standing up from the bottom of the squat. This activates the muscles of the upper thighs and hips that control extension of the legs.
- Keep your chest lifted and spine long during both phases of the squat to ensure that your hips do most of the work.

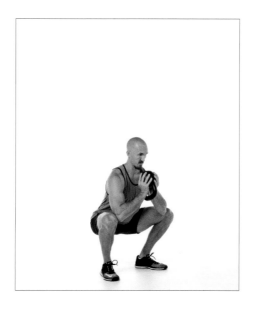

One-Arm High Pull

Benefits

High pulls are a fast, dynamic movement that help you use most of the muscles, fascia, and elastic connective tissues in the legs to increase overall force output. Working at a fast pace can increase overall energy expenditure while enhancing elastic ability and resiliency, which can help reduce the risk of injury from pulls or strains. Learning how to perform the high pull will teach the foundational movement skills for the clean exercise.

Instructions

1. Stand with your feet hip- to shoulder-width apart and hold the kettlebell firmly in your right hand. Keep your spine long and straight as you push your hips back to start a hip hinge. Let your chest drop forward, hinging at your hips, while lowering the kettlebell along the front of your legs.

2. Once you reach the end of the hip hinge, explosively push your feet into the floor and snap your hips forward. This should cause the kettlebell to travel up along the front of your body to approximately chest height as you return to a full, upright position.

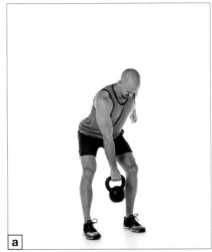

3. The kettlebell should not pause at the top of the lift and instead should fall back into the next repetition. *Note*: The energy to cause the kettlebell to travel up should come from the hips, not your arm. Start the exercise holding the kettlebell in your right hand; halfway through the work interval, switch to your left hand.

Correct Your Form

- This is designed to be a challenging hip exercise that engages the fast-twitch, type II muscle fibers, not an upper-body, arm, or shoulder exercise. The arm guides the path of motion of the kettlebell up along the front of your body and does not provide much strength to move the kettlebell.

- When pushing the hips forward, think about quickly squeezing your glute muscles as you quickly try to press the floor away from you to create the force to move the kettlebell.

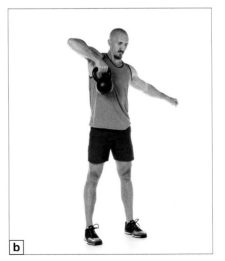

Reverse Crossover Lunge
With Reach to Ground

Benefits

This move takes the muscles that control extension of the hip through a complete ROM, helping increase strength, while alternating lunging action of the legs elevate overall energy expenditure. This lateral movement of the hips can help strengthen all of the muscles responsible for controlling motion at the hip.

Instructions

1. Start in a standing position with your feet hip-width apart, and hold the kettlebell in front of your waist with your right hand. Keep your spine long as you move your right leg behind your left (guiding your right foot toward the seven or eight o'clock position) while sinking into your left hip. As the ball of your right foot hits the ground, hinge forward at your left hip and lower the kettlebell down slightly in front of your left foot. This will create a counterbalance, allowing you to sink a little deeper into your left hip.

2. To return to standing, press your left foot into the ground as you pick up your right leg and place it back in the start position. At the top of the movement when you are standing upright, quickly switch hands and grab the kettlebell with your left hand before alternating legs to move the left leg behind the right while lowering the kettlebell toward the ground with your left hand.

Correct Your Form

- To ensure that your hip muscles are doing most of the work, place your right foot behind you as you use it to step behind the left side of your body. This will ensure that the muscles of the left hip are doing most of the work as you lower yourself during the exercise.

- To increase the level of difficulty, aim a little in front of your foot as you lower the kettlebell toward the floor. This will increase the amount of flexion in the left hip, placing more force into the hip extensor muscles.

- As you return to standing, press your stance foot into the ground and move that hip forward (the left foot and hip in the instructions).

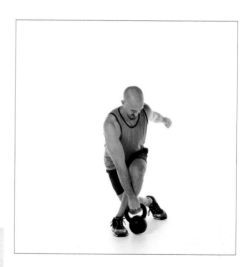

TIP During the first few workouts, focus on learning this exercise so you feel it in your hips.

Two-Hand Swing

Benefits

The swing is an explosive hinging motion that uses the large muscles of the hip extensors to control the movement while also engaging the deep muscles of the core to limit unnecessary movement from the spine. This exercise is energy-expensive while strengthening the muscles along the backs of your hips and thighs.

Instructions

1. Stand with your feet shoulder-width apart and knees slightly bent. Hold a kettlebell with both hands in a palms-down grip, and squeeze the handle in both hands to maintain a firm grip.
2. Keep your spine long, and hinge your hips back behind you while pushing the kettlebell back between your legs under your hips. The motion should look like you're snapping a football.
3. Keep your chest lifted, and quickly push your hips forward and pull your knees back to generate the forward momentum to cause the kettlebell to swing up in front of your body. The strength to move the weight should come from your legs and hips, not your shoulders.
4. Allow the kettlebell to come up to chest height before pulling it back down between your legs to prepare for the next repetition.
5. The fast movement of the kettlebell allows the muscles to work elastically to lengthen during the hip hinge in order and then shorten as you snap your hips forward to initiate the forward momentum.

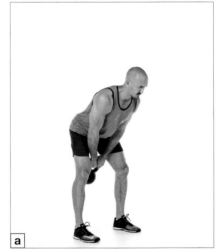

Correct Your Form

- This is a hip exercise. Your spine should remain long and straight during the movement to ensure that the hips are doing the work while your back functions only as a lever as the kettlebell travels in an arc from under your hips to approximately chest height.
- Focus on rapidly pushing your feet into the ground while snapping the hips forward by squeezing your glutes.
- As you learn the movement, think about pulling the kettlebell down under your tailbone; this is where the emphasis of the action should be. The faster you can pull the kettlebell down, the more forcefully you can thrust it upward to approximately chest height.

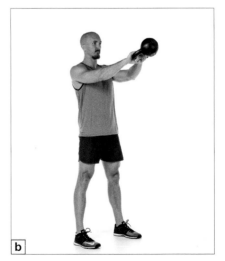

One-Arm Clean

Benefits

This is an explosive movement that uses the larger muscles of the hips and thighs to create the force to move the kettlebell. Learning how to properly clean a kettlebell—that is, catch it so that it rests in the rack position with the arm close to the chest and rib cage—can help improve coordination, motor control, and timing.

Instructions

1. Stand with your feet hip- to shoulder-width apart and hold the kettlebell firmly in your right hand with your arm rotated so that your thumb is pointed toward your body and your pinkie is pointed away from your body. Keep your spine long and straight as you push your hips back to start a hip hinge. Let your chest drop forward while hinging at your hips, and lower the kettlebell along the front of your legs.

2. Once you reach the end of the hip hinge, explosively push your feet into the floor and snap your hips forward; this should cause the kettlebell to travel up along the front of your body. Once it reaches approximately chest height, snap your right elbow toward your rib cage as you drop your right upper arm and shoulder underneath the kettlebell in order to properly catch it as you return to standing in a full, upright position with your knuckles resting along the top of your chest.

3. To lower the kettlebell, quickly drop your right hand and rotate your right thumb to point behind you as you hinge at your hips to lengthen the muscles in preparation for the next repetition.

Correct Your Form

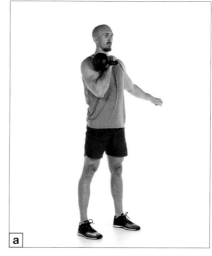

- The key to the clean is to drop your arm under the kettlebell, as opposed to trying to flip the kettlebell over your arm, which is a common—and painful—mistake.

- Emphasize wrist and arm rotation during the clean to properly drop your arm under the kettlebell.

- Your right arm should be rotated in toward your body so that your thumb is pointing directly behind you as you swing the kettlebell under your body with the right arm. When you snap the hips forward to create the momentum to return the kettlebell to the racked position, quickly drop your right elbow toward your rib cage as you rotate the palm of your right hand in toward your chest. This has to happen as one, explosive, fluid movement.

Note: Once you feel yourself become stronger and more efficient with this exercise, link it with the push press (the next exercise) so that you are doing a fluid clean and press with each rep.

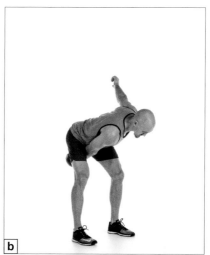

One-Arm Push Press

Benefits

This exercise uses the powerful movement of the hips to generate the momentum to lift the kettlebell up into the air. Performing fast lifts with the larger hip and thigh muscles elevates the overall energy expenditure of the workout.

Instructions

1. Hold a kettlebell in a racked position, with your elbow close to your side and your wrist bent to keep the kettlebell held firmly to the forearm. Keep your spine long as you quickly dip down into your hips before driving both feet into the floor as you snap your hips forward and punch your right arm straight up in the air.

2. As your arm reaches full extension, push back into your hips so you are standing straight and tall with your arm overhead.

3. Slowly lower your right arm by pulling your elbow down to your rib cage to return to the racked position. Use your right arm to complete AMRAP during the work interval, then transition to the left arm for the next work interval.

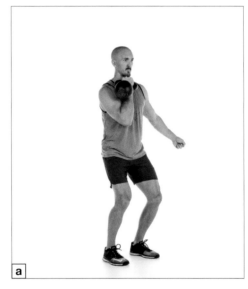

Correct Your Form

- Keep your spine straight and feet planted into the floor to create stability and to enhance the amount of power your hips generate.

- Punch your arm into the air with the palm facing the middle of your body to ensure that the shoulder joint is going through an optimal ROM.

Note: Once you feel yourself become stronger and more efficient with this exercise, link it with the clean (the previous exercise) so that you are doing a fluid clean and press with each rep.

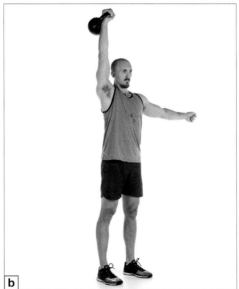

Transverse Plane Lunge With Reach to Ground

Benefits

The hip is a very mobile joint, able to move in all directions. This lunge variation takes the hip through an extensive ROM that includes rotation as well as flexion and extension, helping strengthen most of the muscles responsible for controlling movement at the hip. Reaching for the ground at the end of the lunge lengthens the hip extensor muscles under resistance, which can be one of the most effective strategies for strengthening the tissues.

Instructions

1. Stand with your feet hip-width apart and your arms in front of your body. Hold the kettlebell in your left hand with the palm of your hand facing your body.
2. Press your left foot into the ground with your toes pointed straight ahead in the twelve o'clock position. Squeeze your left thigh; the contraction of the muscles helps protect the knee as the hip rotates.
3. Pick up your right foot and rotate your pelvis to the right so that the right hip faces the three or four o'clock position.
4. Place your right foot on the ground as you shift your weight into the right hip, pushing it directly behind you. Hinge at the hip as you reach down with the left hand to touch the kettlebell to the ground on the inside of the right foot; this increases the amount of flexion in the right hip and rotation in the left hip.
5. As long as your hip is flexed first, you can allow your spine to bend as you reach down with the kettlebell. To return to standing, pull the left hand holding the kettlebell back up and extend your spine as you push off with your right leg. As you push off with your right leg, press your left foot into the floor and bring your foot up so you can return it to the initial position, with both feet facing straight ahead. Alternate legs during the work interval by moving rapidly from right to left.
6. Complete AMRAP during the work interval by alternating right and left legs and right and left arms, respectively.

Correct Your Form

- The front leg should remain so the rotation comes from the hip, not the knee or foot. Pressing your front foot into the ground while squeezing the muscles of the thigh (the left foot and left thigh in the instructions) will ensure this motion.
- The motion for the reach to the ground should come from the hip first, which should flex before the spine bends to complete the motion.
- You can start with a smaller ROM, stepping to the three or nine o'clock positions before opening up the motion to step to the four or eight o'clock positions. Gradually increasing the distance and opening up the ROM can help improve tissue strength and increase overall work rate.

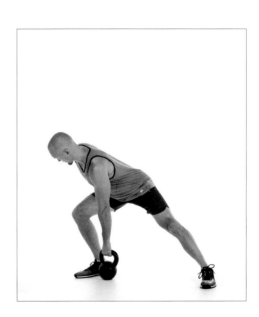

PART III

Get Fit and Stay Fit

6

Designing Your Exercise Program

Time is an extremely precious resource, and no one wants to waste it on an activity that will not provide any enjoyment or a specific return on investment. This is especially true when it comes to exercise; when you make a commitment to an exercise program, you want to know that it can help you achieve your desired outcomes. Almost any type or mode of exercise can provide results if it is done at the appropriate intensity for the necessary amount of time. Where many people go wrong is doing the same types of exercises for too long. Doing the same thing over and over (and over) but expecting different results is one definition of insanity. Following the same program with the same amount of weight or for the same number of repetitions for too long causes the body to adapt to the amount of work, and it will simply stop making changes. In technical terms, this is called *accommodation*; in common gym vernacular, this is known as *hitting a plateau*.

Designing a successful training program can be like planning a vacation: When you want to plan a getaway, you first identify your final destination and then determine the fastest, most affordable way to get there. Sure, you can take the bus to save money, but if you only have a limited amount of vacation time, you probably don't want to waste it getting to your destination. Flying is more expensive, but the benefit is that you will have more time to spend actually being *on* vacation than on getting *to* vacation.

When it comes to planning your program, the first step is to identify a *specific* fitness goal, such as improving mobility, adding strength or lean muscle mass, or enhancing aerobic capacity. It is a good idea to quantify a goal with measurable outcomes. For example, you might want to improve hip mobility to be able to do a deep squat, have the upper-body strength to complete 20 push-ups in a row, or improve your aerobic conditioning in order to reduce the amount of time it takes to get your breath back after a really hard exercise interval.

The second step is to identify the type of exercise program that can help you reach that goal. Just like taking a bus can take longer to get to your vacation spot, designing an inefficient exercise program can result in taking a lot longer to reach a fitness goal. There is a major difference between a training program that just feels really hard and one that can actually produce results. Just because a workout feels challenging doesn't mean that it can make the desired changes to your body.

An extremely common mistake is to begin an exercise program with the hopes of magically changing your body and appearance almost immediately. Here's the good news: Doing more exercise, when combined with other healthy behaviors such as following a good nutrition plan and getting an adequate amount of sleep, can make significant changes to your body. The bad news is that it does not come easy.

Using exercise to change your body requires consistent work and time. When beginning an exercise program, whether it is for the first time or you are returning after a break (why the break happened is not important; what is important is the fact that you are starting to exercise again), remember an old Chinese proverb, "The journey of a thousand miles begins with a single step." Don't start off by trying to do too much at once. Instead, begin slow and gradually build up the intensity of the workouts. Rather than trying to compensate for a period of inactivity in your first couple of exercise sessions, focus on making exercise enjoyable and fun. Regardless of any other short- or long-term goal you may have, it is important to learn how to enjoy the process of exercise

Another common challenge experienced by people who want to get fit is that doing the same exercises with the same amount of weight for an extended period of time can lead to a point where the body no longer experiences any changes. Yes, you are doing some work—and some is better than none—but if your nervous system and muscles are not challenged in new or different ways, they will no longer experience the changes you want. The equipment featured in this book—two-arm resistance bands, kettlebells, medicine balls, stability balls, sandbags, and dumbbells—can provide almost limitless options for challenging your body with exercise.

Some workouts *should* be challenging to stimulate the desired changes you want to make to your body, but the idea that *all* workouts need to be excessively strenuous is a fallacy. Instead of pushing yourself to the point of discomfort with every workout, learn how to use lower-intensity mobility workouts to help you stay active when your schedule gets really busy or to help you recover from the more challenging strength and metabolic conditioning exercise sessions. Yes, harder workouts are necessary to stimulate adaptions in your muscles and physiological systems; however, lower-intensity workouts have the important role of aiding the postexercise recovery process to help alleviate any discomfort the day after a really hard workout (Hausswirth and Mujika 2013). Low- to moderate-intensity mobility workouts can also help reduce muscle tightness and improve blood flow after a long day of limited movement, like being stuck in meetings or sitting in a car or plane. Knowing how to alternate between high- and low-intensity workouts as well as when it might be necessary to scrap a planned HIIT session for some mobility exercises can help you move better while leaving you feeling great for the long run.

Focus on learning to enjoy the process of exercise by knowing when to alternate between low, moderate, and high intensity. On those days when you're feeling great, are well rested, well fueled, and hydrated, you can make a few changes to increase the intensity. Increasing the intensity means doing a few more reps, moving at a faster pace, taking shorter rest breaks, or using a heavier weight. It means doing a *little* more than what you've been doing, not necessarily *a lot* more; do just enough to feel the difference. On the days when you feel tired or sluggish, you'll be surprised at how a low-intensity mobility workout can recharge your batteries and boost your energy levels. Once you start moving a bit, it's highly likely that you will start feeling better, and before long, you'll be moving better and with a little more purpose!

Each workout or exercise session causes a number of short-term responses that lead to long-term changes in the body. The short-term responses take place either during or immediately after a workout, which gradually accumulate into long-term adaptations or changes to the body. An example of an immediate response to a workout is the localized muscle fatigue resulting from applying mechanical forces and depleting the glycogen stored in muscle cells. The long-term adaptations occur after repeated training sessions and consistent adherence to an exercise program. An example of a long-term adaptation is that as the muscles repeatedly exercise to a point of fatigue, using all of the available glycogen for energy, the muscle cells will adapt by storing more glycogen that, in turn, will provide additional energy, allowing you to do more work before reaching fatigue. A secondary benefit from a muscle's ability to store more glycogen is an increase in muscle fiber size because glycogen holds on to water, increasing overall muscle volume. In addition, repeatedly exercising to the point of fatigue can increase the number of type II motor units and muscle fibers recruited for that exercise; over the long run this can increase the ability to engage more muscle motor units for that exercise, leading to an increase in overall force production. Keep in mind that while you will notice an improvement in your quality of movement and start to feel stronger within the first few workouts, it can take six to eight weeks of consistent participation in a program, along with the adoption of other healthy behaviors (e.g., reducing sugary snacks), before any significant changes to your body may take effect.

In the rest of this chapter, we'll examine how to put together individual workouts to maximize your time and effort. Then, a discussion of the concept of periodization will help you understand how best to put workouts together in an organized exercise program to get the results you want. Lastly, we'll discuss the importance of recovery, how to recover from an individual workout so that you're ready for the next session, and how much recovery time you need between workouts so you can avoid overtraining and feel your best.

The Components of a Workout

When cooking a meal, it is possible to throw a bunch of ingredients in a bowl, mix them up, and then pop them in the oven, but unless you follow a systematic manner of how those ingredients are prepared and added to the dish, you may end up with an inedible mess. The purpose of a recipe is to provide a guide for how to organize ingredients to prepare a specific meal. Exercise is the exact same way! If your strategy is just to do a few random exercises that you like or to try to mimic a celebrity's workout without understanding how it's actually affecting your body, the results could be muddled or nonexistent.

It's knowing how and when to perform certain exercises that determines whether they have the desired effect on the body. While the types of equipment or specific exercises might change, the overall structure of a workout should not. Every workout includes three specific components.

The Warm-Up

A warm-up includes low-intensity exercises to elevate the heart rate, raise tissue temperature, and enhance overall activation of the central nervous system (CNS) to prepare the body for the exercises it will perform in the workout. An effective warm-up could be mobility exercises with just your body weight or a light weight. It should take less than 10 minutes and should feature low-intensity movements that replicate the more challenging exercises you will perform later.

Here's an example of a warm-up that can help you properly prepare your body to be ready for exercise.

- Glute bridges: 12 to 15 reps
- High plank: hold for 20 to 40 seconds
- Side plank: hold for 20 to 30 seconds on each side
- Lateral lunges with reach for your opposite foot (e.g., when lunging to your right side, reach for your right foot with your left hand: 8 to 12 on each side)
- Jumping jacks: 12 to 15 reps

Perform these exercises as a circuit, moving from one exercise to the next with minimal rest; rest for about 30 seconds at the end, and complete 2 to 3 circuits. This may seem a little rudimentary, and the jumping jacks definitely add an old school flavor, but this simple little circuit can have you ready to do hard work in 7 to 10 minutes. On those days when your schedule gets absolutely jammed, you can do this circuit on its own to get in a little activity. And remember: When it comes to exercise, a little bit of something is better than a lot of nothing!

What the Science Says: Why Warm Up?

A complete, full-body warm-up provides a number of benefits, including the following:

- *Increased circulation*: Muscles use oxygen and nutrients for fuel. Low-intensity movements as part of a warm-up improve blood flow to muscles, bringing the necessary fuel for the workout. It can take from 8 to 15 minutes to elevate circulation and improve oxygen flow, so be ready to invest that amount of time to adequately prepare your body.
- *Elevated levels of hormones used for energy production*: Epinephrine and norepinephrine (commonly called *adrenaline* because it is produced in the adrenal glands) and cortisol are used to help convert fats and carbohydrates to energy used to fuel muscular contractions. During the warm-up, the body starts increasing production of these hormones so your body has the fuel it needs for the workout.
- *Reduced risk of muscle strains by increasing tissue temperature*: Muscle and connective tissue have more elasticity at higher temperatures, allowing easier, unrestricted motion of joints used in exercise.
- *Activation of the sensory receptors of the CNS*: These receptors are responsible for identifying position changes in the body, which is essential for optimal motor control and coordination during the workout.
- *Improved neural activation of muscle*: This sounds technical, but muscle contractions are initiated by motor units controlled by the CNS. Warm-up exercises with gradually increasing intensity provide the necessary stimulus to the CNS to ensure that the muscle motor units will produce the requisite forces required for the workout.
- *Mental preparation*: A consistent warm-up routine will allow the mind to switch off distracting thoughts such as work, family, or social obligations, and to switch on to focus on the upcoming challenging exercises in the workout.
- *Rehearse movement patterns*: Practice these patterns at a slower, controlled tempo before adding resistance for a core strength workout or increasing speed during a metabolic conditioning workout. Moving at a slower tempo to learn the pattern provides you with the opportunity to correct and improve your form; as your form and technique, improve you will be able to gain strength by additional external resistance or improve metabolic conditioning by moving at a faster tempo with shorter rest intervals.

The Workout

Even though the focus might shift between mobility, metabolic conditioning, and core strength training, each workout contains the same variables: exercise selection, intensity, tempo, repetitions, rest interval, sets, and frequency, all of which were introduced in chapter 2. When you notice a workout becoming easier, that is good

What the Science Says: Increasing or Decreasing Workout Intensity

Making changes to a workout is not that complicated. The following suggestions are easy ways to make simple changes to the variables of exercise program design, which can create an entirely different workout experience to help your body make the desired changes.

Exercise Selection

Think of this as the main component of a dish. If a recipe calls for chicken, you can add different spices to change the taste of the dish. If the workout calls for a squat or lunge movement, keep the exercise the same and adjust the other variables to create a different workout.

Intensity

One of the easiest ways to change a workout is to use a heavier weight. This will limit the amount of repetitions you can perform, but you will engage your muscles differently, which can change the outcome. If you use a lighter weight, you can challenge yourself by changing other variables, such as adding repetitions or moving at a faster tempo.

Repetitions

Remember that for best results, you want to exercise to a point of momentary fatigue. If you increase the intensity, you will complete fewer repetitions to hit fatigue. Reducing the intensity to use a lighter weight will require you to do more repetitions to fatigue.

One easy way to change a workout is to set a countdown timer and perform as many reps as possible in the time allotted. This can be an easy way to measure progress. If you can only complete 15 repetitions the first time you do an exercise for 20 seconds, then when you can complete 20 reps in 20 seconds, you will have made a 33 percent improvement.

Sets

If you want to make your workout harder—and time allows for it—do more sets. If you've been doing two or three sets of a workout, adding an additional set can increase the overload and make a noticeable difference. If you find that you're not properly fatigued after four or five sets of an exercise, use heavier weights or do more reps!

Tempo

Moving at a slower speed can keep the muscle under tension for a longer period of time, which is one strategy for engaging more motor units. Slowing the movement speed so that you are moving for 5 to 10 seconds in each direction can create an entirely different challenge than moving faster. Moving at a fast tempo can be a faster way to reach momentary muscle fatigue, the indicator that all muscle fibers have been recruited in a particular muscle.

Rest Interval

When first starting an exercise program, you may want to give yourself a little break of at least 15 to 30 seconds between each exercise. Moving toward no rest between exercises, or even cutting the rest time in half, can be a fast way to make the workout harder without changing anything else.

news because it means that your body is becoming stronger. But it also means that it is time to change your workout and challenge your body to work a little differently. Just like changing the amount of one or two ingredients can significantly change the outcome of a recipe, adjusting just one or two of the variables of program design can create a different workout.

The Cool-Down

During exercise, the body functions at a heightened state of arousal. The purpose of the cool-down period is to help the body return to its normal operating status, called *homeostasis*. The cool-down is often overlooked, but it is extremely important because it is the time to reduce tension in the working muscles. This allows them to return to their normal resting length, remove metabolic waste from the muscles that generated force during the workout, promote oxygen flow to help repair damaged tissue, and allow the heart rate to return to a normal, resting level. The cool-down helps to kick-start the recovery process, when all of the damaged muscle tissue is repaired and the glycogen used to fuel the exercise is replaced. Think of your cool-down process as the start of the next day's workout session; the more complete the cool-down process, the better prepared you will be for the next time you exercise.

Strategies for Working Out When Time Is a Factor

Whether it's because of work or family obligations, when your schedule gets busy it can be easy to blow off exercise or find things that don't make you work hard. While longer exercise sessions *can* provide more benefits for muscle growth, shorter exercise sessions can be beneficial as long as the intensity is challenging and larger muscles are engaged. Part of maintaining a healthy lifestyle is knowing how to adjust your exercise program to fit the time you have available in your schedule. Even 10 to 30 minutes can provide effective, health-promoting benefits.

Keep this in mind: Up to about two weeks of time off from working out won't have a significant effect on your fitness level, but more time than that—even three or four weeks—without any exercise could result in a loss of strength, cardiorespiratory fitness, or mobility. This is why when times get busy, it is important to exercise when you can—and frequently. Shorter or lower-intensity workouts may not improve strength or make significant changes to your body, but they can help you maintain the changes you've made up to that point.

If you do a shorter workout, don't skip the warm-up and cool-down. It's important to give your body a chance to prep for the activity, then cool down to return to its normal, resting state. The warm-up can simply consist of the exercises you will do in the workout but without weight, or at a slower tempo. The cool-down can include low-intensity bodyweight exercises such as the plank, side plank, and reverse crunches or a couple of stretches to help optimize mobility in a specific joint or muscle group.

Each of the following workout methods can be used when time is limited. These strategies can also be applied to create challenging new workouts when you're looking to make a change in your overall program. If you want to use these formats when you have more time for your workout, simply add more time to the interval or, in the case of Tabata intervals, select different exercises and complete multiple intervals.

Tabata Training

Best for metabolic training, Tabata intervals are based on research by Dr. Izumi Tabata, who observed that 8- to 20-second intervals of extremely high intensity exercise with only 10 seconds of rest in between was enough to increase aerobic efficiency in a workout lasting only 4 minutes. Download a Tabata timer onto a phone or tablet, and select two or four exercises.

- If two exercises are selected, alternate from one to the other over the course of the workout to complete four sets of each exercise.
- If four exercises are selected, alternate between each exercise to perform a total of two sets of each one.

After a good warm-up and when done at the highest intensity possible, meaning exercise to the point of breathlessness in each twenty-second interval, only one cycle of Tabata training, which lasts four minutes, can provide the stimulus to improve aerobic capacity and increase the time to fatigue (Tabata, Ogita, and Miyachi 1996).

Example With Two Exercises

- Squat with forward reach: Complete as many as possible in 20 seconds, then rest for 10 seconds. Alternate with high plank; hold for 20 seconds, then rest for 10 seconds.
- Complete 4 sets of each exercise in a 4-minute Tabata interval.

The following example of a Tabata interval workout is based on using a series of the two-arm resistance band exercises for core strength from chapter 4

Example With Four Exercises

Set a Tabata interval timer (several are available to download for smart phones and tablets) for 4 minutes and prepare to do the following 4 exercises from the core strength workout from chapter 4; do each exercise for 20 seconds, rest for 10 seconds, then switch to the next exercise for a circuit. For the lunge to one-arm pull, do one set with the right arm and left leg and the next with the left arm and right leg. Likewise, for the two-hand forward press, the first time should be done with the left shoulder facing the anchor point, and the second should be done with the right shoulder facing the anchor point.

- Standing crunch
- Lunge to one-arm pull
- Two-hand forward press
- Squat to row

Each exercise will be done twice for 20 seconds in a 4-minute Tabata interval.

Every Minute On the Minute (EMOM)

This set is best for either metabolic conditioning or core strength training. It's a relatively new way to organize a workout. After a complete warm-up, set a timer. At the start of every minute, do a certain number of reps of an exercise. Once you are finished with that number of reps, you have the rest of the minute to rest before you move on to the next exercise.

EMOMs can either focus on only one exercise or alternate between different exercises. One example would be to set a timer for 8 minutes and complete 25 kettlebell swings at the start of every minute; once you complete the 25 swings, you can rest and recover for the remainder of the minute. Another example would be to set a time and alternate between performing an upper-body exercise on the even minutes (starting with 0 when the timer begins) and a lower-body exercise for the odd minutes on the timer.

- Set a timer for 10 minutes and select only one upper-body and one lower-body movement; e.g., dumbbell shoulder presses for the upper-body and alternating lateral lunges for the lower body. Start the timer, on the even minutes, beginning with 0, perform the lateral lunges, on the odd minutes, starting with 1, perform the dumbbell shoulder presses for a total of 5 sets of each exercise.
- Set a timer for 12 minutes and select 4 exercises, such as lower body squat or lunge, upper-body pull, upper-body push, and core exercises (e.g., reverse lunges, dumbbell uppercuts, renegade rows, and inchworm walkouts) for a total of 3 sets of each exercise in 12 minutes.

Ten-Minute Timer: Five Sets of Each Exercise

The following exercises are selected from the bodyweight workout for metabolic conditioning in chapter 5.

- Even minutes (starting at 0): 20 speed squats
- Odd minutes (starting at 1): 10 step-throughs (to each side)

Once all reps are done, the remainder of the minute is a rest interval.

Twelve-Minute Timer: Three Sets of Each Exercise

The following stability ball exercises are selected from chapter 5 on metabolic conditioning. Set a timer for 12 minutes and alternate between each of the following exercises: the first minute (starting with 0), 12 hip bridges to hamstring curls; the second minute (starting with 1), 12 prone hip rolls; the third minute (beginning with 2), 12 roll-outs; and the fourth minute (beginning with 3), 12 Russian twists; then complete the circuit 2 more times in the remaining 8 minutes.

- 12 hip bridges to hamstring curls
- 12 prone hip rolls
- 12 roll-outs
- 12 Russian twists

Once all reps are done, the rest of the minute is a rest interval.

Ladder Sets

Ladder sets can be very effective for metabolic conditioning. After a brief warm-up, set a timer for 6 minutes. For the first interval, do 20 seconds of work followed by 40 seconds of rest, then 30 seconds of work followed by 30 seconds of rest, then 40 seconds of work followed by 20 seconds of rest, which is "climbing the ladder" by performing the shortest to longest workout intervals; once at the proverbial top it will be necessary to repeat the intervals from longest to shortest and climb your way back down the ladder. Select one exercise that will be really challenging to use for each particular ladder set. On the days when time is limited, this is a great way to complete a workout.

For this time-saving workout, select two exercises for two separate ladder sets of 6 minutes each. For the first, use the squat to overhead press (as seen on page 172 of the dumbbell workout for core strength training. Progress from 20 to 30 to 40 seconds then climb back down the ladder with sets of 40, 30, and 20 seconds, respectively. For the second ladder set use kettlebell swings (as seen on page 254 of the kettlebell workout for metabolic conditioning) and follow the same progression up and down the ladder for 6 minutes. Congratulations, that is a lot of exercise in less than 15 minutes, showing that a lot of time is not necessary to do an adequate amount of exercise.

Tri-Sets

Tri-sets are best for core strength training. A tri-set is a series of exercises (usually three but sometimes four) done in a row with little to no rest between each set.

In a tri-set, start with a multijoint movement pattern before moving to single-joint or isolation exercise for a specific muscle. For optimal benefits, do not rest when transitioning from one move to the next. The goal of a tri-set is to completely fatigue a particular muscle or muscle group, which can be one of the fastest ways to create metabolic overload.

The following tri-set is an example of how to re-organize exercises from the bodyweight workout for core strength on page (124) in chapter 4 into a different workout challenge:

- Squat with forward reach: 15 reps
- Reverse lunge with overhead reaches: 12 reps each leg
- Glute bridge: 20 reps

Complete all reps; that is one tri-set. Rest for 30 to 45 seconds. Complete three tri-sets.

The following tri-set is an example of how to re-organize exercises from the sandbag workout for core strength on page 149 in chapter 4 into a different workout challenge:

- Lateral lunge with forward press: 10 reps
- Reverse lunge with rotation: 12 reps
- One-leg hip bridge: 15 reps

Complete all reps on the right leg, then all reps on the left. Rest for 30 to 45 seconds. Complete three to five sets.

30:30

On those days that time is limited but you would still like to complete a relatively challenging metabolic conditioning workout, the 30:30 workout provides an excellent option for how to perform a lot of exercise in a short period of time. The 30:30 workout is so-named because it involves 30 seconds of a moderate- to hard-intensity exercise followed by 30 seconds of rest or active rest with a low-intensity exercise, which is one way to complete a 30:30 workout shown by the kettlebell workout below. A different way is to perform a challenging exercise for 30 seconds followed by a relatively easy, less challenging exercise for 30 seconds so that you are performing an active recovery, continuing to exercise at a low intensity while recovering from a high-intensity exercise, as opposed to a passive recovery where you rest with no bodily movement. The workout below is an example of how to alternate between high-intensity work and lower-intensity active recovery.

The following exercises are selected from the kettlebell workout for core strength on page 174 in chapter 4. Set a timer for 15 minutes and perform each exercise for 30 seconds and then rest for 30 seconds before moving on to the next exercise in the circuit. One full circuit will last five minutes; complete three sets.

- Goblet squat
- Right arm overhead press
- Left arm overhead press
- Right arm bent-over row
- Left arm bent-over row

Set a timer for a specific amount of time, from 8 to 12 (or longer) minutes. Select two to four primary exercises for the intervals of hard work and the same number of secondary, lower-intensity exercises for the intervals of active recovery.

The following exercises are selected from the two-arm resistance band workout for metabolic conditioning on page 234 in chapter 5. The active recovery exercises are chosen from the bodyweight workouts for mobility (found on page 58) and core strength (found on page 124):

- Set a timer for 9 minutes. Perform an exercise for 30 seconds, doing as many reps as possible, followed by 30 seconds of active recovery with a lower-intensity exercise; complete 3 circuits of these 3 exercises.
- Squat to row for 30 seconds, followed by high plank for 30 seconds
- Straight-arm pulldown for 30 seconds, followed by side plank for 15 seconds each side
- Alternating punches for 30 seconds, followed by glute bridge for 30 seconds

With all of the healthy, nutritious foods that you can turn into delicious meals, why would you ever limit yourself to a diet of just peanut butter and jelly sandwiches? If you have been doing the same exercise program for an extended amount of time, that is essentially what you are doing to your muscles: You are restricting them to a limited diet that can impede your ability to experience results from your time spent exercising. Workouts don't need dramatic changes to impose different stimuli on your body. As you have seen so far in this chapter, simply making a few minor adjustments to variables such as repetitions, tempo, and rest interval can provide a significant change to your program. If you know your busy times of the year, such as preparing to present at the annual meeting, budget-planning, getting the kids ready to go back to school, preparing for the end of a semester, hitting a quarterly sales goal, completing a project by an important deadline, or any other time when other parts of your life will interfere with your ability or that can really eat into your ability to make time for exercise, knowing how to use a timer to schedule quick, effective workouts gives you practical solutions to help you maintain the gains from your program.

The Role of Recovery

Exercising applies a stress to the body and is only part of the process required for making the changes you want to see. Yes, exercise is good for you and can provide a number of important benefits, but there is such a thing as too much exercise. Specifically, too much high-intensity exercise without sufficient rest, or working out too many days in a row without allowing for appropriate rest or recovery time, could lead to Overtraining Syndrome (OTS). If you want to use exercise to manage your weight, increase muscle definition, or promote overall good health, it's important to know that OTS could actually result in weight gain, a loss of muscle mass, and a weakened immune system (Wyatt, Donaldson, and Brown 2013; Hausswith and Mujika 2013; Bishop, Jones, and Woods 2008).

The most important part of any workout occurs *after* the workout itself is over. The secret of many of the top strength and performance coaches in the world isn't the specific exercises used in an athlete's workout; it's how the overall program is structured to allow time for optimal recovery between training sessions. While you might not be a professional or competitive athlete, it's a good idea to follow the lead of the top conditioning coaches: If it works for an athlete making a lot of money throwing or kicking a ball, it can probably help you reach your fitness goals.

You may be familiar with the phrases, "Pain is weakness leaving the body" and "No pain, no gain," and have the misguided belief that in order to be effective, exercise must cause extreme discomfort. Exercise should challenge you to work harder than your current abilities, but not every workout has to make you sore to be effective. If you are sore the day after a workout, you may have an accumulation of metabolic by-product (lactic acid and hydrogen ions) in the muscle tissue. Without adequate amounts of rest between sets or workouts, the quality of future efforts becomes compromised, which could increase the risk of developing Delayed Onset Muscle Soreness (DOMS). DOMS creates the perception that exercise is painful, which could provide an excuse for blowing off your next workout. Or, you may feel that muscle soreness is an indicator of a good workout, which isn't necessarily the case.

When you're sore, it might be tempting to skip any physical activity because it doesn't feel great. But elevating your heart rate with low- to moderate-intensity exercise when you're sore the day after a workout can be an effective tactic for promoting a complete recovery. It can take anywhere from 24 to 72 hours to fully recover from an extremely demanding metabolic conditioning workout, but that doesn't call for a day on the couch. Instead, a low-intensity mobility workout can help reduce feelings of soreness and promote optimal recovery. It can be helpful to think of these lower-intensity exercise sessions as regeneration workouts because they help promote both recovery and muscle growth.

When it comes to recovery, your mindset should be: Tomorrow's workout begins at the end of today's workout. Hydration, proper fueling (nutrition), and adequate sleep all play a critical role during the postworkout recovery process. Listed below are specific recovery strategies you can use to ensure that the hard work you put in brings you the results you want. The stark reality is that how you recover can be the difference between getting results or simply spinning your wheels with nothing to show for it. Too many challenging workouts too close together may not allow time for your body to rest, replace lost energy stores, or rebuild new muscle tissue. Don't ever fret about taking a rest day. If you've been working out hard, it is well deserved, and it can do wonders for recharging your batteries, both physiologically and psychologically.

It's important to have a specific strategy for what you do after your workouts. Just as an exercise program is specific to the individual, your recovery should be designed to meet the needs of your workouts. It's important to note that recovery doesn't just mean taking time off to rest. Consider how you can incorporate the following strategies into your workout recovery plan.

Rest

Get a good night's sleep! This is a requisite component of success. On those days when you do an extremely challenging workout, make sure you allow for adequate sleep to promote optimal tissue repair and recovery. Inducing metabolic and mechanical stress in the gym will only go so far in promoting muscle growth. Testosterone (T) and growth hormone (GH) are produced during the REM cycles of sleep, making a full night's rest critical for promoting muscle growth after strength training.

If you're busy with work, travel, or family and are not getting sufficient sleep, adjust your exercise program and do low- to moderate-intensity workouts until you can return to your normal sleep patterns. If you normally love hard-charging workouts, the short-term drop in intensity might not feel like you're really exercising, but your body will appreciate the reduced physical stress load. The danger of too much exercise without proper rest and recovery can lead to injury or illness, both of which could keep you out of the gym for long periods of time.

Postworkout Nutrition

The science of nutrient timing suggests that *when* nutrition is consumed before and after exercise is as, if not more, important than *what* is consumed. Replenish the energy you expended with glycogen from carbohydrates and repair tissue with proteins during the period *after* exercise. This can promote quicker muscle recovery. Consuming a snack or drink with a 3:1 or 4:1 carbohydrate-to-protein ratio within 30 to 45 minutes postexercise can help you recover from the day's activity and get ready for tomorrow's workout. The carbohydrates will increase insulin, which promotes postexercise utilization of proteins for muscle repair.

What the Science Says:
Metabolic Damage Due to OTS

Muscles become stronger during the period *after* training, not during the training session itself. Creating a metabolic overload is essential for stimulating muscle growth, but too much exercise without an appropriate amount of recovery could result in excessive metabolic damage to muscle, fascia, and elastic connective tissue. The following are examples of metabolic damage due to OTS.

Elevated Blood Lactate

When muscles involved in exercise can no longer meet energy demands through aerobic metabolism, they will tap into the adenosine triphosphate phosphocreatine (ATP-PC) and glycolysis energy pathways to produce ATP anaerobically (without oxygen). One by-product of anaerobic metabolism is lactic acid, which can accumulate quickly during high-intensity exercise. The onset of blood lactate (OBLA), commonly called the *lactate threshold* (LT), is a physiological marker of an elevation in blood acidity. It can restrict the production of ATP in muscle cells, leading to fatigue. When you feel that burning sensation in your muscles, it's an indication of OBLA and a sign that it is time for a lower-intensity active recovery interval. However, regular high-intensity interval training (HIIT) can train the body to tolerate working at OBLA as well as improving the ability to quickly remove lactate and other metabolic waste.

Acidosis

Besides lactic acid, anaerobic exercise also elevates levels of hydrogen ions (H+), both of which increase blood acidity and reduce the levels of oxygen and other nutrients available for aerobic energy production. In extreme cases, acidosis can cause severe damage to muscle tissue, resulting in a breakdown of muscle protein called myoglobin. When myoglobin is broken down and subsequently enters the blood stream, this could ultimately lead to rhabdomyolysis. Rhabdomyolysis can inhibit normal function of the kidneys, potentially leading to hospitalization or even death, so it is extremely important to listen to your body and not push physical exertion past your normal comfort levels.

Gluconeogenesis

Protein is normally used to repair tissue damaged during exercise and promote the growth of new muscle. Carbohydrate is converted to glycogen and used for ATP production during anaerobic exercise. Fatty acids require oxygen and take longer to convert to ATP, making them an inefficient energy source for high-intensity exercise. When high-intensity exercise lasts for an extended period of time, the body will convert protein to ATP in a process called gluconeogenesis, reducing the amount of protein available for muscle growth. The process of converting amino acids (the building blocks of protein) to ATP elevates levels of ammonia, further increasing blood acidity and the risk of acidosis.

Flexibility and Tissue Treatment

Most people know that it is important to start a workout with dynamic flexibility exercises and to cool down with static stretching. However, optimal recovery for the body-wide network of fascia and elastic connective tissue goes beyond simply stretching and should include techniques for improving tissue extensibility while reducing tension. Foam rollers, sticks, balls, vibration platforms, static stretching, or massage can be used to apply appropriate pressure or friction to the muscle to improve circulation and break up inelastic collagen fibers, which can accumulate in stress points and limit tissue extensibility. If you run out of time during the workout, it's a good idea to have equipment at home so you can do some tissue work in the evening while relaxing in front of the TV or before bed. Using a foam roller, massage stick, or even a tennis ball doesn't take long and can actually be a good way to wind down the day and prepare for a good night's sleep.

Heat and Cold Treatments

There is a reason why many health clubs have saunas and whirlpools: The heat from these relaxing environments can promote postexercise tissue recovery. Heat increases the body's circulation, which removes metabolic waste products such as H+ while carrying oxygen and other nutrients necessary to repair tissue used during the workout. Another less comfortable but extremely effective option is the use of cold treatments. Ice baths, ice packs, cooling vests, special chairs with pockets for ice packs, or even the use of a cryofreeze chamber are all examples of different options available for applying cold treatment. One benefit of cold treatment is that it can cool down the body's core temperature. This is essential when exercising in hot weather or when exercising two or more times on the same day. A second benefit is that it can reduce inflammation and promote healing in tissue that was used during the workout. The cold from the application of ice to a sore muscle or joint brings more blood to the area, which brings nutrients and oxygen to promote healing.

Compression Clothing

You may have noticed an uptick in the number of people wearing tight compression clothing both during athletic competitions or in the period immediately after completing a race or finishing a game. Evidence indicates that wearing compression clothing after a strenuous activity, whether a hard workout or competition, may help reduce soreness and inflammation to speed up the optimal recovery time. It's not 100 percent clear how compression clothing works to promote recovery. Current hypotheses include that the pressure from the tight clothing can reduce the perception of overall muscle soreness, improve fluid exchange between the capillaries and tissue, or promote venous return to the heart helping to remove metabolic byproduct such as H+ from muscle while promoting the flow of oxygenated blood to augment the tissue repair process (Hausswirth and Mujika 2013; MacRae, Cotter, and Laing 2011). Feel free to try compression garments to see if they help you feel more recovered between workouts.

Understanding how to do exercises to improve mobility, core strength, and metabolic conditioning is the foundation of a long-term exercise program. Knowing why and how to organize your workouts to alternate between various phases of intensity and recovery to allow for optimal adaptation is an equally important part of the foundation. Exercise will not provide its optimal potential unless you give your body the appropriate time to recover between workouts. In the following section, you'll learn how to structure your workouts to allow for optimal recovery and reduce the risk of an overuse injury. Ultimately, this is what keeps you moving forward in reaching your fitness and performance goals.

Periodization

Alternating between core strength, metabolic conditioning, and mobility workouts helps you apply the appropriate amount of stimulus to promote muscle growth and overall performance enhancement without the risk of overtraining. Consistency in the exercises selected for a particular workout can help your body learn the movement patterns so they become a reflexive action, that is, without conscious thought. But realize that the body is a very adaptable machine, and the more it performs the same exercises at the same intensity, the fewer calories it burns to execute those particular movements. *Any* exercise is better than *no* exercise, but following the same routine for too long will not provide the stimulus your body craves to continue making adaptations.

How the physiology of your body's adaptation to exercise is based on hard science; however, planning your workouts over an extended period of time so that you can achieve the desired results is a bit of an art. There's a fine line between staying with the same workout routine for too long, or changing your workouts too frequently. The more often your muscles perform the same movement, the less stimulus they receive, meaning that you will literally just be going through the motions. The same is true if you change workouts too frequently. Yes, the nervous and muscular systems do respond to variation because it challenges them to work differently, but changing too often does not allow for the consistency that is necessary for long-term skill development.

Periodization is the process of organizing an exercise program into phases of higher- and lower-intensity workouts and was developed specifically to maximize the recovery process for athletes preparing for a competition (Bompa and Buzzichelli

What the Science Says: How the Body Becomes More Efficient Performing the Same Exercise Repeatedly

Here's an example of how muscles can do less work performing the same exercises repeatedly: At one point, before I had kids, I used to ride my bike to work a couple times a week. The trip was about nine miles each way, and because there were safe bike lanes, I followed the same route to and from the office. In the morning, when I got to my desk, I would record the time, along with my average heart rate and an estimated number of calories I burned (provided by the heart rate monitor I wore when riding). Over the course of about 14 weeks, I went from burning more than 600 calories to a little less than 500. Nothing changed: My route was the same and, with the exception of shaving off a few minutes for pedaling efficiency or timing the lights right, it was always the same distance. While this was not a formal study, it is an example of how muscles can expend less energy doing the same work. Yes, I got a little quicker and developed more efficiency in my pedaling cadence, but that should not account for that much of a difference. What this shows is that muscles do become more efficient when they are required to perform the same amount of work over a period of time.

2015). An example of a periodized program for professional American football players would be to train to be in football shape before training camps begin in late July and to peak at the highest level of fitness when teams being making a push for the postseason playoffs in late November. Once a professional football team has completed its season, the athletes will have a period of light, non-football-specific activity before beginning the conditioning program to prepare for the next season.

You're not an athlete, you say? Fair enough, but if the science of periodization works to help million-dollar athletes perform their best on the field or court, it can certainly help you get in the best shape possible. The greatest benefit of periodization is that it uses rest as a means of allowing for adaptation to the physically demanding stresses of training.

The science of periodization can provide a systematic way to change the volume and intensity of exercise. The basic exercise movements can be consistent to provide for efficient learning, but the other variables of exercise program design—intensity, reps, sets, rest intervals, and tempo—can be manipulated to create challenging and, more importantly, engaging workouts. Adjusting intensity, reps, and sets is a matter of simply changing the amount of weight or using a different piece of equipment. Intensity can be manipulated not just by the load of the mass but by the direction, height, and speed of the movement. Long-term programs that are dynamic, challenging, fun, and effective can help you reach your goals, whatever they may be.

Linear Periodization

Linear periodization features a gradual progression of exercise intensity that increases over a period of weeks or months. The goal is to peak with the hardest workouts before a specific date, which could be the start of a competitive season or a single competition (Bompa and Buzzichelli 2015). One way to apply the linear model to your program is to change your workouts when the seasons change. As the calendar transitions through spring, summer, fall, and winter, you change your workouts to focus on different goals: strength to mobility to metabolic conditioning based on whether you want to achieve your peak conditioning for your favorite outdoor activities during the summer months or in the winter if cold weather sports are your thing.

Or, you may organize your training around a competition or event. In this case, you want to peak two to three weeks before the start of competition or event. A few days of rest or low-intensity exercise is important immediately before a competitive season in order to allow the body to recover and repair itself before a competitive season begins. If you've ever prepared for a long-distance race where you've gradually increased the distance of your runs building up to the date of the event, you've already followed a linear periodization program.

When applying linear periodization, the volume, intensity, and movement complexity are inversely related. Over the course of the training cycle, as the intensity or complexity of movement gradually increases, the volume or number of repetitions performed should decrease. A linear program can be organized into components based on length of time for each training phase and should include occasional periods of offloading or active rest for optimal adaptation to the training stimulus. The blocks of time are typically organized into the following structures (Bompa and Buzzichelli 2015).

Macrocycle

The macrocycle is the overall time frame for a program designed to achieve a specific, quantifiable performance goal, or a long-term program designed with periods of active rest. A macrocycle may cover a period of months or even years. The point is the overall program should progress to a point of peak conditioning by a specific date or time. For example, members of an Olympic team may be on a four-year training cycle to peak for the next Olympic Games.

Mesocycle

These are smaller units of time that change in training volume, intensity, and complexity on the way to the overall objective of the program. Following the above example, a four-year Olympic macrocycle could be organized into eight six-month blocks of time.

Microcycle

This is the smallest unit of time for organizing a program; it can consist of individual workouts, days, or weeks. In a linear periodization program, each microcycle or mesocycle can become progressively more challenging based on training volume, intensity of the load, or complexity of the movement patterns. A microcycle could also be a specific amount of planned time for optimal rest and recovery from the challenges of the workout program. An Olympic athlete might have 12 two-week microcycles in a six-month mesocycle.

Nonlinear Periodization

Nonlinear, or undulating, periodization uses more frequent variations in training intensity, volume, and movement complexity to allow for workouts that alternate between higher- and lower-intensity days within the same week (Bompa and Buzzichelli 2015). Changing your training stimulus is one way to keep your muscles growing. In a nonlinear plan, Monday might be a high-intensity core strength training day with a kettlebell; Tuesday, a low-intensity metabolic conditioning day with a bodyweight circuit; Wednesday, a moderate-intensity mobility workout; Thursday, a high-intensity anaerobic interval workout with a kettlebell for metabolic conditioning; Friday, a rest day; Saturday, a high-intensity strength day with dumbbells; and Sunday, a long walk followed by a low-intensity mobility workout. Both linear and nonlinear programs recommend taking a few days off every few weeks to allow the body to fully rest and recover from the stresses of the program. And remember, it is important to allow at least 48 hours between high-intensity training sessions for optimal protein resynthesis, muscle glycogen replenishment, and recovery from neuromuscular fatigue.

The nonlinear model applies varying levels of training stress, which can induce metabolic challenges while allowing for rapid adaptations. If you like to exercise every day, nonlinear periodization allows you to change the intensity of training on a more frequent basis so that you can keep training intensity high for one or two sessions per week while allowing for lower-intensity workouts on the other days to reduce the risk of overtraining. This model also allows you to train for multiple events or recreational activities throughout a year, as opposed to a linear model of program design, which is structured to peak at a specific time.

Understanding how to apply periodization for a systematic and progressively challenging application of the variables of exercise program design gives you the ability to change the volume, intensity, and complexity of a program at specific intervals to maximize performance while allowing appropriate levels of rest and recovery for optimal adaptation. That means you can justify your weekend-long TV binges as specific periods of rest to allow your body to make gains, instead of just being lazy and hanging out on the couch.

Applying Periodization to Your Workouts

Whether you follow linear or nonlinear periodization, systematically changing the variables of exercise program design to adjust for intensity and volume is an effective strategy for achieving your goals. It is well-established that physical adaptations to exercise, including muscle growth and definition, depend on the application of these variables in a structured, progressive manner to gradually increase the amount of exercise stimulus to achieve a specific outcome (Bompa and Buzzichelli 2015).

The body will adapt to a specific stimulus after a period of approximately 8 to 12 weeks. Therefore, to help your body make continual changes, it's necessary to adjust your workouts every two to three months. Creating a periodized program can be as simple as switching the types of exercise equipment used, from bodyweight to medicine balls to kettlebells to sandbags to dumbbells to . . . you get the idea. You can keep everything else the same, but changing the type of equipment used will provide a sufficient stimulus for making changes to the body.

For someone who wants to shape up for the summer, here is an example of a year-long exercise program based on changing exercise intensity and volume as the seasons changes. Each season lasts 12 to 13 weeks, which is about the optimal amount of time the body requires to adapt to an exercise stimulus.

January to March, general goal(s):   Foundational preparation for swimsuit season using mobility training, metabolic conditioning, and core strength training.

January

Focus on mobility and metabolic conditioning using medicine ball.

2 workouts per week for a total of 4; the other days of the week focus on normal activities of daily living

February

Maintain metabolic conditioning; add core strength training.

1 mobility workout using body weight, 2 metabolic conditioning workouts using two-arm resistance band, and 2 core strength workouts using body weight

March

Increase intensity of metabolic conditioning to include HIIT; focus on core strength training using dumbbells to promote muscle growth.

1 mobility workout using stability ball, 1 low-intensity metabolic conditioning using bodyweight, 2 HIIT metabolic conditioning circuits using resistance band, and 2 core strength workouts using dumbbells

April to June, general goal(s):   Specific preparation to focus on muscle definition using HIIT metabolic conditioning and core strength training.

April

Focus on mobility to improve ROM using light resistance; metabolic conditioning via circuit training with dumbbells.

2 mobility workouts using dumbbells, 2 metabolic conditioning workouts using dumbbell circuit training, and 2 core strength training workouts using bodyweight

May

Focus on muscle growth with HIIT for metabolic conditioning and dumbbell training for core strength.

1 mobility workout using kettlebell, 2 HIIT metabolic conditioning workouts using kettlebell, and 3 core strength workouts—1 with bodyweight and 2 with dumbbells

June

Alternate between high- and moderate-intensity metabolic conditioning to burn calories and focus on core strength training to the point of fatigue to improve muscular definition.

2 HIIT metabolic conditioning workouts using dumbbells, 1 moderate-intensity metabolic conditioning workout using bodyweight, 2 core strength training workouts with a kettlebell to the point of fatigue, and 1 core strength training workout using bodyweight.

July to September, general goal(s):   Maintain muscle definition using metabolic conditioning and core strength training; participate in 10-kilometer obstacle course race in September.

July

Maintain muscle definition using HIIT and core strength training

2 HIIT metabolic conditioning workouts using bodyweight circuits, 1 moderate-intensity metabolic conditioning using a kettlebell; 2 core strength training workouts using dumbbells, 1 core strength training workout using medicine ball

August

Maintain muscle definition, start training for 10-kilometer obstacle course race.

1 HIIT metabolic conditioning workout using kettlebell, 1 HIIT metabolic conditioning workout using dumbbells, 1 moderate metabolic conditioning workout using bodyweight, 2 core strength training workouts using bodyweight, and 1 core strength training workout using dumbbells.

September

Prepare for 10-kilometer obstacle race at the end of the month.

2 mobility workouts using medicine ball, 2 HIIT metabolic conditioning workouts using bodyweight, 1 HIIT metabolic conditioning workout using dumbbells, and 1 moderate metabolic conditioning workout using stability ball.

October to December, general goal(s):   Focus on mobility; increase strength to prepare for fall and winter chores, including chopping wood and shoveling snow.

October

Allow active rest for body after training hard for obstacle course race.

2 mobility workouts using bodyweight, 1 moderate-intensity metabolic conditioning workout using medicine ball, and 1 core strength training workout using stability ball.

November

Bodyweight training to develop strength without using external resistance.

2 mobility workouts using bodyweight, 2 metabolic conditioning workouts using bodyweight, 1 core strength workout using medicine ball, and 1 core strength workout using bodyweight.

December

Maintain fitness despite end of fiscal year at work and busy holiday season with extended family.

2 mobility workouts using stability ball, 2 metabolic conditioning workouts using kettlebell swings and a Tabata timer, 2 core strength training workouts using dumbbells for 10- to 20-minute EMOMs.

This is by no means the only way to organize a yearly training program, but it should give you some ideas for how you can structure the intensity and exercises within your own workouts throughout an entire calendar year. Planning your exercise program can get you excited about your goals, encourage you to try new activities and workouts to keep things fresh, and help you make fitness and exercise a life-long, enjoyable experience. The next chapter explains how staying active well into your golden years can provide benefits you might not have even thought about yet.

7

Lifetime Programming

Up to this point, you have learned important information about how your body adapts to exercise as well as how to do a variety of workouts to improve mobility, core strength, or metabolic conditioning using only a single piece of equipment. Now it is time to address how to make exercise a lifelong habit and achieve and maintain the long-term benefits of living a healthier lifestyle. Typical fitness goals such as losing weight or improving muscle tone are outcome goals, meaning they are the result of a short-term approach to exercise. As mentioned in the previous chapter, having a process-oriented goal, like learning how to enjoy the process of exercise, can help you to make it a part of your daily habits, which is the real secret to long-term success.

In the short term, following a specific workout program can make some changes to your body, but for the best results, exercise has to become a habit, one that you practice *for the rest of your life,* like brushing your teeth or putting on some clothes before leaving the house. If you have repeatedly gone through phases of starting and stopping workout programs, this can seem overwhelming or even unsurmountable. Have you ever considered that maybe it's time to change your focus? Instead of using exercise as a means of losing weight for some popular culture definition of what a body should look like, why not focus on using exercise as a means to improve your health and enhance your quality of life? One of the most important benefits from regular exercise is that you will have choices for how you live your life. Forget about appearance; the real goal of an exercise program should be to develop the strength to do any activity you're interested in. Improving your fitness can give you the physical ability to do what you want when you want to do it. Said another way, being fit gives you the freedom to do your favorite activities as well as the ability to learn how to do new activities so that you can live your life to its fullest potential.

Find Your Fountain of Youth

The effects of the aging process can greatly diminish the mechanical, metabolic, hormonal, and neural systems that help our muscles control movement. However, regular exercise and physical activity, especially of moderate to high intensity, can help ensure that these systems function at an optimal level of performance as we get older (Taylor and Johnson 2008).

From plastic surgery to Botox injections to anti-aging clinics that specialize in prescribing injections of anabolic steroids, hundreds of millions of dollars are spent every year pursuing the elusive fountain of youth. The harsh reality is that until time travel is invented the aging process cannot be stopped (and getting older certainly beats the alternative). The good news is that a healthy lifestyle that includes high-intensity metabolic conditioning and strength training can help slow down the aging process and be the proverbial fountain of youth. And here's a little secret: Rather than expensive, invasive medical procedures or costly and painful injections, invest your time in moderate to vigorous exercise to minimize those effects of aging. High-intensity strength training and metabolic conditioning programs can be the stimulus to produce the hormones that promote muscle growth (Candow et al. 2011; Godfrey and Blazevich 2004). If you follow the workouts in this book, you can increase the level of difficulty and intensity to the point where exercise can have a significant impact on your quality of life, helping to maintain or retain your youthful energy and appearance.

What's Age Got to Do With It?

We are all familiar with chronological age, which starts the moment we are born and is measured in years. Biological age refers to the condition of tissues and physiological systems; healthy lifestyle habits can help reduce our biological age, meaning that even though an individual could have a chronological age of 65, her biological age could only be 45 (table 7.1). Functional age is a combination of one's functional work capacity and physical ability, and in many cases can be years younger than the actual chronological age (Taylor and Johnson 2008). We all know those individuals whose energy, enthusiasm, physical ability, and overall zest for life are years younger than their actual age. Chances are that those people are probably very active. Being active *is* the true fountain of youth. Being fit means being healthy and having the ability to perform physical tasks, *not* having a particular appearance or shape. The

Table 7.1   **The Benefits of Exercise on the Biological Aging Process**

System(s)	The benefits of exercise on slowing down biological aging
Muscles Fascia Elastic Connective Tissue Skeletal Central Nervous Cognitive	Increase lean muscle mass, especially the type II muscle fibers responsible for force production and definition.
	Improve elasticity and resiliency of fascia and connective tissue, which can help in avoiding muscle strains and pulls.
	Improve dynamic balance and reactive agility.
	Enhance joint range of motion (ROM) for improved mobility.
	Reduce the risk of breaking a bone as the result of a fall by increasing bone mineral density.
	Improve the functional strength and ability to perform a number of common activities of daily life (ADL).
	Enhance production of brain-derived neurotrophic factor (BDNF), the neurotransmitter responsible for producing new brain cells.
Cardiorespiratory Metabolic	Enhance aerobic capacity and $\dot{V}O_2$ max
	Improve mitochondrial density, which can enhance aerobic capacity and improve overall muscular endurance.
	Increase mitochondria in muscle cells to improve cellular health.
	Improve glucose tolerance and metabolism, reducing the risk of developing onset (type II) diabetes.
Endocrine (hormones)	Increase production of the stress hormones cortisol, epinephrine, and norepinephrine, allowing the body to tolerate periods of high stress from a variety of different factors.
	Exercise to the point of momentary muscle fatigue or exercise that creates a significant metabolic overload can increase production of testosterone and growth hormone during the postexercise recovery period.

true sense of being fit is having the energy and ability to enjoy your favorite activities throughout your entire lifespan.

Exercise Throughout the Aging Process

Following an exercise program that includes progressively challenging workouts for both strength (the core strength programs in this book) and power (the metabolic conditioning programs) can help minimize the normal physiological effects of the biological aging process and improve your quality of life.

To provide you with a little extra motivation for starting and adhering to a long-term exercise program, table 7.2 gives an overview of the benefits of exercise during each decade of the adult lifespan.

Note: Cancer and other chronic conditions were specifically omitted from table 7.2 because they can strike at almost any stage of life. While there is no cure for cancer, establishing healthy behaviors and avoiding or limiting certain activities such as smoking, drinking alcohol to excess, and remaining sedentary for extended periods of time can certainly lower the risk of developing it and other conditions. There is no sense wasting any energy worrying about cancer; do your best to be as active as possible and make healthy choices in an attempt to reduce your risk.

Certain Exercise Programs Can Slow Down the Biological Aging Process (Really!)

Being older does not mean you can't do high-intensity exercises. Older adults can and should participate in higher-intensity exercise as long as there are no medical concerns and they follow an appropriate progression of intensity. Strength training can improve the force output of muscles, independent of age and gender, especially when there is a sufficient intensity of exercise (Hakkinen 2011).

Higher-intensity exercises like those done in metabolic conditioning and core strength training programs can promote the production of anabolic hormones that

What the Science Says:
What an Old Car Can Teach You About Your Body

Rebuilding and restoring an old car to like-new condition often requires replacing many worn-out parts and repainting the exterior. Even though medical technology has made important advances in the area of prosthetics, due to cost and the painful recovery process, simply replacing old parts isn't an option as we age. However, gradually progressing the intensity of an exercise program to where you are strength training to a point of momentary fatigue or creating significant metabolic overload can help add new muscle, which can significantly improve your appearance in much the same way that a good paint job can help an older car look like new. In their research on how older males respond to resistance training, Izquierdo and colleagues observed that the skeletal muscle of older adults seems to retain the capacity to experience hypertrophy when the volume, intensity, and duration of the training period are sufficient (Izquierdo et al. 2001).

Just as properly maintaining the engine, waxing the paint, and storing it out of the sun can greatly enhance the longevity of an automobile, exercise programs that stimulate the production of the hormones T, GH, and insulin-like growth factor-1 (IGF-1) can improve our appearance and extend our functional life span as we age.

Table 7.2 **The Benefits of Exercise for Each Decade of Adulthood**

Age	Benefits
20-29	If you're in your 20s, enjoy your youth but realize that the sooner you commit to a healthy lifestyle, the more benefits you will experience throughout your entire adulthood. • Experiment with different workouts to identify your favorite activities, then do them on a regular basis. There is no specific type of exercise that you should be doing, but whichever type you select, make it an important component of your life. The more consistent your physical activity, the better your overall quality of health. • Consider joining a health club, attending classes at a studio, subscribing to an online fitness channel, or purchasing equipment to use at home. When it comes to cost, consider this fact: Either you pay to stay in shape while you're young, or you'll end up spending lots of money over the course of your life dealing with the chronic diseases and health conditions that can result from a sedentary lifestyle. In your 20s, you can likely participate in high-intensity training most days of the week; just remember to make time for mobility training as well. If you make mobility training an integral component of your fitness program now and adopt it as a regular habit, you can reduce the risk of many common overuse injuries that can affect people over the course of the aging process.
30-39	Without regular exercise, both muscular strength and cardiorespiratory efficiency could begin to decline and accelerate the aging process. The biggest challenges during this decade are that your career will be taking off and if you haven't already, you may be starting a family. This is why finding a favorite mode of exercise in your 20s is so important: It will be a regular habit built into your schedule and routine by the time family and career start making more demands on your time. Exercise is so important during this time that if you haven't been successful at following a regular exercise program on your own, you may want to consider hiring a personal trainer or going to a studio with instructor-led workouts. If you have a demanding schedule, it's important to realize that even 15 to 20 minutes of exercise at a time can make a big difference and provide significant health benefits. As you progress through your 30s, you will want to make smarter nutrition choices and plan on going to bed earlier because the right diet combined with proper amounts of sleep are essential for good health. • Without regular exercise, cardiorespiratory efficiency—the ability to efficiently move oxygen around the body—starts to decline, which can increase the risk of developing heart disease. • Without any regular physical activity that challenges the muscles to do physical work, by the time you reach your mid-30s, you could start to experience a loss of muscle mass. • If you're a man, as you reach the later years of this decade, not only will you experience lower levels of testosterone, but if you have excessive amounts of abdominal fat, it could convert what testosterone (T) you do produce into estradiol, a female sex hormone that can promote the growth of breast tissue. • Both strength training, to increase muscle mass, and metabolic conditioning for weight loss are extremely important in this time of life. Both men and women should do strength training because it can elevate levels of human growth hormone (HGH), which can metabolize fat, promote muscle growth, and help skin maintain a youthful appearance. Core strength training workouts that challenge your muscles to work to the point of fatigue can provide significant benefits if they are performed at least 2 or 3 times a week. Metabolic conditioning workouts that leave you almost breathless are important at least 2 or 3 times a week to help ensure optimal function and performance of the cardiorespiratory system. It is also important to make time for walking at least 10 to 15 minutes at a time 2 to 3 times a day (ideally, once in the morning and once during the workday) for overall health benefits.

Age	Benefits
40-49	As you approach your 40s, you may anticipate feeling older. As you progress through this decade, you will no doubt notice that it takes longer to fully recover from high-intensity workouts. If a crazy work or travel schedule causes you to lose a night of sleep, it could affect you for the rest of the week (whereas in your 20s, going without sleep once in a while was no big deal). The biggest change that you might notice is that if you stop exercising for a couple weeks, you will notice an almost immediate drop in your fitness level. This is the age when it is extremely important to maintain consistency in your workouts so you can control the aging process instead of letting it take over your life. • In this decade you're relatively ensconced in your career and family life; while there will be unforeseen challenges, for the most part you have established a consistent routine that includes regular physical activity. • If you find it hard to make time for regular workouts, consider ways that you can add small bouts of exercise to your routine, such as bike commuting to work. Including small activities, such as taking the stairs, using a standing desk at work, or walking during breaks at work. Your daily habits can help you burn an additional couple hundred calories a day, which is essential for healthy weight management. • If you're exercising regularly, congratulations! However, take time for a critical review of your exercise habits. If you follow the same routine for too long, your body adapts, and the exercise, while good, won't have the same effects. • If you're looking for ways to change your routine, consider adding yoga, which can help reduce stress levels while improving mobility, both of which can reduce the risk of disease or injury. • Consider adding at least one high-intensity exercise such as a group cycling, sports conditioning, or kettlebell class to your routine. High-intensity exercise can promote muscle-building hormones while increasing caloric expenditure, both of which are important at this age. It's important to realize that explosive exercises can help improve muscle elasticity, which is reduced during the aging process. Regular strength training exercises make skeletal muscle tissue strong but don't challenge the elastic connective tissue that surrounds it. Adding exercises such as kettlebell swings and plyometric jumps help improve tissue elasticity. • Keep in mind that while some high-intensity exercise is good, it does take longer to recover from challenging activity, so try to limit it to a maximum of 3 times a week, and make sure you are getting plenty of sleep to help promote the recovery process. As you advance through your 40s, it will be important to change your exercise habits on a regular basis so you can continue to introduce new stimuli and challenges to your body. Making small changes such as changing the equipment from dumbbells to a medicine ball or doing sets for an amount of time instead of specific repetitions can provide the necessary stimuli to challenge your body. Continue core strength training and metabolic conditioning
50-59	Exercise is important in all phases of life, but as you hit this decade, regular physical activity is essential for maintaining good health in an effort to avoid conditions such as high cholesterol, heart disease, or arthritis. If you experience any chronic medical conditions, make sure you work with your health care provider to identify the most appropriate types of exercise for your needs. That said, you can continue doing your favorite activities as long as they don't cause you any severe physical discomfort. • In this decade, changing exercise is important not only to keep your muscles working differently but to engage your brain. Make sure to include at least 1 or 2 hard metabolic conditioning workouts a week because exercise that elevates levels of GH can also elevate levels of BDNF, the neurotransmitter responsible for producing new brain cells and improving cognitive function. • Learning new sports or activities can be another way to develop your brain; using your muscles differently can create new neural pathways in your brain, helping improve overall cognitive function. If your kids are out of the house and you have more free time, you can use it to learn a new sport or start a new hobby like dancing or martial arts, which provides essential mental and physical development. • Hopefully your 50s is also when you will have a little more free time and disposable income to take vacations and visit parts of the world you've always wanted to experience. Having the financial freedom to enjoy vacations such as hiking to Machu Picchu, taking a bicycle tour across France, kayaking in New Zealand, or skiing in Switzerland is one thing, but you also want to be fit enough to enjoy those vacations. Even if you cannot afford exotic destinations, you can start cycling and hiking the parks and trails in your area. Identify and participate in any physical activities that you can perform on a frequent basis. Make sure to include at least 1 high-intensity core strength training and metabolic conditioning workout a week for optimal neuroendocrine stimulation.

(continued)

Table 7.2 *(continued)*

Age	Benefits
60-69	When you're young, 60 seems old, but once you've hit your 40s, you will quickly realize it's not, leading many to claim, "Sixty is the new forty!" If you made smart financial decisions when you were younger (which requires an entirely different book altogether), this is the decade in which you will probably retire from your career and decide what you really want to do with your life.
	• It's more important than ever to exercise most days of the week. You can continue to do high-intensity workouts, but it's a smart idea to limit them to 2 days or less in order to allow for optimal recovery. If you enjoy resistance training, this may be the time to start using more machines than free weights so you can experience the numerous benefits of strength training to the point of momentary fatigue while minimizing the risk of injury.
	• If you do retire during this decade, you will have the extra time for your workouts, so continue to experiment with new types of exercises and sports to give your muscles and brain new learning opportunities.
	• Just like young adults in their 20s, taking group classes is a great way to combine physical activity with social time, and, if you're recently retired, they can be an effective way to make new friends. Aqua fitness classes, a good choice at any age, are a good option for exercise because they use a lot of muscle mass while reducing stress on your joints, which is important if you're dealing with any arthritis.
	• If you enjoy being active and want to encourage others to do the same, consider the fact that more and more people are choosing fitness as a second career once they retire from their first. It's possible to earn a fitness certification at any age, and others in the same demographic would appreciate working with someone who understands their specific needs.
	Continue to change your workouts on a regular basis to keep using your muscles in different ways. Improve your physical literacy by using mobility workouts to enhance coordination and develop new movement skills; now's the time to get going! An important benefit of multidirectional mobility and core strength training exercises include strengthened fascia and elastic connective tissues, which help reduce the risk of minor injuries such as muscle strains. In addition, mobility exercises can promote optimal fascial extensibility to help reduce the risk of developing adhesions that can change how joints function.
70-79	If 60 is the new 40, then 70 is the new 50. Oftentimes people in this decade of life can look much younger if fitness has been an integral part of their life for years. (Use that as your motivation for long-term adherence.)
	• Do not let the number slow you down. Continue to participate in your favorite activities, but be smart about it by listening to your body and not forcing it to do any extremely uncomfortable exercise.
	• If you've been a sporadic exerciser up to this point, consider this: Staying fit and strong now can help you maintain your functional independence longer and keep you from having to rely on assisted living.
	• Resistance training is completely appropriate and can help increase lean muscle mass and improve your functional strength for ADLs.
	• If you feel the effects of arthritis, don't let it stop you from cardiorespiratory exercise, but do look for types with reduced impact on your joints.
	• Activities that require you to move your body in all directions, such as tai chi, dance, or yoga, are more important than ever for helping maintain balance and reducing the risk of orthopedic injuries.
	While the workouts in this book were designed specifically for the convenience of exercising at home, in your 70s, besides the social networking, the benefit of joining a health club is access to strength training machines that enhance overall muscular strength with a reduced risk of injury. Just like in your 60s, mobility workouts that focus on multiplanar movements can help improve integrity of your myofascial system, leaving you with more youthful muscles and connective tissue that is more resilient against injury. Finally, resistance training to the point of fatigue will still be important for initiating muscle growth (yes, muscles can still grow at this age) and maintaining optimal physical performance so you can remain functionally independent.

Age	Benefits
80-89	If you make it to your 80s, congratulations because, currently, the average adult life span in the United States is 78 years. No matter your activity level and the number of healthy habits you adhere to, now is the time when you will really start to feel your age, if you haven't already. • Strength training, especially to the point of momentary fatigue, becomes extremely important because it can help you maintain your strength, allowing you to remain functionally independent. Machines are the safest, most effective way to receive this benefit. • If you are considering relocating to a retirement community, look for one with a robust schedule of recreational activities and a well-equipped fitness center so you have plenty of options for exercise. • You are never too old to learn new things, so consider going back to school because social interactions and learning are both great ways to reduce the risk of developing cognitive diseases such as dementia or Alzheimer's. • You can continue to participate in your favorite activities, but respect your age and try not to push your body beyond its limits.
90 +	Keep doing whatever you've been doing because it's working. Whatever physical activity you can do, do it as often as possible. If you're not already doing strength training, ask your medical providers if they can recommend any strength training programs specifically for your age group because you can add muscle mass at any age. If you want to enjoy an active life well into your 90s, it is important that no matter what happens to you, never stop exercising. Even if you can do only a few minutes at a time, regular exercise and physical activity can still provide important health benefits.

provide important anti-aging benefits. Chapter 1 identified a number of hormones produced by the body as a result of exercise; high-intensity exercise is an important stimulus that can elevate the levels of the hormones responsible for promoting muscle growth through all phases of the aging process (Serra et al. 2011; Godfrey and Blazevich 2004).

Exercise not only creates better-functioning muscles but also a brain capable of maintaining its optimal performance throughout the aging process (Chaddock, Voss, and Kramer 2012). Research on the effects of resistance training on older adults and cognitive function has shown that resistance training has a positive effect on cognition, information processing, attention, memory formation, and executive function (Chang et. al 2012). So, as you get older, be sure to include high-intensity exercises and strength training as part of your overall training plan.

Move More

If you complete your workout and then spend the rest of the day doing minimal activity—sitting at a desk or behind the wheel, or laying on the couch, for example—you probably won't see significant changes in your fitness. In fact, sitting too long could undo the exercise you are doing. Unplanned physical activities—movement that you do throughout your day as a part of your ADLs—can have a tremendous effect on your overall health and well-being.

Modernization is both a blessing and a curse. Almost every place, from the modern factory to the home, has been upgraded with easy-to-use machines or appliances. Many aspects of modern technology make life easier, but the downside is that technology reduces your opportunities to be physically active throughout the day. This can lead to weight gain and, even worse, possibly increase the risk of developing chronic diseases, which could reduce your quality of life. Here are some ideas to help you move more throughout the day and make physical activity a part of your active, everyday lifestyle.

Exercise as Part of Your Commute   While this may not be possible in all communities, a number of state and local governments have added bike lanes and multiuse trails in an effort to promote cycling and walking as viable modes of transportation. It may take a little longer and require planning, but a major benefit of walking or cycling to work is that you're burning calories instead of being stuck in traffic burning dollars in the form of wasted gasoline.

Move While Completing Errands   Think about the errands you make or the stores that you visit on a regular basis. How many of them are in relatively close (within two to three miles) proximity to your home? Long popular in Europe, more and more Americans are investing in cargo bikes to be able to perform errands such as dropping kids off or picking up groceries. Investing in a cargo bike or utility cart could allow you to leave the car at home and let you get your daily exercise the next time you need to make a quick run to the store. I love biking to the grocery store because having to fit all of my purchases into a backpack keeps me from buying stuff I don't need.

Stand More   As more companies begin to understand the negative health consequences of sitting for too long, they are investing in stand-up desks for their employees. This allows you to be more active by working while standing up. Standing uses more muscles than sitting, so standing can help burn additional calories. If using a standing desk is not possible, take frequent standing breaks by standing to perform tasks such as making a phone call, typing out a text, or checking your email on a mobile device.

Walk More   Don't use your coffee break to simply go downstairs to the shop in your building; if possible, walk to another coffee shop one or two blocks away. You could even invite a colleague or two so you can have a work-related conversation during the trip. Plus, if multiple people go, you won't stand out as someone who is trying to get out of doing work, and it also encourages a culture of health and movement.

Take the Stairs   As more organizations try to stem health care costs by promoting physical activity at work, they may allow employees to use the stairs once reserved only for emergencies. If you find that you waste time waiting for elevators, ask your office or building manager if it is possible to have access to the stairs. When you're out at the mall or in an airport, use the stairs instead of the escalator. It's always fun to watch peoples' faces when you walk up the stairs next to where they're standing on the escalator, and you're both moving at the same speed.

Park Far Away   Parking near the front of a busy store or shopping mall means being stuck behind people looking for the closest parking spot, or shoppers strolling with no sense of urgency while carrying their purchases out of the store. Parking far from the front of the store serves two benefits: First, you get more activity by walking across the parking lot to your destination, and second, it is easier to leave the lot when you are parked further away from the store entrance, which is a bonus when the stores are busy.

What the Science Says: Benefits of Walking

Walking is one of the most accessible forms of exercise. Making time for brief walking breaks throughout a day can provide numerous health benefits. The body burns approximately 100 calories of energy to walk one mile. The faster you walk, the further you can travel and the more calories you can burn. For example, walking at a 3.0 mile per hour pace means that if you walk for an hour, you can burn approximately 300 calories. Increasing to a 3.5 mile per hour pace results in 350 calories burned, a 15 percent increase.

Regular walking can improve oxygen flow through the body. Walking can increase numbers of mitochondria, the portion of the muscle cells that converts oxygen to energy. More mitochondria means that your body becomes more efficient at converting oxygen to energy.

Taking walking breaks during your workday can help boost your energy levels. Do caffeinated drinks make you jittery? Skip the calories from energy drinks and take a walking break instead. Going for a walk when tired can increase oxygen flow through the body while also increasing levels of cortisol, epinephrine, and norepinephrine, the hormones responsible for elevating energy levels. Energy drinks are designed to elevate these hormones through the use of caffeine or other stimulants, but they also include unnecessary calories.

Reduce the effects of sitting for extended periods of time. Excessive sitting can reduce levels of lipoprotein lipase (LPL), an enzyme critical for fat metabolism. Walking can help sustain levels of LPL, helping metabolize fat into energy.

Make Chores Active No, they're not fun, but chores such as cleaning the kitchen, carrying out the trash, mowing the lawn, or collecting laundry are all opportunities to move more.

Remember the numbers one and five: The human body burns approximately five calories of energy in order to consume one liter of oxygen. It may not seem like taking the stairs or parking far away would make a big difference, but adding little bouts of physical activity to your day can help you increase the need for oxygen and burn additional calories, consequently improving your health. On the flip side, sitting and being sedentary for extended periods of time create a series of negative health outcomes. While regular, planned exercise is the best method of receiving the health-promoting benefits of physical activity, the fact is, on some days it can be hard to schedule the time for a lengthy workout. If you can't make it into the gym or run on your favorite trail, don't despair; brief periods of physical activity throughout the day, especially walking, can offer a big boost to your health.

Into Action

Change doesn't just happen on its own. The body is a very complex and adaptable organism that can adjust to almost any physical stimulus imposed upon it, and this book provides you with plenty of ways to challenge your body in order to improve your quality of life. For the best results, the exercise that you do should be hard enough to make you uncomfortable two to three times a week. This doesn't mean exercise to the point of being in pain; it only needs to be just a little bit harder than you might be used to working. Fitness is having the ability to do what you want to do when you want to do it, and being fit gives you options for what you can do in your life. Fitness *is* freedom. Now, go out and make the most of it.

References

Introduction

Candow, D., P. Chilibeck, S. Abeysekara, and G. Zello. 2011. "Short-Term Heavy Resistance Training Eliminates Age-Related Deficits in Muscle Mass and Strength in Older Males." *Journal of Strength and Conditioning Research* 25, no. 2: 326-333.

Taylor, A., and M. Johnson. 2008. *Physiology of Exercise and Healthy Aging*. Champaign, IL: Human Kinetics.

United States Department of Health and Human Services. 2008. *2008 Physical Activity Guidelines for Americans*. https://health.gov/paguidelines/pdf/paguide.pdf.

Chapter 1

Bubbico, A., and L. Kravitz. 2011. "Muscle Hypertrophy: New Insights and Training Recommendations." *IDEA Fitness Journal* 8, no. 11: 2326-2331.

Candow, D., P. Chilibeck, S. Abeysekara, and G. Zello. 2011. "Short-Term Heavy Resistance Training Eliminates Age-Related Deficits in Muscle Mass and Strength in Older Males." *Journal of Strength and Conditioning Research* 25, no. 2: 326-333.

Haff, T., and T. Triplett. 2016. *Essentials of Strength and Conditioning*. 3rd edition. Champaign, IL: Human Kinetics.

Ingber, D. E. 2003. "Tensegrity II: How Structural Networks Influence Cellular Information Processing Networks." *Journal of Cell Science* 116: 1397-1408.

———. 2004. "The Mechanochemical Basis of Cell and Tissue Regulation." *Mechanics and Chemistry of Biosystems* 1, no. 1: 53-68.

Kenney, W., J. Wilmore, and D. Costill. 2015. *Physiology of Sport and Exercise*. 6th edition. Champaign, IL: Human Kinetics.

Kraemer, W., and N. Ratamess. 2005. "Hormonal Responses and Adaptations to Resistance Exercise and Training." *Sports Med* 35, no. 4: 339-361.

Langevin, H. 2006. "Connective Tissue: A Body-Wide Signaling Network?" *Medical Hypotheses* 66, no. 6: 1074-1077.

Myers, T. 2014. *Anatomy Trains*. 3rd edition. London, UK: Elsevier.

Neumann, D. 2010. *Kinesiology of the Musculoskeletal System*. 2nd edition. St. Louis: Mosby.

Scarr, G. 2014. *Biotensegrity: The Structural Basis for Life*. East Lothian, Scotland: Handspring.

Schleip, R., T. W. Findley, L. Chaitow, and P. A. Huijing. 2012. *Fascia: The Tensional Network of the Human Body*. London: Churchill Livingstone Elsevier.

Schoenfeld, B. 2010. "The Mechanisms of Muscle Hypertrophy and Their Application to Resistance Training." *Journal of Strength and Conditioning Research* 24, no. 10: 2857-2872.

———. 2013. "Potential Mechanisms for a Role of Metabolic Stress in Hypertrophic Adaptations to Resistance Training." *Sports Medicine* 43, no. 3: 179-194.

———. 2016. *Science and Development of Muscle Hypertrophy*. Champaign, IL: Human Kinetics.

Schultz, R. L., and R. Feitis. 1996. *The Endless Web: Fascial Anatomy and Physical Reality*. Berkeley, CA: North Atlantic Books.

Skinner, J., C. Bryant, S. Merrill, and D. Green. 2015. *Medical Exercise Specialist Manual*. San Diego, CA: American Council on Exercise.

Spangenburg, E. 2009. "Changes in Muscle Mass with Mechanical Load: Possible Cellular Mechanisms." *Applied Physiology, Nutrition and Metabolism* 34, no. 3: 328-335.

Taylor, A., and M. Johnson. 2008. *Physiology of Exercise and Healthy Aging*. Champaign, IL: Human Kinetics.

United States Department of Health and Human Services. 2008. *2008 Physical Activity Guidelines for Americans*. https://health.gov/paguidelines/pdf/paguide.pdf.

Verkoshansky, Y., and M. Siff. 2009. *Supertraining*. 6th edition. Rome, Italy: Supertraining Institute.

Vogel, V., and M. Sheetz. 2006. "Local Force and Geometry Sensing Regulate Cell Functions." *Nature Reviews: Molecular Cell Biology* 7, no. 4: 265-275.

Zatsiorsky, V., and W. Kraemer. 2006. *Science and Practice of Strength Training*. 2nd edition. Champaign, IL: Human Kinetics.

Chapter 2

Bishop, P., E. Jones, and K. Woods. 2008. "Recovery from Training: A Brief Review." *Journal of Strength and Conditioning Research* 22, no. 3: 1015-1024.

Contreras, B., and B. Schoenfeld. 2011. "To Crunch or Not to Crunch: An Evidence-Based Examination of Spinal Flexion Exercises, Their Potential Risks and Their Applicability to Program Design." *Strength and Conditioning Journal* 33, no. 4: 8-18.

Haff, G., and N. Triplett, N. 2016. *Essentials of Strength and Conditioning*. 4th edition. Champaign, IL: Human Kinetics.

Hausswirth, C., and I. Mujika. 2013. *Recovery for Performance in Sport*. Champaign, IL: Human Kinetics.

Ingber, D. E. 2003. "Tensegrity II: How Structural Networks Influence Cellular Information Processing Networks." *Journal of Cell Science* 116: 1397-1408.

———. 2004. "The Mechanochemical Basis of Cell and Tissue Regulation." *Mechanics and Chemistry of Biosystems* 1, no. 1: 53-68.

McGill, S. 2010. "Core Training: Evidence Translating to Better Performance and Injury Prevention." *Strength and Conditioning Journal* 32, no. 3: 33-46.

Schleip, R., et al. 2012. *Fascia: The Tensional Network of the Human Body.* London, UK: Elsevier.

Schleip, R., and J. Bayer. 2017. *Fascial Fitness: How to Be Vital, Elastic and Dynamic in Everyday Life and Sport.* Chichester, West Sussex: Lotus.

Schoenfeld, B. 2010. "The Mechanisms of Muscle Hypertrophy and Their Application to Resistance Training." *The Journal of Strength and Conditioning Research* 24, no. 10: 2857-2872.

———. 2013. "Potential Mechanisms for a Role of Metabolic Stress in Hypertrophic Adaptations to Resistance Training." *Sports Medicine* 43, no. 3: 179-194.

Vogel, V., and M. Sheetz. 2006. "Local Force and Geometry Sensing Regulate Cell Functions." *Nature Reviews: Molecular Cell Biology* 7, no. 4: 265-275.

Zatsiorsky and Kraemer. 2006. *Science and Practice of Strength Training.* 2nd edition. Champaign, IL: Human Kinetics.

Chapter 3

Cook, G. 2010. *Movement.* Aptos, CA: On Target Publications.

Gambetta, V. 1998. *The Gambetta Method: Common Sense Training for Athletic Performance.* Sarasota, FL: Gambetta Sports Training Systems.

Ingber, D. E. 2003. "Tensegrity II: How Structural Networks Influence Cellular Information Processing Networks." *Journal of Cell Science* 116: 1397-1408.

Myers, T. 2011. "Fascial Fitness: Training in the Neuro-Myofascial Web." *IDEA Fitness Journal*: 38-45.

———. 2014. *Anatomy Trains.* 3rd edition. London, UK: Elsevier.

Scarr, G. 2014. *Biotensegrity: The Structural Basis of Life.* East Lothian, Scotland: Handspring Publishing.

Schultz, R. L., and R. Feitis. 1996. *The Endless Web: Fascial Anatomy and Physical Reality.* Berkeley, CA: North Atlantic Books.

Verkoshansky, Y., and M. Siff. 2009. *Supertraining.* 6th edition. Rome, Italy: Supertraining Institute.

Chapter 4

Abernathy, B., et al. 2005. *The Biophysical Foundations of Human Movement.* 2nd edition. Champaign, IL: Human Kinetics.

Brown, S., C. Fenwick, A. Karpowicz, and S. McGill. 2009. "Exercises for the Torso Performed in a Standing Posture: Spine and Hip Motion and Motor Patterns and Spine Load." *The Journal of Strength and Conditioning Research 23, no. 2:* 1-10.

Brown, S., C. Fenwick, and S. McGill. 2009. "Comparison of Different Rowing Exercises: Trunk Muscle Activation and Lumbar Spine Motion, Load and Stiffness." *The Journal of Strength and Conditioning Research* 23, no. 2: 350-358.

Contreras, B., and B. Schoenfeld. 2011. "To Crunch or Not to Crunch: An Evidence-Based Examination of Spinal Flexion Exercises, Their Potential Risks and Their Applicability to Program Design." *Strength and Conditioning Journal* 33, no. 4: 8-18.

Cook, Gray. 2010. *Movement: Functional Movement Systems - Screening, Assessment, Corrective Strategies.* Aptas, CA: On Target Publications.

Earls, J. 2014. *Born to Walk: Myofascial Efficiency and the Body in Movement.* Berkeley, CA. North Atlantic Books.

Enoka, R. 2002. *Neuromechanics of Human Movement.* 3rd edition. Champaign, IL: Human Kinetics.

Haff, G., and N. Triplett. 2016. *Essentials of Strength and Conditioning.* 4th edition. Champaign, IL: Human Kinetics.

Hibbs, A., K. Thompson, D. French, A. Wrigley, and I. Spears. 2008. "Optimizing Performance by Improving Core Stability and Core Strength." *Sports Med* 38, no. 12: 996-1008.

Martuscello, J., et. al. 2013. "Sytematic Review of Core Muscle Activity During Physical Fitness Exercises." *The Journal of Strength and Conditioning Research* 27, no. 6: 1684-1698.

McGill, S. 2007. *Low Back Disorders.* 2nd edition. Champaign, IL: Human Kinetics.

———. 2010. "Core Training: Evidence Translating to Better Performance and Injury Prevention." *Strength and Conditioning Journal* 32, no. 3: 33-46.

McGill, S., A. Karpowicz, and C. Fenwick. 2009a. "Ballistic Abdominal Exercises: Muscle Activation Patterns During Three Activities Along the Stability/Mobility Continuum." *The Journal of Strength and Conditioning Research* 23, no. 3: 898-905.

McGill, S., A. Karpowicz, and C. Fenwick. 2009b. "Comparison of Different Strongman Events: Trunk Muscle Activation and Lumbar Spine Motion, Load and Stiffness." *The Journal of Strength and Conditioning Research* 23, no. 4: 1148-1161.

McGill, S., and L. Marshall. 2012. "Kettlebell Swing, Snatch and Bottoms-Up Carry: Back and Hip Muscle Activation, Motion and Low-Back Loads." *The Journal of Strength and Conditioning Research* 26, no. 11: 16-27.

Myers, T. 2014. *Anatomy Trains.* 3rd edition. London: Elsevier.

Neumann, D. 2016. *Kinesiology of the Musculoskeletal System: Foundations for Rehabilitation.* 3rd edition. St. Louis, MO: Elsevier.

Schleip, R., et al. 2012. *Fascia: The Tensional Network of the Human Body*. London, UK: Elsevier.

Taylor, A., and M. Johnson. 2008. *Physiology of Exercise and Healthy Aging*. Champaign, IL: Human Kinetics.

Chapter 5

U.S. Army Physical Readiness Training Information. n.d. Accessed January 1, 2018. www.armyprt.com.

TC 3-22.20 Army Physical Readiness Training

Alcaraz, P., J. Perez-Gomez, M. Chavarrias, and A. Blazevich. 2010. "Similarity in Adaptations to High-Resistance Circuit vs. Traditional Strength Training in Resistance-Trained Men." *Journal of Strength and Conditioning Research* 25, no. 9: 2519-2527.

Borsheim, E., and R. Bahr. 2003. "Effect of Exercise Intensity, Duration and Mode on Post-Exercise Oxygen Consumption." *Sports Medicine* 33, no. 14: 1037-1060.

Boutcher, S. 2011. "High-Intensity Intermittent Exercise and Fat Loss." *Journal of Obesity*. 2011, no. 1: 1-11.

Gibala, M. 2017. *The One-Minute Workout*. New York, NY: Avery.

Gibala, M., and S. McGee. 2008. "Metabolic Adaptations to Short-Term High-Intensity Interval Training: A Little Pain for a Lot of Gain? *Exercise and Sport Sciences Reviews* 36(2): 58-63.

Haff, T., and T. Triplett. 2016. *Essentials of Strength and Conditioning*. 3rd edition. Champaign, IL: Human Kinetics.

Heinrich, K., V. Spencer, N. Fehl, and W. S. Poston. 2012. "Mission Essential Fitness: Comparison of Functional Training to Traditional Army Physical Training." *Military Medicine* 177, no. 10: 1125-1130.

Roy, T., B. Springer, V. McNulty, and N. Butler. 2010. "Physical Fitness." *Military Medicine* 175, no. 85: 14-20.

Schoenfeld, B. 2010. "The Mechanisms of Muscle Hypertrophy and Their Application to Resistance Training." *The Journal of Strength and Conditioning Research* 24, no. 10: 2857-2872.

Schoenfeld, B. 2013. "Potential Mechanisms for a Role of Metabolic Stress in Hypertrophic Adaptations to Resistance Training." *Sports Med* 43 no. 3: 179-194.

Taylor, A. and M. Johnson. 2008. *Physiology of Exercise and Healthy Aging*. Champaign, IL: Human Kinetics.

Chapter 6

Bishop, P., E. Jones, and K. Woods. 2008. "Recovery from Training: A Brief Review." *Journal of Strength and Conditioning Research* 22, no. 3: 1015-1024.

Bompa, T., and C. Buzzichelli. 2015. *Periodization Training for Sports*. 3rd edition. Champaign, IL: Human Kinetics.

Hausswirth, C., and I. Mujika. 2013. *Recovery for Performance in Sport*. Champaign, IL: Human Kinetics.

MacRae, B., J. Cotter, and R. Laing. 2011. "Compression Garments and Exercise: Garment Considerations, Physiology and Performance." *Sports Medicine* 41, no. 10: 1-29.

Tabata, I., F. Ogita, and M. Miyachi. 1996. "Effects of Moderate-Intensity Endurance and High-Intensity Intermittent Training on Anaerobic Capacity and VO2 Max." *Medicine and Science in Sports and Exercise* 28, no. 10: 1327-1330.

Wyatt, F., A. Donaldson, and E. Brown. 2013. "The Overtraining Syndrome: A Meta-Analytic Review." *Journal of Exercise Physiology* 16, no. 2: 12-23.

Chapter 7

Bompa, T., and C. Buzzichelli. 2015. *Periodization Training for Sports*. 3rd edition. Champaign, IL: Human Kinetics.

Candow, D., P. Chilibeck, S. Abeysekara, and G. Zello. 2011. "Short-Term Heavy Resistance Training Eliminates Age-Related Deficits in Muscle Mass and Strength in Older Males." *Journal of Strength and Conditioning Research* 25, no. 2: 326-333.

Chaddock, L., M. Voss, and A. Kramer. 2012. "Physical Activity and Fitness Effects on Cognition and Brain Health in Children and Older Adults." *Kinesiology Review* 12, no. 1: 37-45.

Chang, Y., C. Pan, F. Chen, C. Tsai, and C. Huang. 2012. "Effect of Resistance-Exercise Training on Cognitive Function in Healthy Older Adults: A Review." *Journal of Aging and Physical Activity* 20, no. 4: 497-517.

Godfrey, R., and A. Blazevich. 2004. "Exercise and Growth Hormone in the Aging Individual, with Special Reference to the Exercise-Induced Growth Hormone Response." *International SportMed Journal* 5, no. 4: 246-260.

Hakkinen, K. 2011. "The Aging Neuromuscular System in Men and Women Still Responds to Strength Training." Lecture given at the NSCA National Conference, July 8-11, 2011.

Izquierdo, M., K. Hakkinen, J. Ibanez, M. Garrues, A. Anton, A. Zuniga, and J.L. Larrion. 2001. "Effects of Strength Training on Muscle Power and Serum Hormones in Middle-Aged and Older Men." *Journal of Applied Physiology* 90, no. 4: 1497-1507.

Serra, C., S. Bhasin, F. Tangherlini, E. Barton, M. Ganno, A. Zhang, J. Shansky, H. Vandenburgh, T. Travison, R. Jasuja, and C. Morris. 2011. "The Role of GH and IGF-1 in Mediating Anabolic Effects of Testosterone on Androgen-Responsive Muscle." *Endocrinology* 152, no. 1: 193-206.

Taylor, A., and M. Johnson. 2008. *Physiology of Exercise and Healthy Aging*. Champaign, IL: Human Kinetics.

About the Author

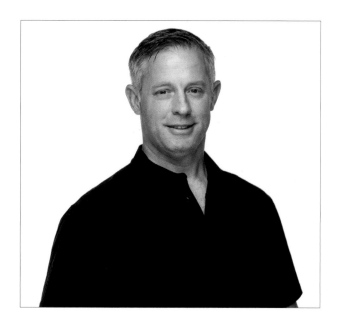

Pete McCall is the owner and president of PMc Fitness Solutions. He is certified as a personal trainer through the American Council on Exercise (ACE) and the National Academy of Sports Medicine (NASM) and also holds a CSCS (Certified Strength and Conditioning Specialist) certification from the National Strength and Conditioning Association (NSCA).

For more than 15 years, McCall has been teaching and writing workshops and courses designed to meet continuing education requirements for certified fitness professionals. He has presented at conferences around the world and is one of only a handful of fitness professionals who has assisted in writing personal training textbooks for both NASM and ACE. He also contributed to the development of ACE's Integrated Fitness Training Model of exercise program design.

Throughout his career, McCall has worked with leading brands and established companies in the fitness industry, including Reebok and 24 Hour Fitness, where he is also a regular contributor to their online magazine, and Core Health & Fitness (the parent company of Nautilus, StairMaster, Star Trac, and Schwinn Indoor Cycling), where he is a master trainer and education content creator. He is a spokesperson for ACE and has been featured as a fitness expert in national publications such as the *Wall Street Journal, New York Times, Washington Post, Los Angeles Times, Men's Health, Shape,* and *Self.*

McCall earned his master's degree in exercise science and health promotion from the California University of Pennsylvania.

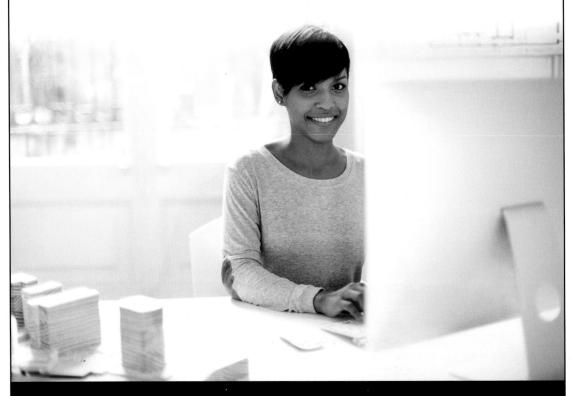
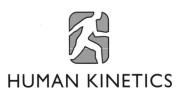